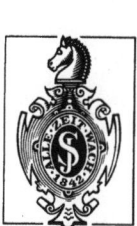

W. Weidner P.O. Madsen H.G. Schiefer (Eds.)

Prostatitis

Etiopathology, Diagnosis and Therapy

With 58 Figures and 52 Tables

Springer-Verlag
Berlin Heidelberg New York London Paris
Tokyo Hong Kong Barcelona Budapest

Prof. Dr. *Wolfgang Weidner*
Urologische Klinik
Klinikum der Justus-Liebig-Universität
Klinikstr. 29
35392 Giessen, Germany

Prof. Dr. *Paul O. Madsen*
Veterans Administration Medical Center
and Department of Surgery
University of Wisconsin School of Medicine
2500 Overlook Terrace
Madison, Wisconsin 53705, USA

Prof. Dr. *Hans Gerd Schiefer*
Institut für Medizinische Mikrobiologie
Klinikum der Justus-Liebig-Universität
Schubertstr. 1
35392 Giessen, Germany

ISBN-13:978-3-642-78183-4   e-ISBN-13:978-3-642-78181-0
DOI: 10.1007/978-3-642-78181-0

Library of Congress Cataloging-in-Publication Data. Prostatitis: etiopathology, diagnosis and therapy/ W. Weidner, P.O. Madsen, H.G. Schiefer (eds.) p. cm. Includes bibliographical references and index. ISBN-13:978-3-642-78183-4 1. Prostatitis. I. Weidner, W. (Wolfgang) II. Madsen, Paul O., 1927–   III. Schiefer, H.G. (Hans Gerd). RC899.P77 1994 616.6′5 – dc20 93–29539

© Springer-Verlag Berlin Heidelberg 1994
Softcover reprint of the hardcover 1st edition 1994

Typesetting: Macmillan India Ltd., Bangalore-25

SPIN: 10083393   31/3130/SPS – 5 4 3 2 1 0 – Printed on acid-free paper

Contributors

Ameye, F.
Department of Urology, University Hospitals Leuven, U.Z. Sint-Pieter,
Brusselsestraat 69, 3000 Leuven, Belgium

Baert, L.
Department of Urology, University Hospitals Leuven, U.Z. Sint-Pieter,
Brusselsestraat 69, 3000 Leuven, Belgium

Blacklock, N.J.
42 Western Way, Alverstoke, Gosport, Hampshire PO12 2NQ, UK

Brähler, E.
Klinik und Poliklinik für Psychotherapie und Psychosomatische Medizin
der Universität, Karl-Tauchnitz-Str. 25, 04107 Leipzig, Germany

Ceri, H.
Department of Biological Sciences, University of Calgary, Calgary,
Alberta T2N 1N4, Canada

Clements, R.
Department of Clinical Radiology, Royal Gwent Hospital, Newport,
Gwent NP9 2UB, UK

De Ridder, D.
Department of Urology, University Hospitals Leuven, U.Z. Sint-Pieter,
Brusselsestraat 69, 3000 Leuven, Belgium

Doble, A.
Department of Urology, Addenbrooke's Hospital, Hills Road,
Cambridge CB2 2QQ, UK

Drescher, P.
Veterans Administration Medical Center and Department of Surgery,
University of Wisconsin School of Medicine, 2500 Overlook Terrace,
Madison, Wisconsin 53705, USA

Frick, J.
Landeskrankenanstalten, Urologische Abteilung, Müllner Hauptstr. 48,
5020 Salzburg, Austria

Gasser, T.C.
Urologische Universitätsklinik, Department für Chirurgie der Universität
Basel, Kantonsspital, 4031 Basel, Switzerland

Griffiths, G.J.
Department of Clinical Radiology, Royal Gwent Hospital, Newport,
Gwent NP9 2UB, UK

Herremans, D.
Department of Urology, University Hospitals Leuven, U.Z. Sint-Pieter,
Brusselsestraat 69, 3000 Leuven, Belgium

Hofstetter, A.G.
Urologische Klinik und Poliklinik der Universität, Klinikum Großhadern,
Marchioninistr. 15, 81377 München, Germany

Kawamura, N.
Department of Urology, Tokai University School of Medicine, Boseidai,
Isehara, Kanagawa 259-11, Japan

Krause, W.
Abteilung für Dermatologie mit Schwerpunkt Andrologie, Medizinisches
Zentrum für Hautkrankheiten der Universität, Deutschhausstr. 9,
35037 Marburg, Germany

Ludwig, M.
Klinik und Poliklinik für Urologie der Universität, Robert-Koch-Str. 40,
37075 Göttingen, Germany

Madsen, P.O.
Veterans Administration Medical Center and Department of Surgery,
University of Wisconsin School of Medicine, 2500 Overlook Terrace,
Madison, Wisconsin 53705, USA

Naber, K.G.
Urologische Klinik, Elisabeth Krankenhaus, Schulgasse 20, 94315 Straubing,
Germany

Nickel, J.C.
Department of Urology, Queen's University, Kingston General Hospital,
Kingston, Ontario K7L 2V7, Canada

Olson, M.E.
Department of Biological Sciences, University of Calgary, Calgary,
Alberta T2N 1N4, Canada

Peeling, W.B.
St. Woolos Hospital, South Gwent Health Unit, 131 Stow Hill, Newport,
Gwent NP9 4SZ, UK

Petrovich, Z.
Department of Urology, University Hospitals Leuven, U.Z. Sint-Pieter,
Brusselsestraat 69, 3000 Leuven, Belgium

Pfau, A.
Department of Urology, Hebrew University – Hadassah Medical Center,
P.O. Box 12000, 91120 Jerusalem, Israel

Schaeffer, A.J.
Department of Urology, Northwestern University Medical School,
303 E. Chicago Avenue, Chicago, Illinois 60611, USA

Schiefer, H.G.
Institut für Medizinische Mikrobiologie der Universität, Schubertstr. 1,
35392 Giessen, Germany

Taylor-Robinson, D.
Division of Sexually Transmitted Diseases, Clinical Research Centre,
Watford Road, Harrow, Middlesex HA1 3UJ, UK

Thin, R.N.T.
Department of Genitourinary Medicine, St. Thomas' Hospital,
London SE1 7EH, UK

Vahlensieck, W. Jr.
Urologische Klinik und Poliklinik der Universität, Klinikum Großhadern,
Marchioninistr. 15, 81377 München, Germany

Van Poppel, H.
Department of Urology, University Hospitals Leuven, U.Z. Sint-Pieter,
Brusselsestraat 69, 3000 Leuven, Belgium

Van Thillo, E.
Department of Urology, University Hospitals Leuven, U.Z. Sint-Pieter,
Brusselsestraat 69, 3000 Leuven, Belgium

Weidner, W.
Urologische Universitätsklinik, Klinikstr. 29, 35392 Giessen, Germany

Preface

Prostatitis syndromes continue to be a major problem in urology. About every second man will experience symptoms of prostatitis during his lifetime. A study by the U.S. National Center for Health Statistics showed that approximately 25% of the men seen for urogenital problems suffer from prostatitis.

What is the intention of this book? Although investigations in recent years, including microbiologic and immunologic ones, have focused on the correct diagnosis of prostatitis, much confusion still remains regarding its correct classification, its etiology, and the evaluation of diagnostic results. Many clinicians, therefore, tend to lump together several diseases of variable type and sequela as prostatitis.

The term "prostatitis" implies an inflammatory disease, but true bacterial infection is detected in only 5%–10% of patients. In fact, most patients reveal no significant bacterial counts in the prostatic fluid. Nonetheless, 40%–60% of these patients suffer from nonbacterial prostatitis, as shown by the fact that the prostatic fluid contains elevated leukocyte counts while common uropathogens are not detected.

Essentially, three clinical types of real inflammatory prostatitis are widely accepted: acute and chronic bacterial and nonbacterial prostatitis. There remains a condition denoted as prostatodynia, covering patients in whom signs of neither inflammation nor infection are found. Multiple extraprostatic disorders are suspected causes of these complaints, e.g., bladder outlet disorders, detrusor hyperreflexia, pelvic floor tension myalgia, interstitial cystitis, urolithiasis, ostitis pubis, and anogenital disorders. Proven data concerning these special problems are rare, and their association to prostatodynia is unclear. The intention of this book is to provide the reader with a clarification of the etiopathogenesis of prostatitis and the competence to exclude the patient with complaints and symptoms of prostatitis but without true prostatic inflammation, i.e., to identify the man suffering from prostatodynia, thus preventing multiple and useless antibiotic trials. Instead, if the diagnosis prostatodynia is clarified, there may be an indication for, among other things, psychodynamic investigation and therapy.

This book concentrates on clinical prostatitis strictu sensu and does not treat the various types of histologically detected inflammation of the prostate, e.g., "prostatitis" associated with benign prostatic hypertrophy. Very rarely, prostatectomy specimens of younger patients or autopsy samples of prostates without evidence of hyperplasia demonstrate inflammatory infiltrates. In men up to the age of 40, prostatitis is mainly located in the peripheral gland, not in the transition zone. Demographic data demonstrate that prostatitis symptoms mostly occur in men over 40 years of age, with decreasing frequency in men beyond the age of 50, in whom chronic recurrent prostatitis is almost exclusively seen in biopsies of hyperplastic prostatic glands. Since inflammatory infiltrates of the prostate must be considered noncharacteristic, we have decided not to include chapters on histology or cytology in consideration of the fact that prostatic biopsies for the morphological diagnosis of prostatitis syndromes are indicated only in cases of clinical suspicion of carcinoma.

The book contains some introductory chapters on basic data, e.g., pathophysiology, host–parasite interactions, anatomy of prostatic infection, and also general considerations of disease-related complaint complexes, psychosomatics, diagnostic management, ultrasonography, and ejaculate analysis. Additionally, the basic conditions of therapy are discussed not only from a pharmacokinetic angle but also considering the development of acceptable animal models, allowing standardized therapeutic trials.

Clinical management of acute and chronic bacterial prostatitis has now been established, following a widely accepted schedule of therapy with a good prognosis for cure. Obviously, the new fluoroquinolones are a significant improvement in therapy, but the urgent question is how to treat patients in whom antibiotic therapy fails. Baert et al. have analyzed this problem, contributing their experience with local therapy and transurethral and open surgery of infected prostatic glands.

Our book also deals with nonbacterial prostatitis. It is our opinion that this complex entity is a major problem as regards its still unknown etiology and missing rational therapy in most cases. In patients with nonbacterial prostatitis, diagnostic efforts should not only concentrate on chlamydial and/or mycoplasmal infections, but on unconventional pathogens, too, in view of the increasing incidence of AIDS and the reestablished significance of parasites as treatable causes of urogenital infections in sexually active men. For practical use, the procedures suggested by Thin seem to us to be a feasible schedule for daily work. The editors would feel satisfied if this monograph could assist the practicing physician to provide optimal diagnosis and treatment to every patient suffering from prostatitis syndromes.

Finally, the editors gratefully acknowledge the continuous efforts and assistance of Mrs. Karoline Karrer in the production of this book.

Giessen, Germany	*W. Weidner*
Madison, Wisconsin, USA	*P.O. Madsen*
Giessen, Germany	*H.G. Schiefer*
January 1994	

Contents

I. Introduction

Classification, Etiology, and Diagnosis of Prostatitis

P.O. Madsen, P. Drescher, and T.C. Gasser

Bacteriological localization studies have been the accepted standard in diagnosis and treatment of prostatitis since Drach et al. (1978) introduced a uniform terminology of diagnosing and classifying prostatitis based on fractionated microscopic examinations as developed by Meares and Stamey (1968). The types of prostatitis recognized at the present time and their clinical features are outlined in Table 1, with an approximate clinical incidence of these various types. An additional acute bacterial prostatitis type is acute nosocomial prostatitis, which is being seen with increased frequency and is often caused by an indwelling catheter (Holt et al. 1992). A better term for nonbacterial prostatitis may be idiopathic prostatitis, implying the uncertainty concerning actual infection in this type of prostatitis.

According to this classification, only acute and chronic bacterial prostatitis were caused by bacterial infection, as demonstrated by positive urine and expressed prostatic secretion (EPS) cultures. The microscopic examination of the expressed prostatic secretion, however, is similar in acute and chronic bacterial prostatitis as well as in nonbacterial prostatitis, showing evidence of inflammation by the presence of numerous white blood cells (WBC) and lipid-laden macrophages. Results of both the microscopic examination of EPS and the bacteriological localization cultures are negative in prostatodynia.

For proper diagnosis, voided urine and prostate secretions are collected and cultured in segmented specimens (Fig. 1). Specimens must be collected with care to prevent bacterial contamination which may lead to misinterpretation of the results. The diagnosis of prostatic infection is confirmed when the quantitative bacterial colony count of the prostatic specimen (EPS and VB3) significantly exceeds those of urethral (VB1) and bladder (VB2) specimens. These examinations often must be repeated, and in the case of cystitis sterilization of the urine, for example, with nitrofurantoin, may be necessary to obtain valid results.

The amount of literature discussing diagnosis and treatment of prostatitis is large. However, information regarding the incidence and the role of reinfection is lacking and controversial. The incidence of acute and chronic bacterial prostatitis is probably very low and the incidence of nonbacterial prostatitis and prostatodynia very high, based on our clinical experience (Table 1). In a study of 600 men attending a prostatitis clinic, Brunner et al. (1983) found that only 5% had bacterial prostatitis, approximately two-thirds nonbacterial prostatitis, and one-third prostatodynia.

Table 1. Clinical features of different forms of prostatitis

Syndrome	History of confirmed UTI	Abnormal on rectal examination	Excessive WBCs in EPS	Positive culture of EPS	Common causative agents	Response to antimicrobials	Approximate clinical incidence
Acute bacterial prostatitis	Yes	Yes	Yes	Yes	Coliform bacteria	Yes	5%–10%
Chronic bacterial prostatitis	±	Yes	Yes	Yes	Coliform bacteria	Yes	5%–10%
Nonbacterial prostatitis	No	±	Yes	No	None, *Chlamydia* (?), *Ureaplasma* (?)	Usually not	40%
Prostatodynia	No	No	No	No	None	No	40%
Nosocomial prostatitis	No	Yes	±	Yes	Coliform bacteria	Yes	?
Rare types	±	Yes	±	±	Fungi Tbc. bacilli Parasites	±	?

EPS, Expressed prostatic secretion, UTI, Urinary tract infection.

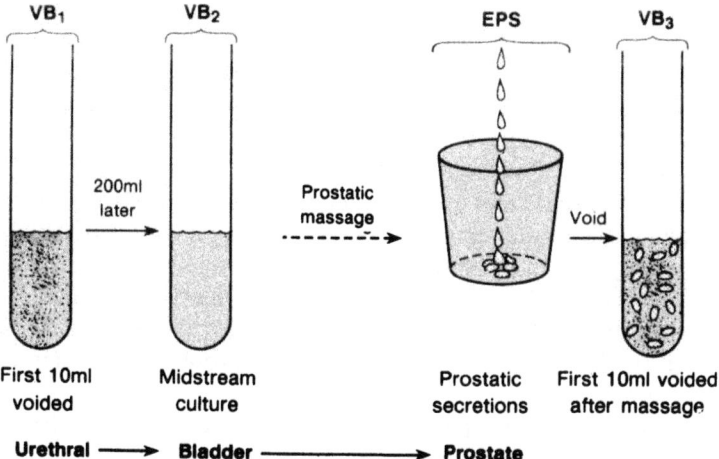

Fig. 1. Urine and prostatic secretions must be cultured in segmented specimens in lower urinary tract localization studies. VB_1, first 10 ml urine voided; VB, midstream urine culture; *EPS*, expressed prostatic secretion; VB_3, 10 ml urine voided immediately after prostatic massage. (Reproduced with permission from Meares and Stamey 1968)

Acute bacterial prostatitis is a well-established clinical entity. It presents with signs and symptoms of an acute septic process, including irritative and obstructive voiding symptoms. Since prostatic massage is contraindicated, the diagnosis depends solely on the results of urine culture and physical examination of the prostate without the benefit of direct microscopic examination of prostatic fluid.

In contrast to the acute form, *chronic bacterial prostatitis* is difficult to diagnose and treat and can vary widely in its clinical presentation. It is a common cause of relapsing urinary tract infections in men. Irritative voiding symptoms (dysuria, urgency, frequency) vary widely among these patients. Perineal, testicular, and low back pain are frequent complaints and can be misleading. Rectal examination discloses no characteristic findings.

The organisms responsible for acute bacterial prostatitis are generally considered to be gram-negative bacteria (Meares and Stamey 1968; Mårdh and Colleen 1975; Smart et al. 1975; Blacklock 1979; Drach and Nolan 1986), although some authors consider gram-positive organisms also to be potential pathogens in prostatitis (Blacklock 1979; Drach and Nolan 1986; Giamarellou et al. 1982; Meares 1992). Investigators who believe in the pathogenicity of gram-positive organisms base their conclusion only on gram-positive cocci in EPS, which being more viscous may contain more urethral contamination than VB1 or VB3, thus leading to false-positive results (Fowler and Mariano 1984; Pfan et al. 1978; Stamey 1980).

According to Meares (1992), gram-positive bacteria are typically localized in the anterior urethra in men and considered as nonpathogens. This is in agreement with Wedren (1989) who found gram-positive bacteria, predominantly *Staphylococcus epidermidis*, in 43% of men with chronic bacterial prostatitis. He further found that antibiotic therapy of prostatitis can eliminate many of the aerobic bacteria in the prostate but might give other bacteria the opportunity to colonize in the prostate. *S. epidermidis* is thus of importance only as an opportunistic organism. There is also evidence (in an in vitro model) of reduced polymorphonuclear leukocyte function in patients with chronic prostatitis caused by *S. epidermidis* (Wedren 1989).

When the patients with acute and chronic bacterial prostatitis are excluded, an ill-defined group of patients, and in fact the largest group, remains. Clinically, they have a wide variety of symptoms referable to the lower back, genitalia, perineum, and rectum. Quite often symptoms from the urinary tract, such as irritative and obstruction symptoms, are predominant. According to the localization studies (Fig. 1), this group is divided into two groups: nonbacterial prostatitis and prostatodynia.

The main criterion to distinguish patients with *nonbacterial prostatitis* from those with prostatodynia is microscopic examination of the prostatic fluid for WBC and lipid-laden macrophages. The validity of using the WBC count in EPS, however, is questionable since it may vary from count to count (Duw 1975), depending on the time from the last ejaculation until the test is performed. The WBC count may increase and remain elevated for several days after ejaculation. Mårdh et al. (1972) suggested that *Chlamydia trachomatis* might be pathogenic in chronic nonbacterial prostatitis. The same authors later doubted their results (Mårdh and Colleen 1975; Mårdh et al. 1978). Poletti et al. (1985) isolated *C. trachomatis* from transrectal aspiration biopsies of the prostate in patients with nonbacterial prostatitis. However, it cannot be ruled out that *C. trachomatis* originated from the rectal flora, and the rectum was not tested for chlamydial infection. *C. trachomatis* has been isolated from rectal mucosa of asymptomatic men (Munday et al. 1981; Quinn et al. 1981; Doble et al. 1989). Doble et al. (1989) were unable to isolate *C. trachomatis* from 50 patients with chronic nonbacterial prostatitis. By transrectal prostatic ultrasound and transperineal biopsy of the abnormal areas of the prostate, *Chlamydia* could not be detected by immunofluorescence, nor was it possible to isolate *C. trachomatis* in McCoy's cell culture, and serum antibodies were not found. Berger et al. (1989) found no evidence of *C. trachomatis* infection among patients referred for symptoms of chronic prostatitis.

Patients with *prostatodynia* present with multiple complaints, which commonly include some combination of pain in the perineum, lower back, and suprapubic areas as well as pain on ejaculation. Dysuria and frequency are generally absent. Rectal examination of the prostate is normal. The diagnosis is made by finding no evidence of inflammation on microscopic examination of EPS, and all negative results upon localization cultures. Since there is no evidence of inflammation in the prostatic fluid of these patients, some studies have indicated that the condition may be caused by detrusor sphincter dyssynergia (Segura et al. 1979; Sinati et al. 1977). Other investigators have shown that prostatodynia may be caused by overactivity of pelvic sympathetic nerves acting at the level of the external urethral sphincter (Barbalias et al. 1983). It should be noted that it is difficult to perform accurate and reproducible urodynamic studies on this group of often very anxious men. Few studies have investigated the efficacy of α-adrenergic blockers in treating these patients (Osborn et al. 1981; Lepor 1990). In a randomized prospective study 27 patients with prostatodynia received either phenoxybenzamine or placebo. Patients receiving phenoxybenzamine had significant relief of irritative symptoms, suggesting that increased smooth muscles tone may be an etiological factor. Since many patients with prostatodynia have associated psychiatric disturbances (Keltikangas-Jarvinen et al. 1989), it is possible that some of the therapeutic benefit of α-blockade may represent a placebo effect.

References

Barbalias GA, Meares Em Jr, Sant GR (1983) Prostatodynia: clinical urodynamics characteristics. J Urol 130:540

Berger RE, Krieger JN, Kessler D et al. (1989) A case controlled study of men with suspected chronic idiopathic prostatitis. J Urol 141:328–331

Blacklock NJ (1979) Prostatitis. Practitioner 223:318–322

Brunner H. Weidner W, Schiefer H-G (1983) Studies of the role of Ureaplasma urealyticum and Mycoplasma hominis in prostatitis. J Infect Dis 147:807

Doble A, Thomas BJ, Walker MM et al. (1989) The role of Chlamydia trachomatis in chronic abacterial prostatitis: a study using ultrasound guided biopsy. J Urol 141:332–333

Drach GW, Nolan PE (1986) Chronic bacterial prostatitis: problems in diagnosis and therapy. Urology 27(2):26–30

Drach TU, Meares EM Jr, Fair WR et al. (1978) Classification of benign diseases associated with prostatic pain: prostatitis and prostatodynia (Letter). J Urol 120:266

Duw D (1975) Trimethoprim sulfamethoxazole in the treatment of chronic prostatitis. Can Med Assoc J 112 Suppl 26

Fowler JE Jr, Mariano M (1984) Difficulties in quantitating the contribution of urethral bacteria to prostatic fluid and seminal fluid cultures. J Urol 132(3):471–473

Giamarellou H, Kosmidis J, Leonidas M et al. (1982) A study of the effectiveness of rifampin in chronic prostatitis caused mainly by Staphylococcus aureus. J Urol 128:321–324

Holt DA, Sinnott JT, Bradley E (1992) Nosocomial prostatitis. Infect Urol 5(5):139–141

Keltikangas-Jarvinen L, Mueller K, Lehtonen T (1989) Illness behavior and personality changes in patients with chronic prostatitis during a two-year follow-up period. Eur Urol 16:181–184

Lepor H (1990) Role of alpha-adrenergic blockers in the treatment of benign prostatic hyperplasia. Prostate Suppl 3:75–84

Mårdh PA, Colleen S (1975) Search for uro-genital tract infections in patients with symptoms of prostatitis. Scand J Urol Nephrol 9:8

Mårdh PA, Colleen S, Holmquist B (1972) Chlamydia in chronic prostatitis. Br Med J 4:361

Mårdh PA, Ripa KT, Colleen S et al. (1978) Role of Chlamydia trachomatis in nonacute prostatitis. Br J Vener Dis 54:330–314

Meares EM (1992) Prostatitis and related disorders. In: Walsh PC, Retik AB, Stamey TA et al. (eds) Campbell's urology, 6th edn. Saunders, Philadelphia, pp 807–822

Meares EM Jr, Stamey TA (1968) Bacteriological localization patterns in bacterial prostatitis and urethritis. Invest Urol 5:492–518

Munday PE, Johnson AP, Thomas BJ et al. (1981) Chlamydia trachomatis proctitis (Correspondence). N Engl J Med 305:1158–1159

Osborn DE, George NJ, Rao PN et al. (1981) Prostatodynia, physical characteristics and rational management with muscle relaxants. Br J Urol 53:621–623

Pfau A, Perlberg S, Shapiro A (1978) The pH of the prostatic fluid in health and disease. Implications of treatment in chronic bacterial prostatitis. J Urol 119:384–387

Poletti F, Medici MC, Alinova A et al. (1985) Isolation of Chlamydia trachomatis from the prostatic cells in patients affected by nonacute abacterial prostatitis. J Urol 134:691–693

Quinn TC, Goodell SE, Mkrtichian E et al. (1981) Chlamydia trachomatis proctitis. N Engl J Med 305:195–200

Segura JW, Opitz JL, Greene LF (1979) Prostatosis, prostatitis or pelvic floor tension myalgia. J Urol 122:168–169

Sinaki M, Merritt JL, Stilwell GK (1977) Tension myalgia of the pelvic floor. Mayo Clin Proc 52:717–722

Smart CJ, Jenkins JD, Lloyd RS (1975) The painful prostate. Br J Urol 47:861–869

Stamey TA (1980) Pathogenesis and treatment of urinary tract infections. Williams and Williams, Baltimore

Wedren H (1989) On chronic prostatitis with special studies of Staphylococcus epidermidis. Scand J Urol Nephrol Suppl 123:1–36

II. Prostatitis: Basic Data

Physiology and Pathophysiology of Prostate Infection

J. Frick

Introduction

The accessory glands of the male genital tract, including the prostate gland, show a wide range of variation and difference in the various species, above all in the anatomy, biochemistry, and function of these organs. For example, while the seminal vesicles are very large, prominent organs, particularly in humans and the rat, these organs do not exist in the cat or dog. However, the prostate gland is found in all mammals, although different species vary greatly in prostate anatomy, biochemistry, and secretion. Prostate pathology also differs in the development of benign as well as malignant changes, and naturally in the occurrence of inflammatory changes in the prostate region. It should be mentioned here that the rat prostate gland is anatomically divided into several distinct lobes, namely dorsal, ventral, and lateral lobes, with these carrying out separate functions. In contrast, the human prostate gland is not divided into separate lobes but into zones. Altogether, however, it has the appearance of an anatomically uniform gland (Fig. 1).

Not only does the anatomy of the prostate gland vary strongly from species to species but also its biochemistry, namely that which the prostate secretes or contributes to the ejaculate (Zanefeld and Tauber 1981). For example, the boar ejaculates a volume of approximately 250 ml, the stud 70 ml, the dog 9 ml, the bull 4 ml, the human 3 ml, and the ram 1 ml. A difference also exists in ejaculate

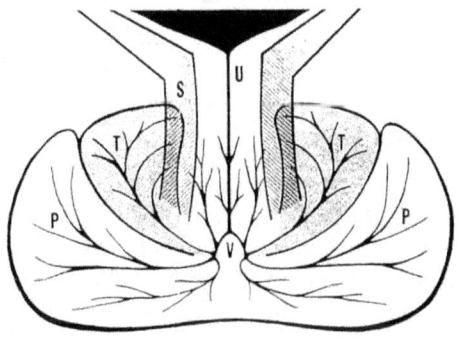

Fig. 1. Schematic representation of the division of the prostate into zones: *T*, transitional zone; *P*, peripheral zone; *U*, periurethral region; *S*, sphincter region. (From McNeal 1981, with permission)

behavior. Human ejaculate first clumps and then dissolves, while in many animals the ejaculate forms a solid lump and is ejaculated in this form. Not only the ejaculate quantity but also its biochemical composition as well as the secretion of proteins and ions differs greatly from species to species (Coffey 1985).

It should be mentioned that among mammals no organ possesses such a wide range of variation in its anatomy and/or biochemistry as does the tissue of the accessory genital glands and, to repeat, this includes the prostate gland (Isaacs et al. 1981). A certain mysticism surrounds the prostate gland and the other accessory genital glands, with great variety and different functions, so that the question must be posed as to whether all this is really necessary – does it make any biological sense? What is the reason for these considerable differences? Are they really necessary for reproduction, or does this diversity play a decisive role in protecting the genital tract from invasion of pathogenic germs? Many things can be interpreted into this diversification. But in all certainty it must be said that there are some things that we simply do not yet understand, and that we will understand only when we learn more about the function and the molecular biologic rules according to which these glands work. We will then have a much better insight than we now have (Niemi et al. 1963; O'Connor and Sinha 1985).

Transport of Biologic Components into and out of the Male Accessory Sex Glands

What biologic material is transported from the serum into the seminal fluid and vice versa? Our knowledge of the transport and exchange of ions, therapeutic substances, or natural products in the secretion of the accessory glands of the male genital apparatus is very limited. It is, however, very important that we especially know more about the transport mechanism of therapeutic substances into these accessory glands particularly to be able to administer the correct therapy for acute or chronic inflammations as well as to achieve effective levels of the individual substances in the target organs (Fair et al. 1973; Fair and Wehner 1979; Fair and Parrish 1981; Stamey et al. 1968).

Androgenic Mechanism of the Prostate Gland

The most important androgen in the human male is testosterone, and as soon as testosterone has reached the prostate cell by diffusion, it is metabolized into other steroids by a series of enzymatic processes. More than 75% of the testosterone is converted into the most important intraprostatic androgen, namely dihydrotestosterone (Bruchovsky and Wilson 1968; Bruchovsky and

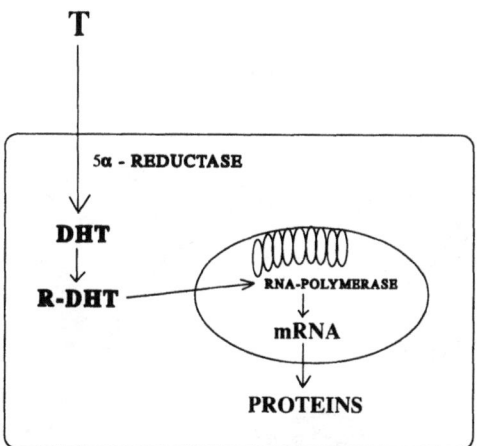

Fig. 2. Androgen metabolism in the prostate cell. *T*, testosterone; *DHT*, dihydrotestosterone; *R-DHT*, DHT receptor complex

Dunstan-Adams 1985; Lasnitzki and Franklin 1972). This transformation of testosterone into dihydrotestosterone takes place under the influence of 5α-reductase. Dihydrotestosterone then binds to the activated androgen receptors in the cell. This hormone receptor complex is finally transformed and transferred into the cell nucleus, where the RNA polymerase is activated and mRNA subsequently synthesized. Thereafter, the mRNA is transported into the cytoplasmatic compartment and begins to convert to secretory proteins (Fig. 2). At a neurologic command, these proteins are secreted into the lumen; this happens during ejaculation. Naturally, there are also other factors that possibly modify the testosterone effect on the prostate cell. A certain cooperation between estrogen and androgen might take place to induce growth of the prostate cell, so that a certain synergistic effect can occur. This has also been seen in several experiments, for example, when castrated dogs were treated with estrogen and dihydrotestosterone, the prostate gland grew to enormous size. Particularly estradiol doubles the prostate's androgen-induced increase in volume. This synergistic effect, however, is not found in the rat (Coffey 1985). Just as there are great differences in the prostate of various species, there are also great differences in the pathology of the prostate.

Pathology of the Prostate Gland

We all know, for example, that in 80% of men the prostate enlarges considerably (hyperplasia) before they become 80 years of age, and that some 25% of men require prostate surgery sometime during their life to eliminate the symptoms of obstruction caused by this excessive prostate growth (Grayhack 1963; Trachtenberg et al. 1981). Judging by statistics compiled in the United States, this condition requires more than 300000 surgical interventions each year and is

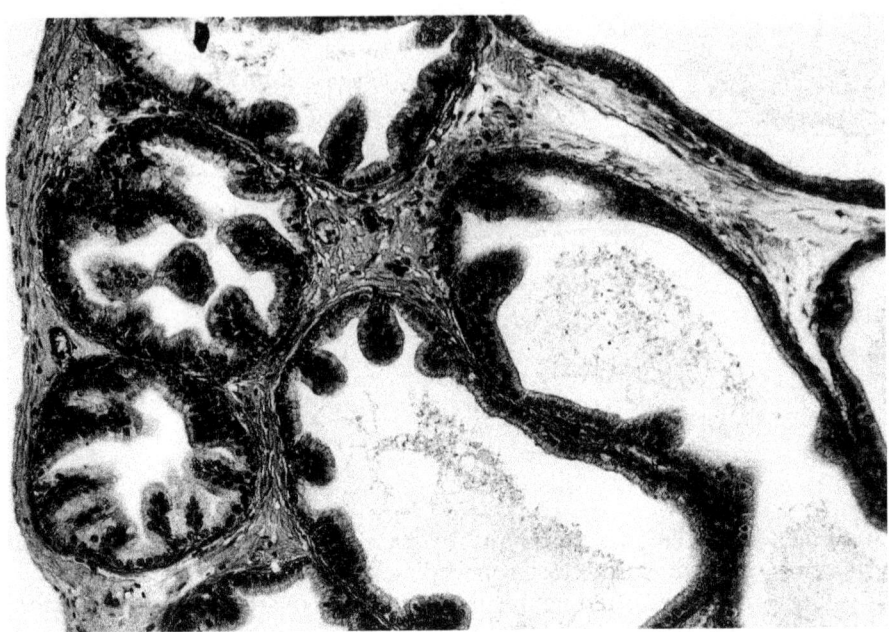

Fig. 3. Histology of the prostate with highly prismatic epithelium of the tubuloalveolar glandular terminals

thus the second most common form of surgery performed in the human male at the moment. This may change in the future as new therapeutic approaches are developed.

The prostate carcinoma, an additional disease, is the most common form of cancer in males over 65 years of age. Today this disease is still not sufficiently recognized at an early stage, a stage when radical surgery can bring about a cure. Today a large majority of patients with a prostate carcinoma still undergo their first prostate examination when metastases have already spread to other organs.

The prostate's specific anatomic structure naturally makes it easily prone to inflammation because of its small glands and narrow gland tubes (Fig. 3). Occlusion of these narrow discharge conduits in the prostate very often causes congestion and secretion stagnation, which in turn can predispose the prostate for acute infection, an acute bacterial prostatitis. This special anatomical feature is of course in the same way responsible for recurrent and chronic prostatitis (Stamey 1989).

Prostate Secretion

Ejaculate volume in the human male is normally approximately 3.0–3.5 ml but ranges from 2 to 6 ml. The ejaculate is composed of two important components.

The first is the spermatozoa and the second the seminal plasma. Both fractions are easily separated by centrifugation. The seminal plasma consists of the secretions from the accessory glands of the male genital apparatus, namely epididymis, vas deferens, ampullae, seminal vesicles, prostate gland, bulbourethral gland (Cowper's gland) and the urethral glands (Littré glands) (Eliasson 1977; Phadke et al. 1973; Polakoski and Kopta 1982). In the ejaculate volume the individual glands contribute approximately the following quantities: seminal vesicle 1.5–2 ml, prostate gland 0.5 ml, and bulbourethral gland and urethral glands 0.1–0.2 ml. These fractions are secreted sequentially during ejaculation (Tsai et al. 1984).

The first fractions of the human ejaculate are rich in spermatozoa and in components from the prostate gland, while the later fractions are rich in products particularly from the seminal vesicles (43). In relation to the other body fluids, the seminal plasma is a somewhat unusual secretion, primarily because of its high concentration of potassium, zinc, citric acid, fructose, and a number of proteins and enzymes, to which certain functions must be ascribed; it is particularly the various enzyme fractions whose role we do not precisely know (Chandler et al. 1977; Dawson et al. 1957; Falk et al. 1980; Jacobs et al. 1979; Mann and Lutwak-Mann 1981; Mattila 1969; Poulos and White 1973; Williams-Ashman et al. 1975). The individual ions and important amines, whose functions we partially know, are discussed below.

Zinc

The high zinc content in the human seminal plasma stems almost exclusively from prostate secretion. The zinc content measures approximately 50 mg per 100 g dry weight (Byar 1974; Chandler et al. 1977; Heathcote and Washington 1973; MacKenzie et al. 1962).

As early as 1921 Bertrand and Vladesco reported that the human prostate gland has the highest zinc content of all tested organs. Various animal experiments have also shown that the zinc content in the prostate gland of many animals is very high, just as in man, and that a very specific zinc absorption occurs in the prostate. Zinc was localized in the human prostate by radioautographic tests performed in the epithelial cells It is also known that zinc levels seen in benign prostate hyperplasia are elevated, while prostate malignancies are accompanied by a reduction in zinc levels.

Many physiologic roles have been postulated for zinc. A specific zinc-binding protein was described, particularly in malignant prostate disease, but it has also been repeatedly emphasized that zinc is a very considerable antibacterial factor in the prostate, as already suggested by the studies by Fair and Wehner (1976). Numerous studies have shown zinc to be one of the important factors effecting a local antibacterial mechanism. One study conducted in 36 healthy men with no bacterial prostatitis showed a zinc content of approximately 350 µg/ml in the prostate secretion, with a very wide range of

150–1000 µg/ml. In contrast, studies have been reported in 61 patients, 15 of whom had documented chronic bacterial prostatitis. In these patients the zinc content had dropped to an average of 50 µg/ml, and the range (0–139 µg/ml) was also depressed compared with healthy study subjects. In vitro studies have also shown that zinc actually evokes an antibacterial effect on gram-positive as well as gram-negative bacteria (Fair and Parrish 1981; Stamey et al. 1968).

The zinc concentration in healthy human seminal plasma (mean 140 mg/ml) is less than half of that found in the normal prostate gland.

Citric Acid

One of the main sources of citrate secretion is the prostate gland, and citrate is one of the most important and most essential anions in human seminal plasma with an average content of 376 mg per 100 ml. The prostate gland is one of the main sources of citric acid, and citric acid is admixed with the seminal fluid. This observation was already made by Huggins, who examined nine human specimens of prostate secretion and found a citric acid content of 480–2688 mg per 100 ml (Huggins and Neal 1942; Huggins 1947). In contrast, he found a very minor citric acid content in the secretion of the seminal vesicle, namely maximum 20 mg citric acid per 100 ml. Citric acid, and very often also the acid phosphatases (see below), have been considered chemical indicators of prostate function. But it has also been seen that the citrate level in the prostate gland is not directly correlated with the plasma testosterone content, as has been repeatedly tested. When the plasma testosterone level is normal or elevated, the citric acid content in the prostate gland would also have to be normal or elevated, and when testosterone is very low, the prostate cells would also have to secrete very little citric acid. This correlation was never established beyond doubt.

Cholesterol

Scott (1945) reported the cholesterol content in human seminal plasma to be approximately 103 mg per 100 ml, with about 83 mg phospholipids per 100 ml. The range for cholesterol content in seminal plasma is, however, relatively large, from 11 to 103 mg per 100 ml. Furthermore, a certain relationship is promoted between cholesterol and the phospholipids in the seminal plasma. White et al. (1976) found that this protects the spermatozoa from temperature shock. The prostate gland is certainly one of the most important sources of the cholesterol found in seminal plasma. It is also believed that cholesterol synthesis in the prostate is elevated in cases of benign prostate hyperplasia (Acevedo et al. 1973).

Spermine

The prostate gland is the main site of secretion of this protein, and the content of spermine in human seminal plasma ranges between 50 and 350 mg per 100 ml. Great interest has always surrounded spermine and other related polyamines in man, for example, spermidine and putrescine. These peptides have been repeatedly associated with growth. The role of spermine has not yet been precisely established, but it is felt that spermines play an important role by protecting the genital tract from infectious agents.

Seminin

Seminin is a proteolytic enzyme with a molecular weight of 30 kDa. Seminin usually appears in the first fraction of a split ejaculate, and it is therefore believed to come from the prostate. This seminal proteinase has no certain fibrinolytic properties, as was once presumed. Today it is believed that seminin influences particularly liquefaction and coagulation of the seminal plasma (Amelar 1962; Tauber and Zanefeld 1976).

Prostaglandin

The most important source of prostaglandins is not the prostate gland but the seminal vesicle. The term prostaglandin is certainly a misnomer, since its discoverer (von Euler 1934) believed that these compounds come from the prostate gland and not from the seminal vesicle. This view was later corrected by Eliasson (1959) in his very precise studies. Thus, this compound should be called seminoglandin instead of prostaglandin, but the original name has survived and has not changed despite the clear scientific evidence. The prostaglandin content of the seminal plasma is about 100–300 μg/ml. Later, it was primarily Bergström et al. (1986), who discovered that a large number of various prostaglandins exist. These authors purified the individual prostaglandins and identified their chemical structure.

There are some 15 different prostaglandins in the seminal fluid alone. The prostaglandins are divided into the main groups A, B, E, and F, according to the structure of the cyclopentane ring. Each of these groups is subdivided according to the position and number of double bonds in the side chains. As we know, these compounds are very potent pharmacologic substances that entail a number of biologic processes. Prostaglandins certainly play an important role in spermatozoa motility and spermatozoa transport, as well as in testicular and penile contraction. Moreover, it is believed that the prostaglandins from the seminal plasma, which are released in the vagina, influence the cervical mucus, increase vaginal secretion, and influence spermatozoa transport in the female genital tract. To date, these effects have not been established with 100% assurance.

Acid Phosphatase and Acid Prostate Phosphatase

Acid prostate phosphatase is a glycoprotein with a molecular weight of 102 kDa (Babson and Read 1959). Both of these enzymes, namely acid phosphatase and prostate acid phosphatase, are expressed in the prostate gland. The seminal plasma contains approximately 800–1500 U/ml acid phosphatase. Both enzymes have long been used to monitor prostate carcinomas, above all the course of very advanced prostate malignancies. Neither of these enzymes play a major role with regard to inflammatory changes in the prostate region. Various studies to date have failed to show that the phosphatases in the prostate gland inhibit or promote inflammation. The most important point has already been mentioned, namely that for many years both factors were the decisive parameters for monitoring the course of advanced prostate carcinomas, until the prostate-specific antigen assumed this role.

Prostate-Specific Antigen

In 1979 Wang et al. reported for the first time on this protein that is expressed by the epithelial cells of the prostate gland. This parameter is a very specific one, and although it is not always successful for early detection of the prostate carcinoma, it is today the standard parameter for monitoring the course of a prostate malignancy, whether after a radical prostatectomy or during endocrine therapy of an advanced, already metastasizing malignancy (Wang et al. 1981). The prostate-specific antigen (PSA) is also a glycoprotein with a molecular weight of 33 kDa. The entire amino acid sequence of this protein is known. With regard to inflammatory changes in the prostate gland, there are no data to show that PSA is influential. Not enough studies have yet been conducted to determine whether changes in PSA expression occur in the case of an acute prostatitis or a chronic, recurrent bacterial prostatitis. Bahnson (1991) reported elevated PSA levels in a patient with a granulomatous prostatitis that developed following instillation of Bacille Calmette-Guérin for a surface bladder tumor. Elevated serum PSA has been reported in isolated cases of patients with prostatitis or a prostate infarction. It is not yet clear, however, exactly what role PSA plays in the inflammatory process.

Immunoglobulins

It is known that immunoglobulins can be demonstrated in the human seminal plasma. IgG values of 7 mg/100 ml and 22 mg/100 ml and IgA values of

0 mg/100 ml and 6 mg/100 ml seminal plasma have been reported. To date, however, no IgM has been discovered in the seminal plasma. The source of these immunoglobulins is not precisely known. Whether or not part of these immuno- globulins is produced in the prostate gland, cannot be reported with certainty. Immunoglobulin levels in the seminal plasma are lower than in plasma, but the possibility exists that these diffuse through the blood seminal plasma barrier, so that this path must also be taken into consideration. What role the immunoglobulins play, and whether they help prevent infections in the region of the accessory glands of the male genital apparatus are not known for sure (Coffey 1985).

Prostate Proteins

In addition to PSA, other proteins are also expressed in the prostate gland. One of these proteins is prostatein, which is composed of several chains, with various molecular weights ranging from 6 to 14 kDa. It is known that the gene for these proteins is under strict androgen control, but it has not yet been discovered what the role of prostatein really is, nor how expression of this protein behaves under inflammatory changes of the prostate gland (Coffey 1985; Isaacs and Shaper 1983; Perry et al. 1985).

Transport of Compounds into the Prostate Secretion

This is a very important aspect, with which we shall deal in more detail below. These transport mechanisms into the prostate secretion are so important because they may contribute to possible new therapies for acute and chronic recurrent prostatitis, and also because new possibilities for chemotherapy are needed, above all for prostate carcinoma.

There are compounds that in the prostate secretion reach a concentration similar to that of the same compound in the blood, or that are sometimes even enriched in the prostate secretion, i.e., the levels in the prostate secretion are higher than in the blood. In general, the transport of compounds into the prostate secretion can be described in the following manner: the substances pass the cell membrane by nonionic diffusion or through the membrane by fat solubility (Hessl and Stamey 1971; Madsen et al. 1978; Stamey et al. 1973). An important role is naturally also played by the pH value of the seminal plasma or the pH value of the prostate secretion. This pH value varies from 6 to 8 in humans, with a mean of 6.6. However, when the prostate gland becomes inflammatory, the pH value of the prostate secretion rises to about 7 or even higher (White 1975). This must be taken into consideration when using certain medications, namely that particular circumstances in the prostate gland create particular pH values. It must also be remembered that the prostate gland contains a very considerable transport force, and that the transport systems in the prostate proceed under a particular hormonal influence. This means that the transport capacity for various substances might be stimulated by androgens and inhibited by estrogens. The compounds that may have a preventive role in regard to inflammatory processes in the prostate are zinc, spermine, and immunoglobulins.

References

Acevedo HF, Campbell EA, Saier EL et al. (1973) Urinary cholesterol. V. Its excretion in men with testicular and prostatic neoplasms. Cancer 32:196–205

Amelar RD (1962) Coagulation, liquefaction and viscosity of human semen. J Urol 87:187–190

Babson AL, Read PA (1959) A new assay for prostatic acid phosphatase in serum. Am J Clin Pathol 32:88–91

Bahnson RR (1991) Elevation of prostate specific antigen from bacillus Calmette-Guérin-induced granulomatous prostatitis. J Urol 146:1368–1369

Bergström S, Carlson LA, Weeks LR (1986) The prostaglandins: a family of biologically active lipids. Pharmacol Rev 20:1–48

Bertrand G, Vladesco R (1921) Prostatic zinc concentration. C R Acad Sci [III] 173:176–179

Bruchovsky N, Dunstan-Adams E (1985) Regulation of 5 alpha-reductase activity in stroma and epithelium of human prostate. In: Bruchovsky N, Chapdelaine A, Neumann F (eds) Regulation of androgen action. Bruckner, Berlin, pp 31–34

Bruchovsky N, Wilson JF (1968) The conversion of testosterone to 5 alpha-androstan-17β-ol-3-one by rat prostate in vivo and in vitro. J Biol Chem 243:2012–2121

Byar DP (1974) Zinc in male sex accessory organs: distribution and hormonal response. In: Brandes D (ed) Male sex accessory organs, structure and function in mammals. Academic, New York, pp 161–171

Chandler JA, Timms BG, Morton MS (1977) Subcellular distribution of zinc in rat prostates studied by X-ray microanalysis. I. Normal prostate. Histochem J 9:103–120

Coffey DS (1985) Biochemistry and physiology of the prostate and seminal vesicles. In: Walsh PC (ed) Campbell's urology, 5th edn. Saunders, Philadelphia, pp 1081–1121

Dawson RMC, Mann T, White LG (1957) Glycerophosphorylcholine and phosphorylcholine in semen and the relationship to choline. Biochemistry 65:627–631

Eliasson R (1959) Studies on prostaglandins. Occurrence, formation, and biological actions. Acta Physiol Scand 158 Suppl 46:1

Eliasson R (1977) Seminal plasma accessory genital glands and fertility. In: Cockett ATK, Urry RL (eds) Male infertility: workup, treatment and research. Grune and Stratton, New York, pp 189–204

Fair WR, Parrish RT (1981) Antibacterial substance in prostatic fluid. In: Murphy GP, Sandberg AA, Karr JP (eds) Prostatic cell: structure and function, part A. Liss, New York, pp 247–264

Fair WR, Wehner N (1976) The prostatic antibacterial factor: identity and significance. Prog Clin Biol Res 6:383–403

Fair WR, Couch J, Wehner N (1973) The purification and assay of the prostatic antibacterial factor (PAF). Biochem Med 8:329–339

Falk JE, Park MH, Chung SI et al. (1980) Polyamines as physiological substrates for transglutaminases. J Biol Chem 255:3695–3700

Grayhack JT (1963) Pituitary factors influencing growth of the prostate. NCI Monogr 12:189–199

Heathcote JG, Washington RJ (1973) Analysis of the zinc binding protein derived from the human benign hypertrophic prostate. J Endocrinol 58:421–423

Hessl JM, Stamey TA (1971) The passage of tetracyclines across epithelial membranes with special references to prostatic epithelium. J Urol 106:253–256

Huggins C (1947) The prostatic secretion. Harvey Lect 42:148

Huggins C, Neal W (1942) Coagulation and liquefaction of semen. Proteolytic enzymes and citrate in prostatic fluid. J Exp Med 76:527–541

Isaacs WB, Shaper JH (1983) Isolation and characterization of the major androgen-dependent glycoprotein of canine prostatic fluid. J Biol Chem 258:6610–6615

Isaacs JT, Barrak ER, Isaacs WB, Coffey DS (1981) The relationship of cellular structure and function. The matrix systems. Prog Clin Biol Res 75A:1–24

Jacobs SG, Pikna D, Lawson RK (1979) Prostatic osteoblastic factor. Invest Urol 17:195–198

Lasnitzki L, Franklin HR (1972) The influence of serum on uptake, conversion and action of testosterone in rat prostate glands in organ culture. J Endocrinol 54:333–342

MacKenzie AR, Hall T, Whitmore WF Jr (1962) Zinc content of expressed human prostatic fluid. Nature 193:72–73

Madsen PO, Baumueller A, Hoyne U (1978) Experimental models for determination of antimicrobials in prostatic tissue, interstitial fluid and secretion. Scand J Infect Dis Suppl 14:145

Mann T, Lutwak-Mann CL (1981) Male reproductive function and semen. Springer, Berlin, Heidelberg, New York

Mattila S (1969) Further studies on the prostatic tissue antigens. Separation of two molecular forms of aminopeptidase. Invest Urol 7:1–9

McNeal JE (1981) The zonal anatomy of the prostate. Prostate 2:35–49

Niemi M, Harkonen M, Larmi TK (1963) Enzymatic histochemistry of human prostate. Arch Pathol 75:528–537

O'Connor T, Sinha DK (1985) Characterization of rat ventral prostatic epithelial cells in collagen gel culture. Prostate 7:305–319

Perry ST, Viskochil DH, Ho KC, Fong K, Stafford DW, Wilson EM, French FS (1985) Androgen receptor binding to the C3 (1) subunit gene of rat prostatein. In: Bruchovsky N, Chapdelaine A, Neumann F (eds) Regulation of androgen action. Bruckner, Berlin, pp 167–173

Phadke AM, Samant NR, Deval SP (1973) Significance of seminal fructose studies in male fertility. Fertil Steril 24:894–903

Polakoski KL, Kopta M (1982) Seminal plasma. In: Zaneveld LJD, Chatterton RT (eds) Biochemistry of mammalian reproduction. Wiley, New York, pp 89–117

Poulos A, White IG (1973) Phospholipids of human spermatozoa and seminal plasma. J Reprod Fertil 35:265–272

Scott WW (1945) Lipids of prostatic fluid, seminal plasma and enlarged prostate gland of man. J Urol 53:712–718

Stamey TA (1989) Urinary infections in males. In: Stamey T (ed) Pathogenesis and treatment of urinary tract infections. Williams and Wilkins, Baltimore, pp 342–429

Stamey TA, Fair WR, Timothy MM, Wehner N (1968) Antibacterial nature of prostatic fluid. Nature 218:44–415

Stamey TA, Bushby SRM, Bragonie J (1973) The concentration of trimethoprim in prostatic fluid: nonionic diffusion or active transport? J Infect Dis 128 Suppl:686

Tauber PF, Zaneveld LJD (1976) Coagulation and liquefaction of human semen. In: Hafez ESE (ed) Human semen and fertility regulation in men. Mosby, St Louis, pp 153–166

Tauber PF, Zaneveld LJD, Propping D, Schumacher GFB (1976) Components of human split ejaculate. II. Enzymes and proteinase inhibitors. J Reprod Fertil 46:165–171

Trachtenberg J, Hicks LL, Walsh PC (1981) Methods for the determination of androgen receptor concentration in human prostatic tissue. Invest Urol 18:349–354

Tsai YC, Harrison HH, Lee C, Daufeld T, Oliver L, Grayhack JT (1984) Systematic characterization of human prostatic fluid proteins with 2-dimensional electrophoresis. Clin Chem 30:2026–2030

von Euler US (1943) Zur Kenntnis der pharmakologischen Wirkungen von Nativsekreten und Extrakten männlicher accessorischer Geschlechtsdrüsen. Arch Pathol Pharmakol 175:78–84

Wang MC, Valenzuela LA, Murphy GP, Chu TM (1979) Purification of a human prostate specific antigen. Invest Urol 17:159–163

Wang MC, Papsidero LM, Kuriyama M, Valenzuela LA, Murphy GP, Chu TM (1981) Prostate antigen: a new potential marker for prostatic cancer. Prostate 2:89–96

White IG, Darin-Bennett A, Poulos A (1976) Lipids of human semen. In: Hafez ESE (ed) Human semen and fertility regulation in men. Mosby, St Louis, pp 144–152

White MA (1975) Changes in pH of expressed prostatic secretion during the course of prostatitis. Proc R Soc Med 68:511–513

Williams-Ashman HG, Corti A, Sheth AR (1975) Formation and functions of aliphatic polyamines in the prostate gland and its secretion. In: Goland M (ed) Normal and abnormal growth of the prostate. Thomas, Springfield, pp 222–239

Zaneveld LJD, Tauber PF (1981) Contributions of prostatic fluid components to the ejaculate. Prog Clin Biol Res 75A:265–277

Host–Parasite Interactions in Prostatitis

H.G. Schiefer

Host Defenses

The male lower urogenital tract is in general fairly well protected against invading pathogens, which have to ascend the long and narrow urethra (Krieger 1984). Here, they meet the dense residual flora of the anterior one third of the male urethra (Bowie et al. 1977; Cohen et al. 1990) and can adhere to urethral epithelial surfaces only by competition for specific adhesion sites, i.e., carbohydrate moieties of glycolipids and proteins. The flushing effect of micturition, the high or low osmolality of urine, its high urea content, low pH, high content of organic acids, and the antiadhesive effects of the mucus layer on uroepithelial cells, of uromucoid (Tamm-Horsfall glycoprotein), and of secreted blood group substances inhibit bacterial colonization and growth (Andriole 1987; Gargan et al. 1993; McNabb and Tomasi 1981; Parkkinen et al. 1988; Sobel and Kaye 1984).

The prostate itself is mechanically further protected by the oblique course of the glandular ducts draining the acini (Blacklock 1981, 1990).

Prostatic secretions contain a lot of mucus (Cohen et al. 1990) which, due to its carbohydrate constituents, is sticky and thus adsorbs bacteria.

Prostatic secretions impede bacterial infection by their high content of antibacterial substances (Coffey 1992; Colleen and Mårdh 1990; Daniels and Grayhack 1990).

Zinc is found in high concentrations in prostatic tissue and secretions (Sugarman 1983) and is believed to be the active component of prostatic antibacterial factor. The mean level in prostatic fluid is 240 μg Zn/ml (4.8 mM), i.e., 200–300 times the normal serum level. On the one hand, zinc is a constituent of over 100 mammalian metalloenzymes which become active with zinc incorporation. All organisms need zinc, with bacteria generally requiring less (10^{-10}–10^{-7} M for growth, and 10^{-7}–10^{-5} M for optimal growth) than eukaryotic cells. At zinc concentrations close to those normally found in human serum, bacteria display characteristics associated with increased virulence. On the other hand, the high zinc concentrations in the millimolar range of the normal prostate and prostatic secretions toxically suppress bacterial growth. Zinc inhibits the growth of most urinary pathogens, *Chlamydia trachomatis*, *Candida* spp, herpesviruses, and *Trichomonas vaginalis*. Millimolar or higher concentrations of zinc clump bacteria, and large clumps of bacteria offer phagocytic cells an easier target. Concentrations of zinc between 10^{-5} and 10^{-3} M decrease bacterial sugar transport, amino acid uptake, and electron transfer. Inhibition is probably mediated, at least in part, by the binding of zinc to sulfhydryl or histidine residues and subsequent inhibition of enzyme functions; however, at concentrations greater than 0.1 mM, zinc also inhibits essential defense functions such as phagocytosis and thus may contribute to the chronic course of some prostatic infections (Sugarman 1983).

Polyamines such as spermine and spermidine, found in high concentrations in prostatic fluid, are cidal to many bacteria (Coffey 1992; Daniels and Grayhack 1990; Tabor et al. 1961). Structurally, spermidine and spermine can be considered derivatives of 1,4-butanediamine, as indicated in the following formulae (Bachrach 1970):

$$NH_3^+-(CH_2)_3-NH-(CH_2)_4-NH_3^+$$

Spermidine, N-(3-aminopropyl)-1,4-butanediamine

$$NH_3^+-(CH_2)_3-NH-(CH_2)_4-NH-(CH_2)_3-NH_3^+$$

Spermine, N,N'-bis(3-aminopropyl)-1,4-butanediamine

Polyamines occur ubiquitously in tissues at high concentrations and are involved in physiologic processes such as cell proliferation and growth. They can serve as growth factors for eukaryotic cells and bacteria. The level of spermine in normal human seminal plasma ranges from 0.5 to 3.5 mg/ml, originating primarily from the prostate, which is the richest source of spermine in the body. Spermine binds strongly to negatively charged molecules such as phosphate ions, nucleic acids, and phospholipids. Spermine itself does not inhibit the multiplication of bacteria.

However, oxidative products of spermine and spermidine formed via bacterial metabolism or an amine oxidase found in plasma are active antibacterial factors (Bachrach 1970). The structure of oxidized spermine is:

$$OHC-(CH_2)_2-NH-(CH_2)_4-NH-(CH_2)_2-CHO$$

Oxidized spermine, N,N'-bis(3-propionaldehyde)-1,4-butanediamine

Oxidized spermine inhibits the growth of many bacteria, e.g., *Staphylococcus aureus, Escherichia coli, Neisseria gonorrhoeae, Mycobacterium tuberculosis*, and viruses. Oxidized polyamines inhibit the synthesis of nucleic acids immediately; protein synthesis is inhibited after a lag period.

The bacteriolytic enzyme lysozyme occurs in prostatic secretions (Colleen and Mårdh 1990). It hydrolyzes a specific glycoside bond in the polyglycan chain of the murein sacculus, yielding the disaccharide N-acetylglucosamine–N-acetyl-muramic acid. It is primarily active against gram-positive bacteria whereas gram-negatives, due to the barrier presented by their outer membrane, are destroyed only after damage of this outer membrane.

Immunoglobulins are present in human prostatic secretions (Coffey 1992; Daniels and Grayhack 1990; Krieger 1984; Meares 1992; Shortliffe 1986).

Published data on immunoglobulin concentrations in prostatic secretions vary greatly, which may be due to technical differences in measuring immunoglobulin levels or to the methods used to collect prostatic fluid. Further variation may be attributed to the selection of males studied. Using strict criteria to define "normal" men with healthy prostate (no symptoms attributed to the prostate, no history of urinary tract infections, normal prostatic fluid, no evidence of gram-negative bacteria in the lower urinary tract bacterial localization), Shortliffe (1986) determined immunoglobulins in prostatic fluids to consist of 14.9 $\pm$ 8.5 mg immunoglobulin G (IgG) and 4.2 $\pm$ 2.7 mg immunoglobulin A (IgA) per 100 ml. Immunoglobulin M (IgM) levels are very low and often not detected. IgG are considered to be prostatically secreted humoral antibodies which, in pooled sera, contain a lot of antibodies directed against common uropathogens, e.g., *E. coli* serotypes 04, 06, 025, and 075 (Dierdorf and Schiwek 1991).

Production of local immunoglobulins by the prostate is regarded as an important defense mechanism (McNabb and Tomasi 1981) of the gland. Antigen-specific antibody coating of bacteria was shown in patients suffering from prostatitis. The antigen-specific antibody response in prostatic secretions, predominantly secretory IgA, is significantly greater than serologic response. Elevation of antigen-specific IgA in expressed prostatic secretions may persist longer than the elevation of either the prostatic IgG antigen-specific antibodies or the serum antigen-specific antibody levels (Shortliffe 1986).

Expressed prostatic fluid contains considerable amounts of the C3 component of complement, being present at 1.8 mg/100 ml (Coffey 1992; Daniels and Grayhack 1990).

An iron-binding protein, lactoferrin, is found in prostatic fluid and may slow bacterial growth by competing for this essential metal (Coffey 1992; Daniels and Grayhack 1990; McNabb and Tomasi 1981).

Cellular immune processes are operative in the prostate (Hargreave et al. 1986). Polymorphonuclear leukocytes and macrophages are scarce in normal prostatic secretions: up to ten leukocytes per high-power field ($\times 1000$) in expressed prostatic secretions are considered normal. T cells of the suppressor/cytotoxic type are present within the prostatic epithelium, while the majority of T cells of the helper/inducer subset are found within the interstitium. Seminal plasma has immunosuppressive effects and has been shown to suppress T and B lymphocytes, natural killer cells, macrophages, and neutrophils. The presence of immunosuppressive cells and soluble factors may minimize sensitization to sperm autoantigens, but a negative consequence of this might be an impaired response against invading pathogens.

Patients with prostatitis exhibit changes in the constituents of prostatic secretions, i.e., depressed levels of zinc, prostatic antibacterial factor, and spermine, and increased pH values. One might hypothesize that alterations of prostatic secretory functions due to unknown mechanisms might facilitate bacterial invasion and prostatic inflammation. However, it is unclear whether prostatic secretory dysfunction is a cause or consequence of bacterial infection (Meares 1990, 1992).

Bacterial Infection

Most pathogens causing prostatitis, i.e., the common uropathogens such as
E. coli and other *Enterobacteriaceae* species, *Pseudomonas aeruginosa*, and
Enterococcus spp, reach the prostate by reflux of infected urine into the prostatic
ducts (Meares 1990, 1992). By ascending infection from the urethra, *Staphylococcus saprophyticus* and sexually transmitted microorganisms such as *Neisseria
gonorrhoeae, Ureaplasma urealyticum, Chlamydia trachomatis*, and *Trichomonas
vaginalis* infect the prostate. Hematogenous spread and concomitant prostatic
infection occur during generalized infections, e.g., by *Mycobacterium tuberculosis* and by fungi such as *Cryptococcus neoformans* and *Coccidioides immitis*,
especially in cases of immunosuppression. Infections extending from the surrounding tissues occur during schistosomiasis.

Essential pathogenetic factors contributing to *E. coli* infection of the urogenital tract have been studied in some detail (Schoolnik 1989; Svanborg Edén et al.
1988). Similar pathomechanisms may also be effective in other gram-negative
bacteria.

Analysis of uropathogenic *E. coli* proved that the serotypes 04, 08, 025,
050, and 075 prevail in urinary tract infections (O'Hanley et al. 1985). Uropathogenic *E. coli* are resistant to the bactericidal activity of human serum, produce a
cytotoxic hemolysin, colicin V, aerobactin, and cytotoxic necrotizing factors
(Falbo et al. 1992).

Several urogenital pathogens, i.e., *Neisseria gonorrhoeae, Proteus* species,
and *Ureaplasma urealyticum*, produce human IgA 1-specific proteases (Loomes
et al. 1992; Spooner et al. 1992), thus inducing local paralysis of immune defense
mechanisms and facilitating bacterial colonization and penetration through the
mucosal barrier.

Using filamentous adhesins (fimbriae), *E. coli* attach to carbohydrate structures on uroepithelial surfaces (Krogfelt 1991; Schaeffer 1990). Fimbriae are
protein polymers composed of about 1000 identical subunits per fimbria. They
have a diameter of 2–7 nm and a length of 0.2–20 μm. *E. coli* fimbriae have been
divided into two broad categories based on their hemagglutination properties
(Andriole 1987; Schaeffer 1990; Sobel and Kaye 1984). Fimbriae whose agglutination with erythrocytes is inhibited by coincubation with D-mannose are
designated mannose sensitive (MS or type 1 fimbriae). All the rest are termed
mannose resistant (MR or non-mannose-sensitive fimbriae). MR fimbriae have
different carbohydrate specificities: type P fimbriae bind to galactose–galactose
residues on glycolipids or – proteins; type S fimbriae bind to N-acetylneuraminic acid – 2,3-galactose; type M fimbriae bind to structures with galactose, N-
acetylgalactosamine, N-acetylneuraminic acid, and terminal serine residues;
type G fimbriae bind to terminal N-acetyl-D-glucosamine residues; and type X
fimbriae bind to as yet unidentified carbohydrate structures (Krogfelt 1991).

Due to different carbohydrate structures on the host cells of the urogenital
tract, *E. coli* with type 1 fimbriae prefer to bind to epithelial cells of the bladder,

and less to cells of the renal pelvis or tubuli, and are mainly found in patients with cystitis. In contrast, *E. coli* with type P fimbriae preferentially bind to cells of the renal pelvis and tubuli, thus inducing pyelonephritis. More than 90% of pyelonephritogenic *E. coli* possess type P fimbriae, whereas less than 20% of *E. coli* isolated from patients with lower urogenital tract infections have type P fimbriae. *E. coli* with type P fimbriae efficiently escape host defense mechanisms, since they are not bound by phagocytes (Svanborg Edén et al. 1988; Virkola et al. 1988).

The adhesive mechanisms of gram-positive bacteria, e.g., *Enterococcus* spp, are less clear, and several mechanisms of adhesion have been detected. Gram-positive bacteria bind to N-acetylneuraminic acids of glycoproteins, to galactosamine or β-galactoside residues, or to fibronectin-rich cells, using their teichoic or lipoteichoic acids. An adhesin called aggregation substance, which enables cell–cell contact between bacteria, mediates adhesion of enterococci to eukaryotic cells. The adhesin is of proteinaceous nature, is located on the surface of the bacteria, and can be seen as hairlike structures using an electron microscope (Andriole 1987; Hasty et al. 1992; Kreft et al. 1992; Teti et al. 1987).

It is unknown whether analogous binding mechanisms operate in binding *E. coli* to prostatic epithelial cells. A recent report of immunohistologic studies on peanut (*Arachis hypogaea*) lectin-binding sites on prostatic epithelial cells (Wernert et al. 1986) is presumably pertinent to this problem. Using *Arachis hypogaea* lectin, corresponding carbohydrate structures, i.e., β-D-galactose residues, were seen on the surfaces of prostatic epithelial cells and, thus, may be assumed to be readily accessible for binding *E. coli* with type P fimbriae, similar to binding to uroepithelial cells. However, mere bacterial invasion into the gland may be sufficient for prostatic infection.

Nevertheless, invasion and attachment of bacteria are followed by mucosal inflammation, presumably induced by lipid A, cytotoxic hemolysin, and cytotoxic necrotizing factors of the directly adhering gram-negative bacteria, which subsequently might invade the mucosa (Falbo et al. 1992; Svanborg Edén 1988).

The kinetics and sequelae of the ensuing inflammatory process in the prostate has been studied in more detail in animal models of prostatitis induced in small rodents (Jantos et al. 1990). Inoculation of uropathogenic *E. coli* into the bladder of *Mastomys natalensis* induced severe prostatitis. Histologic and microbiologic courses of the prostatic infection strongly resembled human disease, and acute bacterial prostatitis was followed by the development of chronic bacterial and nonbacterial prostatitis.

The prostates of all animals killed within the initial 3 days were infected. *E. coli* was cultured in numbers ranging from 10^3 to 10^{11} colony-forming units (CFU) per gram tissue. Later on, the rate of infection was found to decline, but self-limitation of the infection was not observed, since 6 months after infection the prostates of some animals were still infected (range, $10^2–10^9$ CFU/g; Jantos et al. 1990).

Antilipopolysaccharide antibodies were first detected at day 3 after infection in the infected animals. From day 6 through to the end of the study, antibody response was observed in 98% of animals. Titers rose rapidly during the second week and remained at high levels within the first month. After 2–6 months, titers returned to low levels (Jantos et al. 1990).

Histopathologically, in the infected animals at day 1 after infection, emigration of inflammatory cells from the vessels of the prostatic stroma was noted. Two days after infection, the epithelium of the prostatic acini was heavily infiltrated with neutrophil granulocytes and showed local destruction and desquamation. The lumen was filled with an exudate of neutrophil granulocytes. In the stroma, a moderate infiltration of plasma cells, lymphocytes, and occasionally neutrophils was seen. Subsequently, an increase of periacinar and intraluminal inflammation was noted. The lumina became dilated and filled with numerous granulocytes, macrophages, and cellular debris. The epithelial lining was almost completely destroyed, and abscesses had formed. At 15 days, wide areas of the prostatic tissue were replaced by granulation tissue. Remaining acini were filled with purulent exudate. The epithelium had lost its secretory activity and was cuboid in shape. At 2 and 3 months, histology showed a granulomatous inflammation; focal epithelial regeneration was also seen. In all animals killed 6 months after infection, inflammatory changes were still present. Most of the epithelium was regenerated and showed localized hyperplasia and metaplasia. The surrounding stroma was filled with an infiltrate consisting of plasma cells and lymphocytes. In animals with sterile prostatic specimens, some scattered intraluminal leukocytes were observed, while in the animals that were still infected, the lumina of some acini were dilated and filled with neutrophils. No major morphologic differences in the histologic pattern of inflammation were noted between animals with positive and negative bacterial cultures (Jantos et al. 1990).

An interesting observation for understanding the pathogenesis of chronic bacterial prostatitis was the demonstration of a glycocalix which enclosed and protected bacterial microcolonies within the prostatic acini and ducts. The immune system presumably does not recognize the causative bacteria, because they are embedded within the glycocalix. On the other hand, antibodies raised against the glycocalix might induce chronic inflammation within the prostate (Costerton 1984; Nickel et al. 1990).

Morphology of Prostatitis

There is no accepted histologic classification of prostatitis in general use at the present time (Helpap 1989). Histologic evidence of prostatic inflammation is often present in surgical and autopsy material. Inflammatory lesions are found in up to 40% of adult prostates and inflammatory changes are detected in about 50% of noninfected prostates, suggesting the possibility of a noninfectious etiology of prostatic inflammation.

In a series of 162 cases of surgically resected hyperplastic prostates, the incidence of inflammation was 98%. Six morphologic patterns of inflammation were described (Kohnen and Drach 1979):

1. Segregated glandular inflammation is the most frequently encountered lesion and is considered the basic morphologic unit of prostatitis. It is characterized by a central dilated gland or duct and a segregated inflammatory response. The lumen of the gland is filled with secretory material, cellular debris, foamy macrophages, and neutrophils. Most of the epithelium is nonsecretory. A narrow band of lymphocytes and plasma cells surrounds each gland.
2. Periglandular inflammation exhibits a band or nodular focus of lymphocytes and plasma cells adjacent to a gland or duct, with the lumen free of inflammatory cells.
3. In diffuse stromal inflammation, sheets, clusters, and rows of lymphocytes, plasma cells, and some neutrophils dissect between stromal cells. The inflammatory infiltrate lacks circumferential orientation around glands or ducts.
4. The pattern of isolated stromal lymphoid nodules is characterized by nodular aggregates of lymphocytes and plasma cells in the stroma, mostly in close proximity to a vein.
5. Acute necrotizing inflammation is characterized by a dense infiltrate of neutrophils and extensive tissue necrosis, leading to abscess formation.
6. The nodular lesion of localized granulomatous inflammation is composed of macrophages or epithelioid cells, multinucleated giant cells, lymphocytes, and plasma cells. Fibroblastic proliferation at the periphery of the lesion leads to concentric layers of fibrous tissue being deposited.

No significant morphologic differences were found among groups of cases with positive and negative results of bacterial cultures.

Risk Factors for Prostatitis

Several predisposing, exogenous and endogenous factors favor an increased incidence of lower urinary tract infections in general and prostatitis in particular (Andriole 1984, 1985; Kunin 1984; Sobel and Kaye 1985):

1. Incomplete emptying of the urinary bladder caused by mechanical obstruction (stricture, stenosis, calculi) and neurologic defects (diabetic neuropathy, paralysis, spinal cord injury)
2. Advanced age (obstructive uropathy, reduction of prostatic antibacterial factor, reduced uromucoid)
3. Instrumental manipulation
4. Indwelling urethral catheter (breakdown of the mucus layer, facilitated bacterial ascension)
5. Diabetes mellitus (bacterial multiplication favored by high glucose levels, reduced granulocyte function)

References

Andriole VT (1984) Genitourinary infections in the patient at risk: an overview. Am J Med 76 (5A):155–157

Andriole VT (1987) Urinary tract infections: recent developments. J Inf Dis 156:865–869

Bachrach U (1970) Metabolism and function of spermine and related polyamines. Annu Rev Microbiol 24:109–134

Blacklock NJ (1981) Prostatitis: pathogenesis, clinical features and management. In: Hendry WF (ed) Recent advances in urology/andrology 3. Churchill Livingstone, New York, pp 185–197

Blacklock NJ (1990) The prostate. Surgical anatomy. In: Chisholm GD, Fair WR (eds) Scientific foundations of urology, 3rd edn. Heinemann, Oxford, Year Book, Chicago, pp 340–350

Bowie WR, Pollock HM, Forsyth PS, Floyd JF, Alexander ER, Wang SP, Holmes KK (1977) Bacteriology of the urethra in normal men and men with nongonococcal urethritis. J Clin Microbiol 6:482–488

Coffey DS (1992) The molecular biology, endocrinology, and physiology of the prostate and seminal vesicles. In: Walsh PC, Retik AB, Stamey TA, Vaughan ED (eds) Campbell's urology, 6th edn, vol 1. Saunders, Philadelphia, pp 221–266

Cohen MS, Weber RD, Mårdh PA (1990) Genitourinary mucosal defenses. In: Holmes KK, Mårdh PA, Sparling PF, Wiesner PJ (eds) Sexually transmitted diseases, 2nd edn. McGraw-Hill, New York, pp 117–127

Colleen S, Mårdh PA (1990) Prostatitis. In: Holmes KK, Mårdh PA, Sparling PF, Wiesner PJ (eds) Sexually transmitted diseases, 2nd edn. McGraw-Hill, New York, pp 653–661

Costerton JW (1984) The etiology and persistence of cryptic bacterial infections: a hypothesis. Rev Inf Dis 6:S608–S616

Daniels GF, Grayhack JT (1990) Physiology of prostatic secretions. In: Chisholm GD, Fair WR (eds) Scientific foundations of urology, 3rd edn. Heinemann, Oxford, Year Book, Chicago, pp 351–358

Dierdorf RE, Schiwek DR (1991) Intravenöse Immunglobuline. Grundlagen und klinische Befunde. Sandoz, Basel

Falbo V, Famiglietti M, Caprioli A (1992) Gene block encoding production of cytotoxic necrotizing factor 1 and hemolysin in Escherichia coli isolates from extraintestinal infections. Infect Immun 60:2182–2187

Gargan RA, Hamilton-Miller JMT, Brumfitt W (1993) Effect of pH and osmolality on in vitro phagocytosis and killing by neutrophils in urine. Infect Immun 61:8–12

Hargreave TB, James K, Chisholm GD, El Demiry M, Szymaniec S, Harvey J, Ritchie AWS (1986) Mechanisms of immunity within the prostate and male genital tract. In: Weidner W, Brunner H, Krause W, Rothauge CF (eds) Therapy of prostatitis. Klinische und experimentelle Urologie 11. Zuckschwerdt, Munich, pp 123–126

Hasty DL, Ofek I, Courtney HS, Doyle RJ (1992) Multiple adhesins of streptococci. Infect Immun 60:2147–2152

Helpap B (1989) Pathologie der ableitenden Harnwege und der Prostata. Springer, Berlin Heidelberg New York

Jantos C, Altmannsberger M, Weidner W, Schiefer HG (1990) Acute and chronic bacterial prostatitis due to E. coli. Description of an animal model. Urol Res 18:207–211

Kohnen PW, Drach GW (1979) Pattern of inflammation in prostatic hyperplasia: a histologic and bacteriologic study. J Urol 121:755–760

Kreft B, Marre R, Schramm U, Wirth R (1992) Aggregation substance of Enterococcus faecalis mediates adhesion to cultured renal tubular cells. Infect Immun 60:25–30

Krieger JN (1984) Prostatitis syndromes: pathophysiology, differential diagnosis, and treatment. Sex Transm Dis 11:100–112

Krogfelt KA (1991) Bacterial adhesion: genetics, biogenesis, and role in pathogenesis of fimbrial adhesins of Escherichia coli. Rev Inf Dis 13:721–735

Kunin CM (1984) Genitourinary infections in the patient at risk: extrinsic risk factors. Am J Med 76 (5A):131–139

Loomes LM, Senior BW, Kerr MA (1992) Proteinases of Proteus spp: purification, properties, and detection in urine of infected patients. Infect Immun 60:2267–2273

McNabb PC, Tomasi TB (1981) Host defense mechanisms at mucosal surfaces. Annu Rev Microbiol 35:477–496

Meares EM (1990) Prostatitis. In: Chisholm GD, Fair WR (eds) Scientific foundations of urology, 3rd edn. Heinemann, Oxford, Year Book, Chicago, pp 373–378

Meares EM (1992) Prostatitis and related disorders. In: Walsh PC, Retik AB, Stamey TA, Vaughan ED (eds) Campbell's urology, 6th edn, vol 1. Saunders, Philadelphia, pp 807–822

Nickel JC, Olson ME, Barabas A, Benediktsson H, Dasgupta MK, Costerton JW (1990) Pathogenesis of chronic bacterial prostatitis in an animal model. Br J Urol 66:47–54

O'Hanley P, Low D, Romero I, Lark D, Vosti K, Falkow S, Schoolnik G (1985) Gal–Gal binding and hemolysin phenotypes and genotypes associated with uropathogenic Escherichia coli. New Engl J Med 313:414–420

Parkkinen J, Virkola R, Korhonen TK (1988) Identification of factors in human urine that inhibit the binding of Escherichia coli adhesins. Infect Immun 56:2623–2630

Schaeffer AJ (1990) Role of bacterial adherence in urinary tract infections. In: Chisholm GD, Fair WR (eds) Scientific foundations of urology. Heinemann, Oxford, Year Book, Chicago, pp 123–130

Schoolnik GK (1989) How Escherichia coli infects the urinary tract. New Engl J Med 320:804–805

Shortliffe LMD (1986) Characterization of prostatic mucosal immunity to enterobacterial infections. In: Weidner W, Brunner H, Krause W, Rothauge CF (eds) Therapy of prostatitis. Klinische und experimentelle Urologie 11. Zuckschwerdt, Munich, pp 118–122

Sobel JD, Kaye D (1984) Host factors in the pathogenesis of urinary tract infections. Am J Med 76 (5A):122–130

Sobel JD, Kaye D (1985) Reduced uromucoid excretion in the elderly. J Inf Dis 152:653

Spooner RK, Russell WC, Thirkell D (1992) Characterization of the immunoglobulin A protease of Ureaplasma urealyticum. Infect Immun 60:2544–2546

Sugarman B (1983) Zinc and infection. Rev Inf Dis 5:137–147

Svanborg Edén C, Hausson S, Jodal U, Lidin-Janson G, Lincoln K, Linder H, Lomberg H, de Man P, Marild S, Martinell J, Plos K, Sandberg T, Stenqvist K (1988) Host–parasite interaction in the urinary tract. J Inf Dis 157:421–426

Tabor H, Tabor CW, Rosenthal SM (1961) The biochemistry of the polyamines: spermidine and spermine. Annu Rev Biochem 30:579–604

Teti G, Chiofalo MS, Tomasello F, Fava C, Mastroeni P (1987) Mediation of Staphylococcus saprophyticus adherence to uroepithelial cells by lipoteichoic acid. Infect Immun 55:839–842

Virkola R, Westerlund B, Holthöfer H, Parkkinen J, Kekomäki M, Korhonen TK (1988) Binding characteristics of Escherichia coli adhesins in human urinary bladder. Infect Immun 56:2615–2622

Wernert N, Goebbels R, Seitz G, Dhom G (1986) Immunohistochemical demonstration of peanut agglutinin (PNA) binding sites in prostatic carcinomas before and after antiandrogenic treatment. Verh Dt Ges Path 70:329–331

The Anatomy of the Prostate: Relationship with Prostatic Infection*

N.J. Blacklock

Introduction

The prostate which is involved in prostatitis is the functional prostate still largely unaffected by the age-related changes of benign prostatic hyperplasia. Prostatitis is a sexually acquired infection, whatever the organism, and therefore occurs in the more sexually active phase of life. It tends to commence in the latter part of the second decade in adolescence.

Anatomical Factors

The gland which is anatomically the one involved has been described by McNeal (1972) and others as comprising a central zone at the base of the gland and a peripheral zone towards the apex; the peripheral zone comprises two thirds of the gland mass (Fig. 1). The primitive duct entities within the embryo are recognisable at the 120 mm stage, with a group of ducts originating above the seminal colliculus giving rise eventually to the central zone acini and a group below the colliculus which develop into the peripheral zone. The central zone is closely associated with other Wolffian-derived structures such as the seminal vesicles and distal vas deferens, and it is noteworthy that the central zone encloses the lower part of the vesicles and the ejaculatory ducts. This part of the gland is developmentally homologous to the paraurethral glands of the female, and the acinar epithelium of the central zone has fewer androgen receptors and appears less androgen dependent than the epithelium of the peripheral zone; the acini develop from the otherwise undifferentiated fibromuscular stroma before puberty unlike those of the peripheral zone, which are much more androgen dependent and await the stimulus of puberty before development. The central zone is separated entirely from the urethra by the preprostatic sphincter muscle,

---

* Due to unforeseen circumstances, Prof. Blacklock was unable to attend the Sils-Maria Symposium Prostatitis; however, he has kindly placed his planned contribution at our disposal, which was previously published in *Infection*, Vol. 19, Suppl. 3, © MMV Medizin Verlag GmbH München.

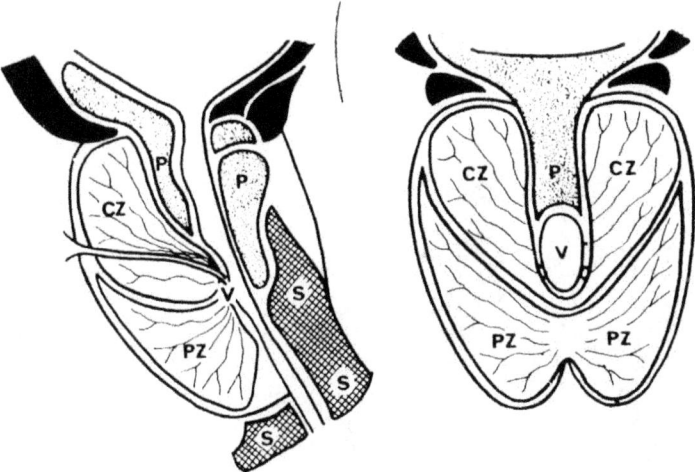

Fig. 1. Sagittal (*left*) and coronal (*right*) sections of the prostate; *p*, pre-prostatic sphincter; *cz*, central zone; *pz*, peripheral zone; *s*, striated sphincter of the urethra; *v*, verumontanum

which is a prolongation downwards from the deep trigone and internal sphincter. This terminates at the level of the verumontanum, and below this level the peripheral zone comes much more directly into contact with the urethra. The ducts of the central zone are characteristically obliquely inclined to the long axis of the urethra and enter the urethra at the lower margin of the preprostatic sphincter posteriorly just above and on either side of the verumontanum. The entry of these ducts is valvular and this contrasts with the mode of entry of the peripheral zone ducts perpendicular to or obliquely against the line of flow down the prostatic urethra (Fig. 2). A possible reason for the configuration of these ducts is that this is a mechanism to produce turbulence within the prostatic urethra as a mixing chamber at the time of ejaculation to ensure mixture of the four separate constituents of seminal fluid which come together for the first time in this location.

These and other anatomical features are directly related to the natural history of prostatitis as well as factors associated with the dynamic nature of the prostatic urethra and its related sphincters.

The prostate is infected by the ascent of organisms from the lower urethra. This implies an earlier stage of usually asymptomatic colonisation of the lower urethra. Ascent from the lower urethra is by direct extension at least as far as the upper bulbous urethra. Thereafter, organisms may be lifted upwards into the prostatic urethra by the turbulence produced in the otherwise linear flow of the column of urine at the level of the external sphincter. This is the result of the greater rigidity and slight narrowing of the urethra at this point, and this turbulence may be increased in states wherein the external sphincter is not completely relaxed at the time of urination. Mayo and Hinman (1973) elegantly

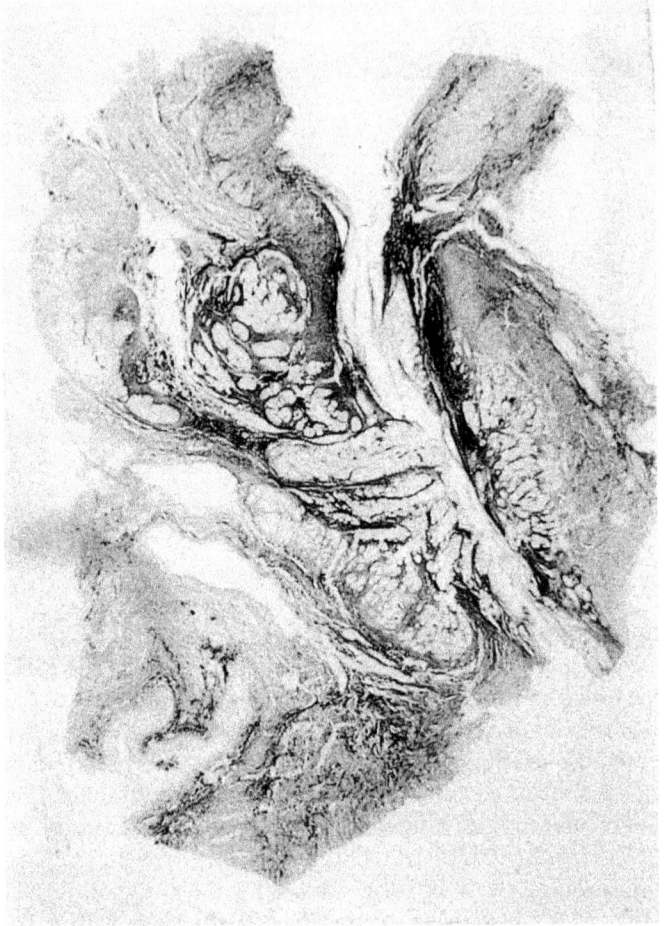

Fig. 2. Sagittal section of the prostate showing direction of entry of central and peripheral zone ducts into urethra (Van Gieson stain)

demonstrated the occurrence of this type of ascent in experimental studies in the female. Whether by this means or by direct extension, organisms gain access to the lower prostatic urethra, where there is easy access to the ducts of the peripheral zone. Any increase in intraurethral pressure, however transient, will encourage reflux of urine, and organisms, if present, into these ducts in preference to the ducts of the central zone whose oblique entry into the urethra is almost valvular in nature; pressure rise within the prostatic urethra might therefore be expected to occlude central zone ducts and prevent such reflux. This may account for the much greater incidence of prostatitis within the peripheral zone.

The course of the peripheral zone ducts through this part of the gland is an additional factor of anatomical importance in the natural history of the disease. They pass posteriorly and then curve laterally and ultimately anteriorly within the substance of the gland (Fig. 3). These ducts are therefore vulnerable to

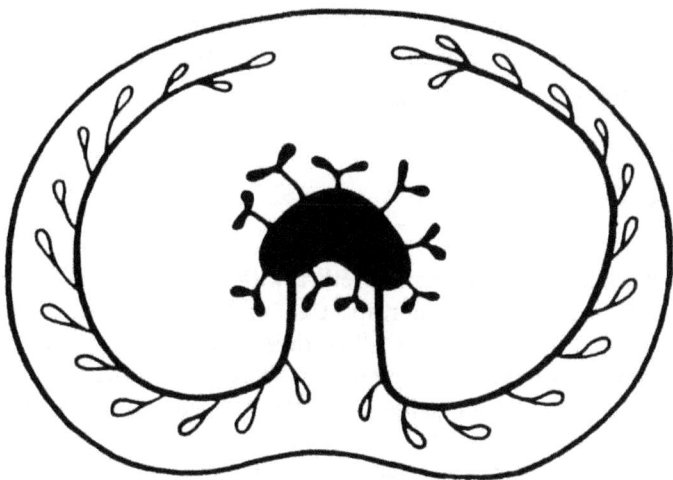

Fig. 3. Diagram of course of peripheral zone ducts to the prostate

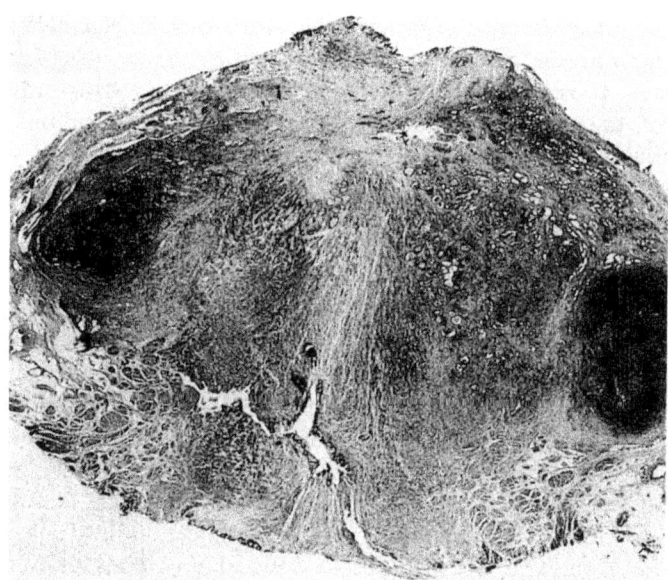

Fig. 4. Section of prostate showing peripheral loculi of infection within the gland

occlusion by oedema or scarring, such that loculation of infection and its products is possible. This is a risk if, at the outset, treatment of the acute infection is inadequate or ineffective. When this occurs, there is the likelihood of chronicity and recrudescence of acute episodes from residual pockets of infection within the periphery of the gland (Fig. 4). In states of compromised immunity, abscess formation may occur in these sites. This duct morphology and the realisation of the likely sequel to inappropriate or inadequate antibiotic treatment emphasises the importance of effective therapy at the earliest possible stage following recognition of prostatitis.

Dynamic Factors

The dynamic characteristics of the prostatic urethra with its related sphincters give rise to a number of possibilities in respect to pressure rise within the prostatic urethra during urination and at other times. In normal urination, synchronously with the contraction of the detrusor, there is relaxation first of the internal sphincter and, almost immediately, of the external sphincter. Any pressure rise within the prostatic urethra is minimal and transient.

The internal and preprostatic sphincters are richly innervated by α-adrenergic nerve endings and respond to noradrenergic stimulation, resulting in closure. Both the muscle of the prostatic capsule, the individual acinar smooth muscle and muscles surrounding the prostatic ducts, the ejaculatory ducts, the vas and the seminal vesicles are also richly endowed with adrenergic nerve endings, so that the same noradrenergic stimulation results in ejaculation. Reflux of the ejaculate into the bladder is thus prevented by the closure of the preprostatic sphincter. It is noteworthy that ejaculation in the structurally normal gland achieves the most effective emptying of acini and ducts, and this is far more effective than any attempt to evacuate acinar and duct content by prostatic massage. Good management of prostatitis should therefore include advice on early resumption of normal sexual activity after the acute phase of treatment, using a condom if necessary to minimise cross-infection of the spouse or sexual partner.

The external sphincter complex is largely voluntary, although there is an α-adrenergically innervated inner sleeve of involuntary muscle. This sphincter is part of the pelvic floor, and its innervation is therefore otherwise somatic, as is that part of the pelvic floor musculature which surrounds the anus. It is for this reason that sphincter induced micturitional disturbances are so frequently accompanied by anal complaints. Noradrenergic stimulation as in anxiety and apprehension, whilst resulting in general increase in somatic muscle tension, may specifically affect the peri-urethral and peri-anal sphincters and result in disturbances of micturition. This is usually most noticeable as diminution in urine flow rate and detrusor irritability. This has been termed the "anxious bladder" syndrome, and is characterised by a variably raised urethral pressure profile with low bladder pressure at the same time (1979). Within the urethra, the increase in urethral pressure at the time of urination resultant on the failure of complete relaxation of the external sphincter encourages reflux into the peripheral zone ducts and, if organisms are present within the prostatic urethra, this may give rise to prostatitis. Intra-prostatic duct reflux has been visualised during micturating cysto-urethrography (Fig. 5), and there is confirmation of urinary reflux into prostatic acini and ducts by the composition of prostatic calculi, whose constituents are so often uriniferous in origin. These dynamic factors link the mood and personality of the individual with a predisposition to this particular infection and is an interesting example of the influence of the psyche on the soma. It is also the basis for our understanding of the condition of prostatodynia – the syndrome of prostatic, genital and anal pain and variable micturitional disturbances in the absence of objective evidence of prostatic inflammation. An understanding of the mechanism provides the rationale of management of such cases by reassurance and muscle relaxant therapy.

Normal urination is terminated by closure of the external sphincter and the rapid milk-back of urine remaining in the prostatic urethra into the bladder by the action of the striated muscle of the urethra. This muscle can be rudimentary in some men and is best represented in male animals which have territorial instincts, i.e. the fox, wolf, dog and cat. Its purpose is to conserve urine in the

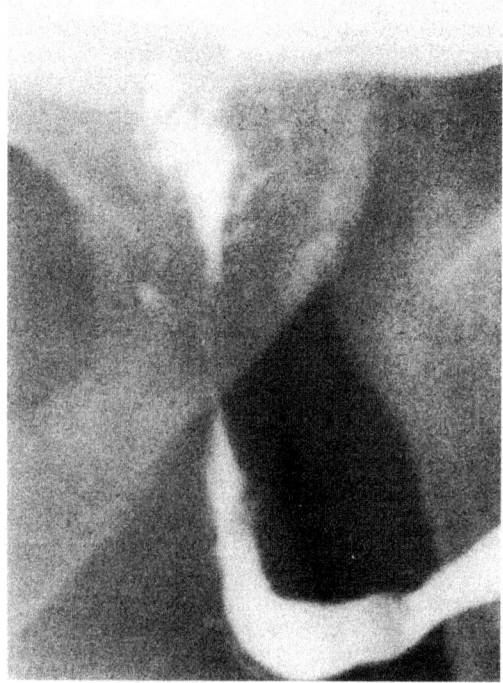

Fig. 5. Micturating cysto-urethrogram. Reflux of contrast has occurred into some of the main prostatic ducts on each side

course of the marking out of territorial acquisition or its maintenance by "spotting" with urine. It is, therefore, an atavistic structure. Following milk-back, the bladder neck is closed. The prostatic urethra is therefore occluded at its upper and lower extremities. In this situation, any sudden rises in intra-abdominal pressure or jolting of the body as in cycling and in jogging will be transmitted to the closed prostatic urethra, and any residual prostatic urethral content may in these circumstances be forced into the prostatic ducts. This phenomenon can account for the occurrence and refractory nature of prostatitis in some sportsmen and, to a lesser extent, in those who spend long hours in the driving seat of heavy goods vehicles.

In the absence of actual infection, it is entirely conceivable that urinary constituents may set up minor inflammatory reaction within the prostate and account for minor urinary symptoms manifested by some men in these occupations.

If the internal sphincter is compromised surgically by bladder neck resection or by neurogenic disease, the prostatic urethra remains in communication with the bladder at all times and is therefore subject to pressure changes within it. These pressures may originate intrinsically within the bladder or be transmitted from the abdominal cavity. Reflux is even more likely in these circumstances and is demonstrable by cystography (Fig. 6). The prostate is therefore continually at risk of infection and reinfection. Any operation which compromises the internal sphincter is therefore contra-indicated in patients who have manifested the tendency to prostatitis.

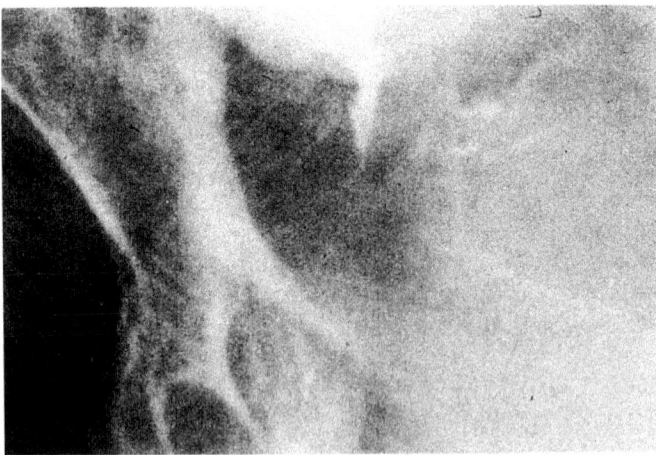

Fig. 6. Cystogram in patient following compromise of the bladder neck by transurethral resection. There is direct communication between the bladder and the prostatic urethra and reflux of contrast is seen in the prostatic ducts

Related Factors

Studies have defined the immunological reaction of the prostatic tissues to infection. Immunoglobulins G, A and M have been found in the prostatic fluid and immune complexes have also been demonstrated within the basement membrane of the acinar and ductal epithelial cells and in the periacinar tissues, the latter suggesting circulating immune complexes. These may be produced in response to microbial species of one form or another or to their by-products and perhaps even to urinary constituents. Recent work has shown that the organisms within the prostatic acini and ducts can respond to adversity in this environment induced by antibiotics or the immune response by forming glycocalix-enclosed microcolonies. This exopolysaccharide film can protect the bacteria from the effects of antibiotic and the host defence mechanisms, so permitting their persistence within the gland (1990). Whilst loculation of organisms within the gland due to duct obstruction by oedema or fibrosis occurs in chronic prostatitis, this glycocalix formation can also explain the phenomenon of chronic prostatitis with recrudescence at intervals. The glycocalix-enclosed bacteria are closely adherent to the acinar and duct epithelium and therefore difficult to dislodge by prostatic massage. Not only will this mechanical feature encourage the persistence of infection, but it can also account for the failure to culture microorganisms at the time of investigation, so giving rise to an apparent non-infective or non-bacterial prostatitis. The release from these enclosed colonies of small numbers of planktonic organisms may accompany flare-ups of infection, at which time the organism in small numbers may be recoverable. Glycocalix-enclosed bacteria may also explain the reduced chemotactic response of leucocytes which has been shown in some studies using organisms from patients with prostatitis.

These new observations provide a further challenge in the management of this difficult disease and a further stimulus to greater efficiency in antibiotic treatment. A full understanding of the anatomical features of prostatitis and related predisposing factors is important in overall effective management.

References

McNeal J (1972) The prostate and prostatic urethra: a morphologic synthesis. J Urol 107:1008

Mayo ME, Hinman F (1973) Role of midurethral high pressure zone in spontaneous bacterial ascent. J Urol 109:268

George NJR, Slade N (1979) Hesitancy and poor stream in neurologically normal younger men without outflow tract obstruction. Br J Urol 51:506

Nickel JC, Olson ME, Barabas A, Benediktsson A, Dasgupta MK, Costerton JW (1990) Pathogenesis of chronic bacterial prostatitis in an animal model. Br J Urol 66:47

Complaint Complexes
and Psychosomatic Aspects

E. Brähler

In spite of refined diagnostic methods, over half the patients with prostatitis symptoms today are given the diagnosis prostatodynia, because no evidence of a relevant, objective, bacteriological finding can be found (see Brähler and Weidner 1989). It must be assumed that psychopathological or neurotic mechanisms are involved in symptom development, making it especially important to register the symptoms of this group of patients with extreme care. This is partly because the symptoms play a particular role in the diagnosis of prostatitis, but also partly because many of the symptoms involved show a gradual transition into the area of psychosomatic or psychoneurotic complaints.

Symptoms and Complaint Complexes

Apart from the urological differential diagnosis, the symptoms of chronic prostatitis are identical. We differentiate between typical inflammatory symptoms, disturbances arising in the genital region, in micturation, in sexual functioning and in the anorectal area, and diffuse, generalized symptoms, frequently rheumatic in nature (Table 1; see Brähler and Weidner 1989; Ludwig et al. 1992; Weidner 1984).

First Junker (1969) and then Brähler et al. (1986) constructed complaints lists for recording subjective prostatitis-related complaints. Table 2 shows the most frequent prostatitis-related complaints registered in patients with chronic prostatitis, reported independently of the differential diagnosis (Brähler et al. 1986). Studies by Deinhart (1993) and Pott et al. (1991) came up with very similar results. Junker (1969) and Janssen et al. (1983) registered certain complaints even more frequently, but this may be due to their using different criteria in sample selection.

Among patients with chronic prostatitis we find that generalized physical complaints are registered even more frequently than prostatitis-related complaints. Table 3 shows the 11 complaints in the Giessen Subjective Complaints List (Giessener Beschwerdebogen; Brähler and Scheer 1983) which were reported by over 50% of patients, regardless of their specific urological diagnosis (Brähler et al. 1986). Similar results are reported by Deinhart (1993). In other words, unrelated to urological diagnosis, patients with chronic prostatitis suffer

Table 1. Symptoms of chronic and prostatitis and prostatodynia

Inflammatory symptoms	Diffuse disorders in the genital area	Micturation disorders	Sexual dysfunctioning	Disorders in anorectal area	General symptoms
Burning pain in the urethra, hemospermia, pyospermia	Sensation of pressure on the pubic bone and perineum; twinging pains in the testes and epididymis; pain in the penis, groin, and lower abdomen; prostatospermatorrhea	Dysuria, pollakisuria, nocturia, terminal dribbling, strangury, dorsolateral pains	Disturbances in libido, appetence, erection and ejaculation, and emotional relationships	Sensations of burning and itching around the anus; feeling of pressure on the rectum	Conjunctivitis, pains in limbs, backache

Table 2. Most frequent subjective prostatitis-related complaints

Dribbling after urination	48.8%
Getting up in the night to urinate	48.8%
Twinges and pains in the groin	48.0%
Involuntary erections in the night	45.5%
Pain in the testes	44.7%
Burning pain in the urethra after urination	43.5%
Delay at begin of urination	43.1%
Itching of the anus after bowel movement	39.8%
Pain in the bladder area	36.6%
Burning pain in the urethra during urination	35.8%
Failure to erect in spite of sexual desire	34.1%
Tenderness in urethra after urination	34.1%
Feeling of pressure and pain in the area between anus and testes	33.3%

Table 3. General physical complaints most frequently reported by patients with chronic prostatitis

Backache	68.3%
Excessive sweating	68.3%
Tiredness	61.0%
Cold feet	58.5%
Pain in joints or limbs	58.5%
Pain in the neck	57.7%
Headache	57.7%
Exhaustion	52.8%
Disturbed sleep	52.0%
Tired legs	52.0%
Sensation of pressure in the abdomen	50.4%

from a whole series of general bodily complaints significantly more frequently than average men of their age in the general population. Diederichs (1986) defines hypochondria as a typical characteristic of men with abnormal prostata diagnoses and relates this to a central disturbance in their body experience.

However as may be judged by an outside observer, these additional body complaints cause the patient so much discomfort that they cannot be ignored as relevant factors detracting from his overall quality of life (see Gross 1991).

Systematic Measurement of Complaints

To objectify subjective bodily complaints, it is advisable to use questionnaires whose responses can be converted into scales. Scales have the advantage over single items that they produce far more reliable results. Brähler and Weidner

(1986) created a prostatitis questionnaire from which they extracted four complexes of complaints. However, only two of these could be confirmed in a replica study by Deinhart (1993) to the extent that they can now be regarded as fulfilling the standard quality criteria most satisfactorily. One of these two scales ("prostatitis complaints") contains 18 items referring to complaints in the anal and urogenital area and represents the "true " prostatitis symptoms (Table 4).

Questions concerning these items all ask for responses reflecting the degree of subjective discomfort experienced for each complaint (not at all, 0; slightly, 1; somewhat, 2; considerably, 3; very much, 4), so that on scale 1 scores can range from 0 to 68. With this scale chronic prostatitis can be diagnosed very reliably with regard to subjective complaints (Cronbach test, $\alpha = 0.91$; split-half correla-

Table 4. Complaint complexes in systematic measurement of chronic prostatitis and related neurotic symptoms

Scale 1: prostatitis complaints

Burning in the urethra after urination
Pain/twinges in the groin
Pressure/pain in the area between anus and testes
Heavy sensation in the rectum
Pain in the bladder after urinating
Feeling of pressure in the pubic area
Burning pain in the urethra when urinating
Feeling of pressure/pain in the anus
Itching at the tip of the penis
Pressure/pain in the anus after bowel movement

Itching of anus after bowel movement
Painful ejaculations
Pain in the testes
Tenderness in urethra after urinating
Pain around the bladder
Urgency to urinate
Constipation
Pains in the abdomen

Scale 2: disorders in sexual functioning

Pain in the penis
Premature ejaculation before or directly after penetration
Inability to erect in spite of sexual desire
Premature ejaculation on erection
Premature ejaculation without erection
Reduced sexual excitability

Scale 3: exhaustion

Generalized weakness
Excessive need for sleep
Tendency to rapid exhaustion
Sleepiness
Feeling of numbness/dazedness
Lethargy

Scale 4: pain in limbs

Pain in limbs or joints
Backache
Pain in neck or shoulders
Headache
Heavy or tired legs
Feeling of pressure in head

tion test, $r_{12} = 0.80$; test-5-year-retest, $r_{tt} = 0.72$). This scale is comparable to the various scales that have been developed to record the symptoms of benign prostata hyperplasia (see Effert and Ackermann 1992; Barry et al. 1992a, b) and exceeds their internal consistency scores (Barry et al. 1992a). Scale 2, with 6 items, comprises secondary neurotic symptoms related to sexuality. Here, too, the reliability is very high ($\alpha = 0.82$, $r_{12} = 0.77$, $r_{tt} = 0.66$). On this scale, as on scales 3 and 4, scores between 0 and 24 are possible. Scale 3 reflects generalized, concomitant symptoms of a neurotic nature ($\alpha = 0.70$, $r_{12} = 0.70$, $r_{tt} = 0.56$). As Scale 3 is taken from the Giessen Subjective Complaints List, representative and illness-related standard scores are available. The same applies to Scale 4, which relates to pains in limbs ($\alpha = 0.77$, $r_{12} = 0.55$, $r_{tt} = 0.66$). Scales 3 and 4 are valid and reliable indicators for quality of life and are preferable to the type of quality of life index which is based on only one item (e.g., in Effert and Ackermann 1992).

Chronic Development of Complaints

Catamneses on the long-term development of subjective complaints in chronic prostatitis are rare. Relatively short-term studies on therapeutic success have been carried out on small or selected samples by Weidner et al. (1991) and Rugendorff et al. (1992). Using interviews and psychological tests to collect data on 40 patients, Keltikangas-Järvinen et al. (1989) found that, where symptoms persisted, anxiety, stress, and sexual problems increased during a 2-year period of observation, as did the fear of contracting cancer or a venereal disease. At the same time, social activities were reduced. In 38% of patients, the symptoms improved over the 2 years and in 62% they became worse.

In 1993, Deinhart published the results of a 5-year catamnesis on illness development in 95 patients with chronic prostatitis. In the two urological complaint complexes, "prostatitis complaints" and "disorders in sexual functioning" (see Table 4), no general decrease in the degree or intensity of complaints could be found.

However, the development in the degree of complaints varies greatly between individuals and covers a wide range, with improvements in 51% of patients, including considerable or complete recovery, and a worsening of symptoms in 49% of patients; in some cases, symptoms persisted or increased to a striking degree. In other words, the illness frequently takes a chronic course with continued subjective discomfort. This pattern applies equally to both subgroups (infectious prostatitis and prostatodynia). Results such as these provide confirmation for the thesis that both diagnostic groups are in fact very similar and may well have an almost identical etiology.

In spite of treatment with antibiotics, the patients with infectious prostatitis showed no significant improvement in symptoms. This raises serious doubts as to the value of this form of treatment. There were no indications of a marked persistence of prostatitis-related symptoms in patients with existing neurotic or general psychosomatic complaints.

The interaction between increases or decreases in recorded prostatitis-related complaints and the scale "exhaustion" (see Table 4) was minimal. There is similarly no connection between prostatitis-related complaints and age or diagnosis of patient.

However, a comparison between the diagnostic subgroups with respect to the development of their overall quality of life over time revealed a striking divergence between the two groups. Whereas the patients with infectious prostatitis on the whole showed a slight reduction in complaints, those with prostatodynia registered a significant increase in complaints on the scales "exhaustion" and "pain in limbs" (see Table 4), so that at the end of 5 years both groups differed considerably in the two areas that reflect neurotic and generalized psychosomatic physical complaints. For prostatodynia patients, the psychoneurotic or psychosomatic components of their illness increase, i.e., the quality of their life declines, while the emotional state of those with infectious prostatitis appears to improve even if their urological complaints remain largely unchanged, i.e., the quality of their life has improved. A possible explanation for this is that the information that treatment with antibiotics has been successful, i.e., that at least the laboratory results have improved, has a certain positive influence on the course of the illness for these patients.

In contrast, the prostatodynia patients received neither adequate treatment for their complaints nor the encouragement mentioned above so that, in comparison to patients with infectious prostatitis, they feel more strongly that their illness is not being taken seriously and that they have been left to cope with their symptoms alone. Where the urological symptoms persist, this can very well result in a further increase and generalization of the depressive tendencies which find expression in increased psychosomatic complaints. This group of patients would greatly benefit from access to psychotherapy, for example, as part of a program of psychosomatic care arranged by their doctor in the context of his or her practice.

Psychosomatic Aspects

The etiology of chronic prostatitis has still not been satisfactorily elucidated. The traditional models that have persisted for so long, such as congenital weakness of the nervous system, external noxa such as mechanical vibrations or stress, alcohol abuse, masturbation, coitus interruptus, and sexual perversions, and iatrogenic breeding of prostataneurosis, have not been confirmed in any of the empirical studies on the subject to date. However, in numerous recent studies, the psychological abnormalities in patients with prostatitis have been more closely described and personality factors and structures analyzed in detail (see the review of research in Junk-Overbeck and Pott 1989; Brunner and Girshausen 1989). In these studies, it has repeatedly been established that a majority of patients with chronic prostatitis have certain psychological disorders in common, which may, however, be described in different terms, depending upon the methodological and theoretical approach of the author. Thus, we come across terms like "psychosomatic patient," "psychosomatic structures," "psychoneurotics," "alexithymia patients," "borderline personalities" (Keltikangas-Järvinen et al. 1981), "narcissistic personality," "hypochondriac," "male identity disorder" and others. The patients are characterized as "emotionally instable, depressed, aggressively inhibited, compulsive" individuals, who "have problems in relationships, are vulnerable to narcissistic injury and anxious," with "typically feminine self-images, emotional instability and introversion." The factor "depression" plays a major role in all of these descriptions: in a number of studies the patients show a marked tendency to exhaustion and pains in limbs, which can be interpreted as physical correlates of affective depression (Junk-Overbeck et al. 1988; Brähler and Weidner 1986; Deinhart 1993).

However, a specific personality structure or psychodynamic configuration typical for patients with this urological disease, such as was postulated by Alexander (1971) for psychosomatic patients, could not be identified in any of these studies.

Similarly, there is no evidence of a sexual origin of prostatitis. In spite of very exact data collection, Esk (1985) found nothing unusual in the sexual anamneses of these patients. However, in the course of a 2-year observation, Keltinkangas-Järvinen et al. (1981, 1989) did find that a number of patients reported impotence, bisexuality, homosexuality, latent homosexuality and sexual problems that either existed prior to or developed in the course of illness.

Furthermore, with respect to their relationships with their partners, these patients have been diagnosed as revealing a "psychosomatic defense syndrome in partner conflicts" or "an oral collusion pattern" in relationships (Willi 1975) and "deep-lying or patent relationship problems," as diagnosed by Riedel and Brähler (1983).

Miller (1988) made the stress reported by his patients (overwork, exhaustion, anxiety) responsible for the development of prostatitis and treated them with a stress management therapy program. All attempts at differentiating between patients with a positive bacteriological result and those without, using psychodynamic or psychometric methods, have failed so far. The hypothesis that patients with prostatodynia show more psychoneurotic tendencies than those with a positive urological diagnosis has also had to be rejected (e.g., Janssen et al. 1983; Junker 1969; Brähler et al. 1986; Deinhart 1993; Junk-Overbeck et al. 1988).

All in all, it would appear that all attempts to differentiate between a more organic and a more neurotic origin are not justified in the case of chronic prostatitis. Here, psychological factors clearly play a role in both types of diagnosis. It has been demonstrated that patients with infectious prostatitis have

as abnormally high scores for neurotic and generalized psychosomatic complaints (compared to healthy subjects) as those with prostatodynia (Brähler and
Weidner 1986). Furthermore, it has also been shown that antibiotic therapy may
cause a positive urological finding to disappear, but this is no guarantee that the
prostatitis complaints will improve correspondingly. Similarly, an undiscovered
infection may well play a role in prostatodynia, since antibiotic treatment can
also be successful with these patients (Pavone-Macaluso et al. 1991).

It becomes clear that in the case of chronic prostatitis, it is more useful to
assume complex psychosomatic and somatopsychic interactions than to seek
simple causal explanations (Brähler and Weidner 1989). For example, one
plausible hypothesis is that emotional depression and chronic persistence of
prostatitis symptoms influence each other (Junk-Overbeck et al. 1988).

Since in all cases, regardless of the urologically differential diagnosis, the
therapeutic success rate is very low (de la Rosette et al. 1992a, b; Deinhart 1993),
the therapist must be content with reducing the patient's anxiety and trying to
help him cope with his symptoms and live with his illness as best he can. This
can at least prevent a worsening of his condition, for example, through an
iatrogenic fixation on isolated symptoms, and can protect the patient from
unnecessary suffering in consequence.

If their disease becomes chronic, it would appear that particularly patients
with the diagnosis prostatodynia are in danger of suffering a substantial
impairment in their overall quality of life (Deinhart 1993).

References

Alexander F (1971) Psychosomatische Medizin, De Gruyter, Berlin
Barry et al. (1992a) Correlation of the American Urological Association symptom index with self-
    administered versions of the Madsen-Iversen, Boyarsky and Maine Medical Assessment
    Program symptom indexes. J Urol 148, 11:1558–1563
Barry et al. (1992b) The American Urological Association symptom index for benign prostatic
    hyperplasia. J Urol 148, 11:1549–1557
Brähler E, Brunner A, Girshausen C, Weidner W (1986) Psychosomatic and somatopsychological
    aspects of chronic prostatitis. In: Weidner W, Brunner H, Krause W, Rothauge CF (eds)
    Therapy of prostatitis. Klinische und experimentelle Urologie 11. Zuckschwerdt, Munich
Brähler E, Scheer JW (1983) Der Gießener Beschwerdebogen – Testhandbuch. Bern, Huber
Brähler E, Weidner W (1986) Testpsychologische Untersuchungen zum Beschwerdebild von
    Patienten mit chronischer Prostatitis oder Prostatadynie. Urologe A 25:97–100
Brähler E, Weidner W (1989) Psychosomatische Aspekte der chronischen Prostatitis. Psychomed
    1:244–247
Brunner A Girshausen C (1989) Die Erfassung von Beschwerdekomplexen bei Patienten mit
    chronischer Prostatitis und Prostatadynie. Dissertation, Gießen
Deinhart M (1993) Krankheitsverlauf bei der chronischen Prostatitis – Eine 5-Jahres-Katamnese.
    Dissertation, Gießen
Diederichs P (1986) Psychosomatische Störungen des männlichen Urogenitaltrakts. In: Brähler E,
    Meyer A (eds) Partnerschaft, Sexualität und Fruchtbarkeit. Springer, Berlin Heidelberg New
    York

Effert P, Ackermann R (1992) Klinische Manifestation und Indikation zur Therapie der benignen Prostatahyperplasie. Urologe A 31:135–141

Esk PC (1985) Prostatakongestion und Prostatitis. pmi, Frankfurt

Gross M (1991) Psychometrische Eigenschaften zweier Fragebogen zur Erfassung der psychischen Dimension der Lebensqualität. In: Bullinger M, Ludwig M, von Steinbüchel N (eds) Lebensqualität bei kardiovaskulären Erkrankungen. Hogrefe, Göttingen

Janssen PL, Kukahn R, Spieler KH, Weissbach L (1983) Zur Psychosomatik der chronischen Prostatitis. In: Brunner H, Krause W, Rothauge CF, Weidner W (eds) Chronische Prostatitis. Schattauer, Stuttgart, p 265

Junker H (1969) Psychopathologische Untersuchungen über Patienten mit chronisch abakterieller Prostatitis einschließlich. Kongestionsprostatitis. Dissertation, Gießen

Junk-Overbeck M, Pott W (1989) Empirische Untersuchungen zur Psychosomatik der chronischen Prostatitis. Dissertation, Gießen

Junk-Overbeck M, Pott W, Pauli U (1988) Empirische Untersuchungen zur Psychosomatik der chronischen Prostatitis. In: Brähler E, Meyer A (eds) Partnerschaft, Sexualität und Fruchtbarkeit. Springer, Berlin Heidelberg New York, pp 217–234

Keltikangas-Järvinen L, Järvinen H, Lehtonen T (1981) Psychic disturbances in patients with chronic prostatitis. Ann Clin Res 13:45–49

Keltikangas-Järvinen L, Mueller K, Lehtonen T (1989) Illness behavior and personality changes in patients with chronic prostatitis during a two-year follow-up period. Eur Urol 16 (3):181–184

Ludwig M, Schroeder-Printzen I, Weidner W (1992) Diagnostik und Therapie der chronischen Prostatitis. In: Vahlensieck W, Rutishauser G (eds) Benigne Prostatopathien. Thieme, Stuttgart, pp 55–62

Miller HC (1988) Stress prostatitis. Urology 32 (6):507–510

Pavone-Macaluso M et al. (1991) Prostatitis, prostatosis and prostalgia. Psychogenic or organic disease? Scand J Urol Nephrol Suppl 138:77–82

Pott W, Junk-Overbeck M, Wirsching M (1991) Chronisch bakterielle Prostatitis – Prostatodynie. Die Differenzierung aus psychosomatischer Sicht. Z Psychosomat Med Psychoanalyse 37:157–171

Riedell H, Brähler E (1983) Prostatitis und Ehepaarbeziehung. In: Brunner H, Krause W, Rothauge CF, Weidner W (eds) Chronische Prostatitis. Schattauer, Stuttgart

Rosette de la et al. (1992a) Results of a questionnaire among Dutch urologists and general practitioners. Concerning diagnostics and treatment of patients with prostatitis syndromes. Eur Urol 22:14–19

Rosette de la et al. (1992b) Research in 'prostatitis syndromes': the use of alfuzosin (a new α_1-receptor-blocking agent) in patients mainly presenting with micturition complaints of an irritative nature and confirmed urodynamic abnormalities. Eur Urol 22:222–227

Rugendorff EW, Weidner W, Ebeling L, Buck AC (1992) Behandlungsergebnisse mit Pollenextrakt (Cernilton N) bei Prostatodynie und chronischer Prostatitis. In: Vahlensieck W, Rutishauser G (eds) Benigne prostatopathien. Thieme, Stuttgart, pp 76–83

Weidner W (1984) Moderne Prostatitisdiagnostik. In: Schmiedt E, Altwein JE, Bauer HW (eds) Klinische und experimentelle Urologie, vol 7. Zuckschwerdt, Munich

Weidner W, Schiefer HG, Brähler E (1991) Refractory chronic bacterial prostatitis: a re-evaluation of Ciprofloxacin treatment after a median followup of 30 months. J Urol 146:350–352

Willi J (1975) Die Zweierbeziehung. Rowohlt, Reinbek

Diagnostic Management in Chronic Prostatitis

W. Weidner and M. Ludwig

Introduction

The term "prostatitis" is not a definite nosologic entity, but includes various inflammatory and noninflammatory conditions affecting the prostate. A widely accepted clinical classification system (Drach et al. 1978) has been developed based on the standardized sequential bacteriologic localization technique introduced by Meares and Stamey in 1968, including analysis of expressed prostatic secretions (EPS) for evidence of increased numbers of leukocytes (Table 1). Although this classification system must be considered an outstanding breakthrough in the rational approach to classifying patients with prostatic inflammation, we still do not fully understand all the complexities of prostatic disease, in particular the etiology and pathogenesis of nonbacterial prostatitis. This may be due to the fact that our diagnostic procedures are still inadequate for many patients. Careful attention should therefore be given to the diagnostic sensitivity and specifity of our examinations and to the exact classification of the inflammation.

Table 1. Classification of chronic prostatitis

	Evidence of inflammation in EPS (PML, Macrophages)	Positive culture		Etiologic bacteria	Rectal examination (prostate)
		(EPS)	(Bladder)		
Chronic bacterial prostatitis	+	+	(+)	Enterobacteriaceae spp. Enterococcus spp. Pseudomonas spp. S. saprophyticus	Normal
"Nonbacterial" prostatitis	+	0	0	?	Normal
Prostatodynia	0	0	0	0	Normal

Definition and Classification of Prostatic Inflammation

Patients suffering from bacterial and nonbacterial prostatitis (NBP) present inflammatory cellular reactions in EPS as summarized in Table 1. Normally, as part of the standardized localization technique (Meares and Stamey 1968), one drop of EPS is counted for polymorphonuclear leukocytes (PML), which are an indication of inflammation. Available data suggest that white blood cells are rarely present in normal prostatic fluid (Schaeffer 1990). After exclusion of an inflammatory urethral reaction, between two and five white blood cells per high-power field (hpf) are the upper limit for "normal" (Anderson and Weller 1979; Schaeffer 1990). Although in some "normal" cases, higher numbers of leukocytes in EPS may be found, it seems to us to be a practical suggestion to consider $\geq$ 10 PML/hpf indicative of prostatitis (Drach et al. 1978). When using a more sensitive method of quantifying leukocytes, by counting in a Fuchs-Rosenthal chamber, an upper limit of 1000 PML/μl has been suggested (Anderson and Weller 1979). This approximates to the number of 15 PML/hpf, recently quoted by Meares as being indicative (Meares 1990).

In our group, an increased number of granulocytes in urine after prostatic massage (VB3) was taken to be the first cellular indication of prostatitis, if the first and midstream urine were free of leukocytes; $\geq$ 10 granulocytes in the sediment of VB3 may be highly indicative and comparable to elevated leukocyte numbers in EPS (Table 2; Weidner and Ebner 1985).

Anderson and Weller (1979) reported increased severity of clinical symptoms with increased numbers of granulocytes and fat-laden macrophages, which are claimed to be a further typical cytologic sign of inflammation (Fig. 1). For cytologic differentiation, special staining techniques are necessary; we prefer Papanicolaou staining for safe identification of inflammatory elements.

Table 3 summarizes our schedule for the simple evaluation of an inflammatory response in expressed prostatic secretions.

Table 2. Comparison of numbers of granulocytes in VB3 with numbers of leukocytes in EPS ($n = 73$)

Granulocytes in VB3 ($\times$ 400)	Leukocytes in EPS (HPF, $\times$ 1000)		
	< 10	10–20	> 20
− 2	46	−	−
− 4	3	4	−
$\geq$ 10	1	12	7

EPS, expressed prostatic secretions; HPF, high-power field; VB3, postmassage bladder urine

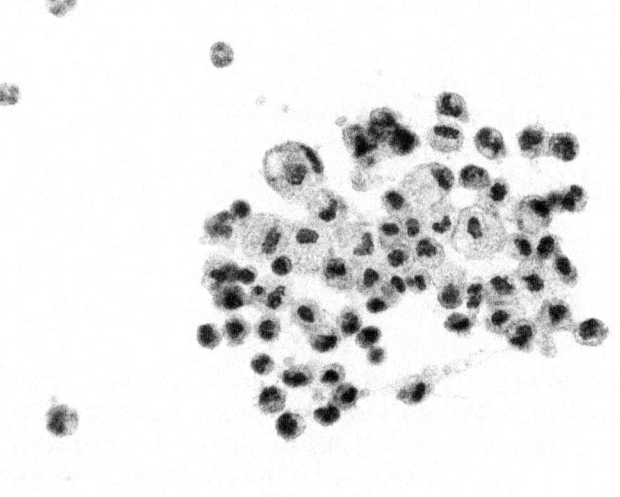

Fig. 1. PML and macrophages in a smear of EPS (Papanicolaou/ × 400)

Table 3. White cells in the diagnosis of prostatitis

Material	Parameter	Threshold	Pathologic finding
VB3	White cells (× 400)	> 4	⩾ 10
EPS	White cells/HPF (× 1000)	10–20	> 20

VB3, post-massage bladder urine; EPS, expressed prostatic secretion; HPF, high-power field

Diagnosis of Prostatic Infection

The diagnostic method of choice is the so-called "four-specimen-test" (Meares and Stamey 1968), in which approximately equal urine samples are quantitatively compared before and after prostate massage, also including EPS. The so-called "*prostatitis histogram*" of quantifiable pathogens is the criterion for the diagnosis. The determining factor is the tenfold higher concentration of pathogens in the VB3, as compared to the first voided urine (VB1). With this method, chronic bacterial prostatitis (CBP) can be clearly diagnosed.

The following pathogen concentrations are common (CFU/ml; Weidner 1984):

- First urine (10–15 ml; VB1) $< 10^3$
- Midstream urine/second urine sample (10–15 ml; VB2) $< 10^3$
- Drop of prostatic secretions   (EPS) $\geqslant 10^4$
- Urine voided after massage (10–15 ml; VB3) $\geqslant 10^3$

Nitrofurantoin Test

As a prerequisite for establishing a prostatitis histogram, a urinary tract infection must be definitely excluded. In individual cases, treatment with nitrofurantoin prior to the localization test facilitates the correct diagnosis. Nitrofurantoin is only effective in the urinary tract; it does not diffuse into the parenchymatous organs or into prostatic secretions. In this way, pathogenetic microorganisms from infected prostatic secretions can be isolated but the midstream urine cleared by high antibiotic urine levels. Nitrofurantoin treatment, 100 mg for 4 days, is followed by a second four-specimen test, which allows correct inflammatory localization to the prostate gland.

In *cases of urethritis*, midstream and post-massage urine may also be contaminated with high concentrations of pathogens which stem from the anterior urethra. However, such (non-gonococcal) urethritis is almost exclusively caused by *Chlamydia trachomatis* or *Mycoplasma*. Other gram-positive bacterial pathogens, e.g. streptococci, can be disregarded as etiologic agents in the diagnostic workup of patients with prostatitis.

Chronic Bacterial Prostatitis

Bacteria causing both acute and CBP are identical in species, serotype, and incidence to those causing common urinary tract infections, with *Escherichia coli* predominating. The data from two recent studies underline that prostatitis is an important, but uncommon, bacterial infectious disease (Krieger and McGonagle 1989; Weidner et al. 1991a). In these carefully performed examinations of patients with a history of chronic prostatitis, 5% (Weidner et al. 1991a) to 9% (Krieger and McGonagle 1989) met the criteria of CBP, the prostatitis histogram of the four-specimen-test being used as the determining factor. In one study (Krieger and McGonagle 1989) the analysis of the inflammatory response with respect to infections by gram-positive or gram-negative bacteria only revealed a mean of 44 PML/hpf in cases of enterobacterial infections, while patients in whom only gram-positive bacteria were found, also localized to the prostate, had normal leukocyte counts in EPS.

Our studies (Weidner et al. 1991a) gave similar results, but in two cases *Staphylococcus saprophyticus* was found in typical numbers (prostatitis constellation) with a concomitant leukocytic reaction in EPS. Recent data from Nickel and Costerton (1992) underline the implication of the last-mentioned bacterial species in prostatitis with positive cultures of *S. saprophyticus* in EPS and positive perineal needle biopsies of prostatic tissue.

Clinical Features

Unlike acute bacterial prostatitis, which is easily diagnosed by acute symptoms and clinical findings, the history and physical examination of patients with CBP/NBP may only suggest the diagnosis, but most signs and symptoms of CBP, NBP and prostatodynia are identical (Table 1).

The *clinical features* of CBP are highly variable (Table 4). Although some men develop chronic prostatitis, following an initial bout of acute bacterial prostatitis, many have no history of acute prostatitis. Especially in men over the age of 40, recurrent epididymitis is often noted. Although a tender, spongy prostate is often found, these findings are not specifically diagnostic of CBP (Weidner 1984).

Symptoms

Symptoms include typical inflammatory signs, but also voiding disturbances and signs of sexual dysfunction (Weidner 1984). Symptoms and complaint complexes have been evaluated in the book and by Brähler and Weidner (1986) in a highly sophisticated way, thus providing the possibility in the future of asking for typical "true" prostatitis symptoms, using a special questionnaire.

Table 4. Symptoms in patients with the prostatitis syndrome (after Weidner 1984)

Leading symptoms	
Typical signs of inflammation	Burning in the urethra during voiding; discharge, prostatorrhea; pyospermia
Diffuse anogenital symptoms	Pressure behind pubic bone; perineal pressure; tension in testes and epididymes; penile pain; inguinal pain; anorectal dysaesthesia; lower abdominal discomfort
Voiding disturbances	Difficult urination; stranguria; frequency; nocturia
Sexual dysfunction	Loss of libido; erectile dysfunction; ejaculatory dysfunction (pain during or after orgasm)
Other symptoms	Myalgia

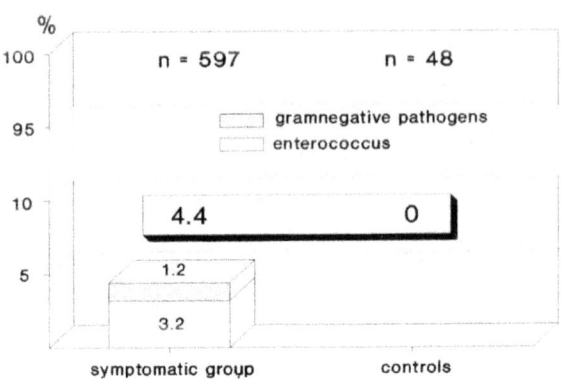

Fig. 2. Significant bacteriuria in chronic prostatitis.

The hallmark of CBP is *relapsing bacteriuria*, in which the same pathogen is found repeatedly. In a prospective study, we compared the results of the four-specimen technique in a group of 597 patients with symptoms of chronic prostatitis with the findings of 48 men without symptoms. Before examination, urinary tract infection, urethritis, and acute bacterial prostatitis were excluded in all patients. Whereas significant bacteriuria could not be found in any case in the control group, it was verified in 26 (4.4%) patients of the symptomatic group, in spite of normal leukocyte and bacteria counts before examination. The relevant pathogenetic spectrum consisted of gram-negative bacteria and enterococci (Fig. 2). These data refer to all patients with symptoms of prostatitis. With regard to all patients with CBP 25% reveal periods of significant bacteriuria.

Classification and Bacteriological Diagnosis

To properly identify the site of inflammation, the clinician has to analyze one drop of EPS for increased numbers of white blood cells and lipid-laden macrophages. Provided the urethral and midstream urine samples show low numbers of PML, over 10 PML/hpf in EPS is considered diagnostic of prostatic inflammation.

Diagnosis of CBP must be confirmed by *quantitative bacteriologic localization studies* (see above). The question is whether this technique really provides useful information for *every* patient suspected of having chronic prostatitis. Considering that between 50% (Weidner et al. 1991a) and 80% (Krieger and McGonagle 1989) of patients with symptoms of prostatitis attending a special outpatient clinic suffer from prostatodynia, we presently limit this examination to those patients in whom repeated evidence of increased leukocyte numbers in EPS has been established.

Ejaculate Analysis

An ejaculate analysis is also done in these men to get further information about whether the inflamed prostate is part of a generalized infection of the male accessory glands. It should be kept in mind that for correct bacteriologic evaluation of ejaculate specimens, a urethral inflammation or bladder infection must be ruled out; only then does the bacteriologic study of semen specimens give significant results, that is to say, evidence of bacteriospermia (> 10^3 cfu/ml in half of the patients with CBP in contrast to 6.8% with NBP); with only one exception, bacterial species isolated from the ejaculate were identical to those from EPS (Weidner et al. 1991b). Positive antibody coated bacteria test (ACB-test) was demonstrated in 31 men of the CBP group (96.9%), in three men of the NBP group (3%), in nine men of the prostatodynia group (6.3%) and in none of the controls (Weidner 1991b). These results underline the biological significance of bacteriospermia in men with CBP and its lack of importance in NBP and prostatodynia.

Prostatic Secretory Dysfunction

Alterations in the composition of prostatic secretions have been assumed to be diagnostic in patients with prostatitis (Meares 1990). In CBP, these alterations are sufficiently distinct to suggest an accompanying generalized secretory dysfunction of the gland. An overview is given in Fig. 3. Particularly the decrease of zinc and the zinc-containing prostatic antibacterial factor (PAF), both known to be highly bactericidal, have been accused of playing an important role in the pathogenesis of bacterial prostatitis. However, until now, it has not been proved that these alterations are a cause and not merely a consequence of inflammation.

The prostate gland is known to be capable of *a systemic* and *local immune response* to invading micro-organisms. In CBP that has been cured by antibiotic therapy, antigen-specific IgA in prostatic secretions – particularly secretory IgA – is elevated for almost 2 years, and antigen-specific IgG for 6 months, before both immunoglobulins slowly decrease to the previous values. In patients

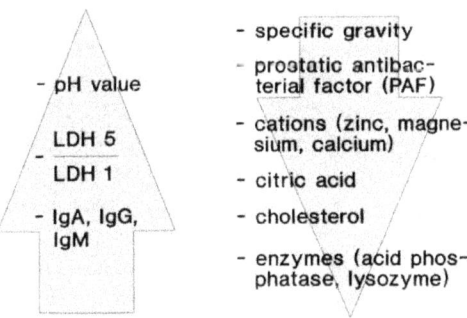

Fig. 3. Prostatic secretory dysfunction in chronic bacterial prostatitis

with failure of medical treatment, both parameters remain persistently elevated (Shortliffe et al. 1981). Relevant serum elevations of immunoglobulins could not be discovered. In NBP, significant elevations of immunoglobulins could not be verified (Shortliffe et al. 1992).

In our view, only increased EPS pH (> 7.8) provides an additional pointer in the clinical workup of CBP (Weidner 1992).

Nonbacterial Prostatitis (Abacterial Prostatitis)

Obviously the most common form of the prostatitis syndrome NBP is an inflammation of the prostate of unknown cause. Patients with NBP have many of the symptoms seen in CBP, e.g., increased leukocytes and macrophages in EPS, but no positive cultures of common uropathogens. There is no history of relapsing urinary tract infection. Current evidence suggests that NBP is either an infectious disease caused by as yet unidentified (uncommon, fastidious) pathogens or a noninfectious form of prostatic inflammation.

During the last decade, *Chlamydia trachomatis* and *Ureaplasma urealyticum* have been discussed as being etiologically involved in NBP. We consider the role of *C. trachomatis* debatable. Although these microorganisms can be isolated by urethral swabbing more frequently in patients with NBP than in controls, it is impossible to discriminate between urethral colonization and prostatic infection (Weidner and Schiefer 1986). Recently, Bruce and Reid (1989) reported on a new attempt to exclude urethral contamination. Chlamydial elementary bodies were stained by direct immunofluorescence in prostatic secretions, and chlamydial infection of the prostate was diagnosed in cases of chlamydia-free urethral specimens. A further promising approach to better understanding may be provided by directly measuring IgG and IgA response in prostatic secretions, combined with direct immunofluorescence (Tsunekawa and Kumamoto 1989). In fulfilling one of Koch's postulates, some authors have tried to establish chlamydial infection of prostatic epithelial cells directly in prostatic tissue taken under sterile conditions from patients with NBP, with diametrically different results (Abdelatif et al. 1991; Doble et al. 1991; Poletti et al. 1985; Pust et al. 1986; Shurbaji et al. 1988; Weidner 1991a) (Table 5). One reason for these discrepancies may be the different techniques used for taking prostatic material. Via transrectal aspiration biopsy, open operation, and transurethral resection of the prostate, tissue is available both from the peripheral gland and from the prostatic urethra; in perineal biopsies done in our study (Weidner et al. 1991a) and by Doble et al. (1989) tissue was only taken from the peripheral prostatic lobes. In other words, tissue from transrectal biopsy or transurethral resection of the prostate also contains epithelia of the prostatic urethra, which may have been infected in the course of urethral infection.

Similarly, the role of *U. urealyticum* in NBP has still not been settled. These microorganisms are part of the normal male urethral flora (Bowie et al. 1977).

Table 5. Biopsy studies in NBP and detection of chlamydial infections of the prostate gland

Study	Positive chlamydial findings				
	Patients (n)	Prostatic urethra (n)	Prostate (n)	Type of operation	Chlamydial detection
Poletti et al. (1985)	30	Not done	10	Transrectal biopsy	Culture
Pust et al. (1986)	32	6	1	Urethral and perineal biopsy	Immunofluorescence
Shurbaji et al. (1988)	16	Not done	5	TUR-P, open operation	Immunohistochemistry
Abdelatif et al. (1991)	23	Not done	7	TUR-P	In situ hybridization
Weidner et al. (1991a)	22	4	None	Perineal ultrasonically guided biopsy	Culture
Doble et al. (1989)	50	Not done	None	Perineal ultrasonically guided biopsy	Culture, immunofluorescence

NBP, nonbacterial prostatitis; TUR-P, transurethral resection of prostate

Therefore, quantification of *U. urealyticum* is obligatory. Numbers below 10^3 cfu/ml in first urine samples are considered normal urethral colonization (Bowie et al. 1977; Brunner et al. 1983). However, there has been a recent report (Berger et al. 1989) of higher numbers in the first urine samples of healthy men, which is contradictory to other authors. More conflicting are the studies done on patients with NBP. Three relevant investigations were carried out on patients with NBP, demonstrating a typical prostatitis pattern of ureaplasmas in EPS (Table 6) as a hint for localization of these pathogens to the prostate (Brunner et al. 1983; Meseguer et al. 1986; Weidner et al. 1980). These data are in contrast to the findings of Berger et al. (1989), who found no evidence of ureaplasmas in EPS of men with NBP. These conflicting data need commenting on. Studies confirming the pathogenic role of ureaplasmas in NBP analyze patients with significantly increased leukocyte numbers in EPS, whereas in Berger's study (1989), the majority of patients had no cytologic signs of prostatitis. Furthermore, in the data from Hofstetter (1973) there was a good correlation between excessive numbers of ureaplasmas and increased numbers of leukocytes in EPS: in 15 cases, a perineal biopsy from the prostate was performed, and in 12/15 cases, *U. urealyticum* were cultivated from tissue taken aseptically.

In conclusion, at present there are many hints indicating that *C. trachomatis* and/or *U. urealyticum* may ascend to the prostate; on the other hand, there is no conclusive answer as to whether these microorganisms are really involved in prostatitis. Recently, Shortliffe et al. (1992) conducted an important study, analyzing IgA antibodies against *C. trachomatis* and *U. urealyticum* in EPS. They did not find any antibody differences between men with CBP, NBP and prostatodynia, in cases where urethritis was clinically excluded. Assaying the EPS for IgG antibodies against *U. urealyticum*, titers were detectable in 11 of 38 men (29%) with NBP, in none with CBP and in one with prostatodynia. Nevertheless the differences were not significant. The authors conclude that even though the data show that more men with detectable prostatic fluid titers are available in NBP, the titers are low and do not represent an active process. We

Table 6. Evidence of "ureaplasma-associated" (U +) urogenital infections in men with prostatitis

Study	Total (*n*)	U + (*n*) (%)	Titer VB1 (cfu/ml)	U + (EPS/VB3) (*n*) (%)	Titre EPS/VB3 (cfu/ml)
Weidner et al. (1980)	187	103 (55.1)	$< 10^3$	36 (19.3)	$5 \times 10^4/4\text{--}7 \times 10^3$
Brunner et al. (1983)	597	51 (8.5)		82 (13.7)	
		49	$< 10^3$	49	$> 10^3$
		2	$> 10^3$	31	$> 10^4$
Meseguer et al. (1986)	131	?	?	8 (6.1)	5×10^4
Berger et al. (1989)	30	2 (7)	1×10^3	0	–

think that further subtle localization studies are needed, including immuno-cytologic and immunohistological techniques, combined with a search for local antibody response in EPS.

Prostatourethritis

At the moment, routine culture for *C. trachomatis* and *U. urealyticum* is only recommended when urethritis is suspected. One key for better understanding of ascending infections to the prostate gland is certainly to rule out urethritis when NBP is suspected. New data provide evidence of chemotactic activity of *Chlamydia* in urethral exudate, questionably triggering a local inflammatory reaction even after eradication of the microorganisms (Lomas et al. 1993). These data are underlined by the findings of our group (Weidner et al. 1991b) that peroxidase-positive leukocytes in semen are significantly increased in chlamy-dia-infected patients with positive urethral swabbing.

Further research into noninfectious prostatitis is urgently needed. Reflux of sterile urine into the prostatic ducts may sustain inflammation (Hellstrom et al. 1987; Kirby et al. 1982); biopsies taken from men with prostatitis with noted deposition of antibodies and complement in the tissue as compared to a non-prostatitis group give further hints for an immunologic cause of prostatitis (Doble et al. 1991). A host response against prostatic invasion by spermatozoa has been claimed as another important stimulus for sterile inflammation (McClinton et al. 1990), data well in accordance with Blacklock's (1991) findings of a disturbed (nonlaminar) urinary flow, sustaining a reflux into the prostatic ducts in many cases of prostatitis. Nevertheless, all these data cannot be collected in routinely performed diagnostic procedures.

Further Diagnostic Workup

Urodynamics

The *evaluation of the bladder-emptying process* by flow-rate measurement and subsequent measurement of the residual urine by ultrasonography is a man-datory diagnostic step in patients with prostatitis-like symptoms. This diag-nostic workup should include a voiding cystourethrogram, if necessary. Changes in the area of the bladder neck, resulting from congenital or acquired pathological changes in the urethra with disturbances of the laminar urinary flow may cause prostatitis-like symptoms such as alguria, difficult micturition and spontaneous urethral secretions (Weidner 1984).

Urodynamically effective changes are found in approximately 33%–43% of patients with prostatitis-like symptoms (Fig. 4). If the flow-rate measurement is

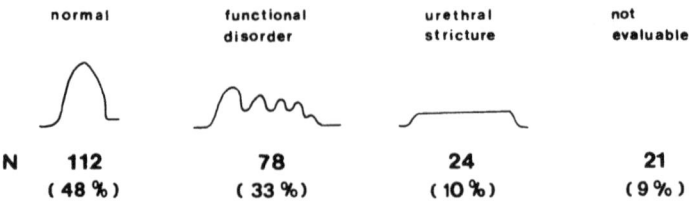

normal	functional disorder	urethral stricture	not evaluable
N 112	78	24	21
(48 %)	(33 %)	(10 %)	(9 %)

Fig. 4. Voiding pattern in 235 men with prostatitis

definitely abnormal, urethrocystoscopy and voiding cystourethrogram should be performed to differentiate between functional disturbances and anatomical changes (e.g., bladder neck sclerosis, benign prostatic hyperplasia, urethral stricture). Urethrocystoscopy often reveals visible inflammatory changes in posterior urethra ("urethritis posterior"). To evaluate neurological alterations in the detrusor and urethral function in patients with abnormal uroflow, a filling cystometry should be performed (Hellstrom et al. 1987).

Transrectal Prostatic Sonography

Prostatic calculi are known to increase with growing age and occur independently of the kind of prostatic disease. They are estimated to originate through thickened prostatic secretions and through reflux of urine. Clinically, two kinds of prostatic calcifications are distinguishable: the solitary type is characterized by a discrete dot or region facultatively accompanied by an acoustic shadow; diffuse type calcifications are described as a larger, irregularly formed mass or line and are known to include large parts of the prostate gland and, in the case of infection, are referred to as "prostatitis calcarea." The detection of prostatic calculi in chronic prostatitis is of clinical importance, because they are regarded as being one of the main causes of therapeutic failure. They hinder the diffusion of antibiotics through the prostate gland tissue and, therefore, by serving as a nidus for pathogens, lead to recurrent prostatic infections.

In a prospective study, we compared the sonographic findings in 88 patients with CBP and NBP with the results of 53 men with prostatodynia. With regards to the frequency of prostatic calcifications (Fig. 5), solitary calculi indicated no significant difference between the two groups, whereas a significant accumulation of the total number of calculi and of diffuse type calcifications could be demonstrated. As both patient groups were of the same mean age, these results cannot be sufficiently explained by a difference in physiological prostate secretion activity. As urodynamically effective flow disturbances of morphological or functional origin are found in 30%–40% of all patients with symptoms of chronic prostatitis, prostatic calcifications may be explained by urinary reflux, caused by laminar flow disturbances. Whether these calculi are of any pathogenetic importance in prostatodynia is not known.

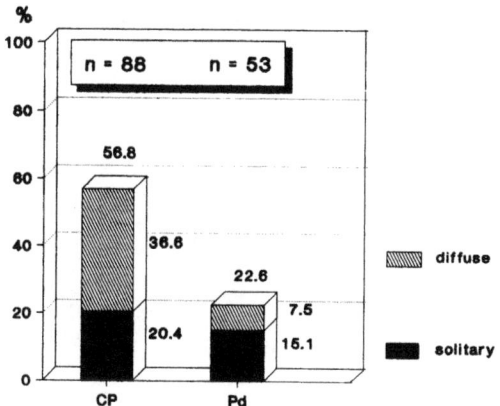

Fig. 5. Distribution of prostatic calcifications in chronic prostatitis (*CP*) and prostatodynia (*Pd*)

Biopsy

Some attempts have also been made to clarify the diagnosis by perineal biopsy of "typical" prostatic areas under ultrasonographic guide, to get a *specific histology* and *to evaluate particular microorganisms* in order to reach an adequate diagnosis (Doble et al. 1989; Weidner and Schiefer 1986). The question is whether there are really "typical inflammatory findings" under transrectal ultrasonography (Christiansen and Purvis 1991). At present, we do not believe in such findings. We think that any kind of biopsy for histology is not helpful in the diagnosis, because foci of chronic inflammation are often present in prostatic tissue, particularly in association with prostatic calculi, nodular hyperplasia and adenocarcinoma (Weiss and Mills 1989). Following the experience of Helpap (1992), the so-called chronic prostatitis associated with paraurethral nodular prostatic hyperplasia has no significance "as an independent disease, with the possible exception of acute exacerbation." In cases without benign prostatic hyperplasia (BPH), periglandular prostatitis may occur in a moderate form in up to 24% of patients and in a severe form in up to 13.5%, data which are not very different from the BPH-findings. To us, these findings do not underline any necessity to prove clinical suspicion of prostatitis by biopsy and histological or cytologic examination.

The only indication for biopsy is to rule out *granulomatous prostatitis* when palpatory findings are suspicious for carcinoma. It must be recognized, however, that a combination of carcinoma and granulomatous prostatitis may exist, requiring multiple biopsies (Helpap 1992).

Prostatovesiculitis

The seminal vesicles can be figured near the upper prostatic pole and often stretch out as far as the lateral bladder regions. Under transrectal prostatic

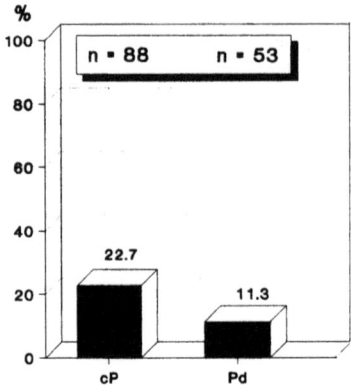

Fig. 6. Distribution of seminal vesicle asymmetry in chronic prostatitis (*CP*) and prostatodynia (*Pd*)

sonography they show a wide variety of size and shape. Size, internal echodensity, and configuration are widely accepted as evaluation criteria. Their size is assumed to depend mainly on the period of sexual abstinence and on prostatic size. As physiological factors do not influence the appearance of just one gland, symmetry in all evaluation criteria is a prerequisite for considering them as normal. In our above-mentioned study (see Fig. 5), a significant accumulation of seminal gland asymmetry in chronic prostatitis was detected (Fig. 6).

Asymmetry in the case of inflammation is considered to be either a consequence of enlargement due to ductal obstruction of the infected gland or a result of seminal vesicle shrinking by obliteration. It indicates participation of the lower urogenital tract in the inflammatory process, particularly in prostatitis (Weidner et al. 1991c). Further causes of asymmetry play a minor role; especially local congenital abnormalities like aplasia or hypoplasia have been described, as has cystic malformation associated with upper urogenital tract abnormalities. As a further cause of asymmetry, hemorrhage into or around the gland, mainly in cases of severe hypertension and coagulation disorders, has been reported.

It must be emphasized that seminal gland alterations in chronic prostatitis do not prove inflammation, but indicate vesicle gland involvement in the inflammatory process in the sense of prostatovesiculitis.

Further Diagnostic Procedures

An objective correlate to inflammation, either increased white cells or a positive microbiological result, can only be found in 50% of patients with typical prostatitis-like symptoms. Prostatodynia is therefore a diagnosis of exclusion. Because of the uncertain etiology, no uniform treatment strategies exist. From a urological standpoint it appears relevant to *diagnose* and to *treat* concomitant *functional bladder-emptying disturbances* very early. A treatment trial with prazosin 1 mg orally every day may be indicated. The doses may be increased to 2 mg orally twice daily. To reduce the undesirable side effects of α-adrenergic blockade, the medication should be taken in the evening at bedtime. If this medication is not sufficient, diazepam may be given in a dosage of 2–5 mg orally three times every day. Using this concept, investigators have achieved a symptom-free state, with regard to bladder-emptying problems, in approximately 50% of patients, thus excluding these men from further microbiological investigations. Patients with *anogenital symptoms complex* should be referred to a proctologist to evaluate pathologic changes in the anal area and initiate appropriate concomitant treatment.

Many possible causes of prostatodynia have been discussed in the past. However, none of them could be scientifically proven to be etiologically responsible. Despite the fact that patients with prostatitis demonstrate *psychological and behavioral differences* when compared with the normal population, no significant psychopathological differences between the various diagnostic groups with prostatitis-like syndromes have been identified (Weidner 1984). Patients can therefore not be assigned a diagnosis based on psychosomatic symptoms. In particular patients with objective urologic findings often show also evidence of psychosomatic problems. Equally, patients with prostatodynia show evidence of a "psychosomatic personality," meaning that during the initial interview they are rather reluctant to enter into emotional contact with the physician. This separates these patients from patients with true bacterial prostatitis (Brähler and Weidner 1986).

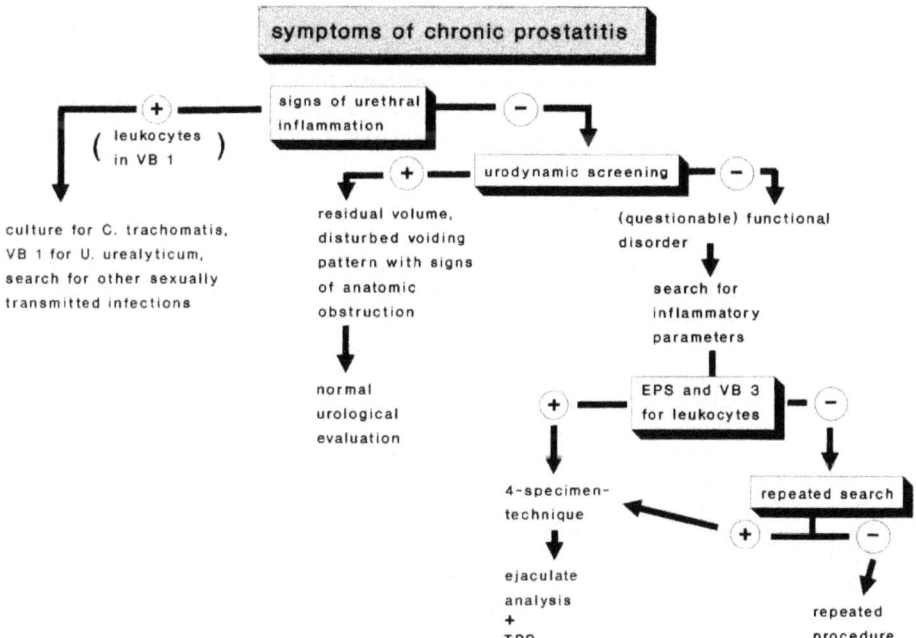

Fig. 7. Algorithm of diagnostic approach to chronic prostatitis

Since antibiotic treatment is found to be ineffective, but likely to cause fixation of the patient on nonexistent somatic causes for his problems, such *probative antibiotic therapy* should not be conducted for diagnosis.

Conclusions

Standardized diagnostic procedures, including microbiological and cytologic examinations of expressed prostatic secretions, are prerequisites for a correct classification of prostatitis syndromes. Figure 7 presents an algorithm of our diagnostic approach.

References

Abdelatif OMA, Chandler FW, McGuire BS (1991) Chlamydia trachomatis in chronic abacterial prostatitis: demonstration by colorimetric in situ hybridization. Hum Pathol 22:41–44

Anderson RU, Weller C (1979) Prostatic secretion leucocyte studies in non-bacterial prostatitis (prostatosis). J Urol 121:292–294

Berger RE, Krieger JN, Kessler D, Ireton RC, Cose C, Holmes KK, Roberts PL (1989) Case control study of men with suspected chronic idiopathic prostatitis. J Urol 141:328–329

Blacklock NJ (1991) The anatomy of the prostate: relationship with prostatic infection. Infection [Suppl 3] 19:111–114

Bowie WR, Wang S-P, Alexander ER, Floyd J, Forsyth P, Pollock HM, Lin J-S, Buchanan TM, Holmes KK (1977) Etiology of nongonococcal urethritis. J Clin Invest 59:735–737

Brähler E, Weidner W (1986) Testpsychologische Untersuchungen zum Beschwerdebild von Patienten mit chronischer Prostatitis oder Prostatodynie. Urologe A 25:97–100

Bruce AW, Reid G (1989) Prostatitis associated with C. trachomatis in six patients. J Urol 142:1006–1007

Brunner H, Weidner W, Schiefer HG (1983) Studies on the role of Ureaplasma urealyticum and Mycoplasma hominis in prostatitis. J Infect Dis 147:807–813

Christiansen E, Purvis K (1991) Diagnosis of chronic abacterial prostato-vesiculitis by rectal ultrasonography in relation to symptoms and findings. Br J Urol 67:173–176

Doble A, Thomas BJ, Walker MM, Harris JRW, O'N Witherow R, Taylor-Robinson C (1989) The role of Chlamydia trachomatis in chronic abacterial prostatitis: a study using ultrasound guided biopsy. J Urol 141:332–333

Doble A, Walker MM, Harris JRW, Taylor-Robinson D, Witherow R (1991) Intraprostatic antibody deposition in chronic abacterial prostatitis. Br J Urol 65:598–605

Drach GW, Meares EM Jr, Fair WR, Stamey TA (1978) Classification of benign disease associated with prostatic pain: prostatitis or prostatodynia? J Urol 120:266

Hellstrom WJG, Schmidt RA, Lue TF, Tanagho EA (1987) Neuromuscular dysfunction in non-bacterial prostatitis. Urology 30:183–187

Helpap B (1992) Pathology of chronic non-specific prostatitis. In: Vahlensieck W, Rutishauser G (eds) Benign prostate diseases. Thieme, Stuttgart, pp 33–48

Hofstetter A (1973) Mykoplasmen bei entzündlichen Erkrankungen des Urogenitaltraktes. Infection 1:247–250

Kirby RS, Lowe D, Bultitude MJ, Shuttleworth KED (1982) Intraprostatic urinary reflux: an etiologic factor in abacterial prostatitis. Br J Urol 54:729–731

Krieger JN, McGonagle LA (1989) Diagnostic considerations and interpretation of microbiological findings for evaluation of chronic prostatitis. J Clin Microbiol 27:2240–2244

Lomas DA, Natin D, Stockley RA, Shahmanesh M (1993) Chemotactic activity of urethral secretions in men with urethritis and the effect of treatment. J Infect Dis 167:233–236

McClinton S, Eremin O, Miller JD (1990) Inflammatory infiltrate in prostatic hyperplasia – evidence of a host response to intraprostatic spermatozoa? Br J Urol 55:606–610

Meseguer MA, de Rafael L, Ferrer MM, Allona A, Baquero F, Sanz I (1986) Ureaplasma urealyticum counts and other laboratory findings in male urologic disorders. In: Weidner W, Brunner H, Krause W, Rothauge CW (eds) Therapy of prostatitis. München, Zuckschwerdt, pp 110–113

Meares EM Jr (1990) Prostatitis. In: Chisholm GT, Fair WR (eds) Scientific foundations of urology, 3rd edn. London, Heinemann, pp 373–378

Meares EM Jr, Stamey TA (1968) Bacteriologic localization patterns in bacterial prostatitis and urethritis. Invest Urol 5:492–518

Nickel JC, Costerton JW (1992) Coagulase-negative Staphylococcus in chronic prostatitis. J Urol 147:398–401

Poletti F, Medici MC, Alinovi A, Menozzi MG, Sacchini P, Stagni G, Toni M, Benoldi D (1985): Isolation of C. trachomatis from the prostatic cells in patients affected by nonacute abacterial prostatitis. J. Urol 134:691–692

Pust R, Schäfer R, Stumpf Ch, Leitenberger A, Engstfeld JE, Meier-Ewert H (1986) Urethritis posterior. In: Weidner W, Brunner H, Krause W, Rothauge CF (eds) Therapy of prostatitis. München, Zuckschwerdt, pp 102–109

Schaeffer AJ (1990) Diagnosis and treatment of prostatic infection. Urology [Suppl] 36:13–17

Shortliffe LMD, Wehner N, Stamey TA (1981) Use of a solid-phase radioimmunoassay and formalin-fixed whole bacterial antigen in the detection of antigen-specific immunoglobulin in prostatic fluid. J Clin Invest 67:790–799

Shortliffe LMD, Sellers RG, Schachter J (1992) The characterization of nonbacterial prostatitis: search for an etiology. J Urol 148:1461–1466

Shurbaji MS, Gupta PK, Myers J (1988) Immunohistochemical demonstration of chlamydial antigens in association with prostatitis. Modern Pathol 1:348–351

Tsunekawa T, Kumamoto Y (1989) Chlamydia trachomatis Ig-A. J Jpn Assoc Infect Dis 3:130–132

Weidner W: Moderne Prostatitisdiagnostik. Bd. 7 der Reihe Klinische und experimentelle Urologie Zuckschwerdt München 1984

Weidner W (1992) Prostatitis-diagnostic criteria, classification of patients and recommendations for therapeutic trials. Infection 20 [Suppl 3]:227–231

Weidner W, Ebner H (1985) Cytological analysis of urine after prostatic massage (VB 3) – a new technique for a discriminating diagnosis of prostatitis. In: Brunner H, Krause W, Rothauge CF, Weidner W (eds) Chronic prostatitis. Clinical, microbiological, cytological and immunological aspects of inflammation. Schattauer 1985, 141–151

Weidner W, Schiefer HG (1986) Reisolation of Chlamydia trachomatis from the prostatic cells in patients affected by nonacute abacterial prostatitis (letter to the editor). J Urol 136:690

Weidner W, Brunner H, Krause W (1980) Quantitative culture of Ureaplasma urealyticum in patients with chronic prostatitis or prostatosis. J Urol 123:622–623 (1980)

Weidner W, Schiefer HG, Krauss H, Jantos C, Friedrich HJ, Altmannsberger M (1991a) Chronic prostatitis; a thorough search for etiologically involved microorganisms in 1461 patients. Infection 19 [Suppl 3]:119–125

Weidner W, Jantos C, Schiefer HG, Haidl G, Friedrich HJ (1991b) Semen parameters in men with and without proven chronic prostatitis. Arch Androl 26:173–183

Weidner W, Jantos Ch, Schuhmacher F, Schiefer HG, Meyhöfer W (1991c) Recurrent haemospermia – underlying urogenital anomalies and efficacy of imaging procedures. Br J Urol 67:317–323

Weiss MA, Mills SE (1989) Lesions of the prostate and seminal vesicles. In: Weiss MA, Mills SE (eds) Atlas of genitourinary tract disorders. Gower, Singapore

Ultrasonographic Features of Prostatitis

R. Clements, G.J. Griffiths, and W.B. Peeling

A clinical diagnosis of prostatitis is often made by the urologist but is often not confirmed by objective laboratory or radiological evidence. Prostatitis is not one disease but occurs in several distinct forms or syndromes, and the common types of prostatitis may be divided into acute (ABP) and chronic bacterial prostatitis (CBP), non-bacterial prostatitis (NBP) and prostatodynia. This classification is based on obtaining evidence of bacterial infection localised to the prostate, and inflammatory cells in the expressed prostatic secretions (EPS). Bacterial prostatitis is associated with bacteriuria. In cases of CBP the persistent presence of the pathogenic organism leads to recurrent bacteriuria, whilst in patients with NBP or prostatodynia bacteriuria rarely (if ever) occurs. Patients with CBP and NBP have excess fat-containing macrophages and leukocytes in their prostatic secretions whilst patients with prostatodynia have prostatic secretions without such evidence of inflammation.

Acute Bacterial Prostatitis

The clinical features of ABP include fever, low back pain and perineal pain, generalised malaise and arthralgia coupled with urinary symptoms such as frequency, nocturia, dysuria, and outflow tract obstruction. Digital rectal examination usually reveals an enlarged, markedly tender prostate. The causative organism may often be identified by culture of the voided bladder urine. Prostatic microabscesses may occur early in the disease process, and large abscesses may be a late complication. The exact pathogenesis of ABP is uncertain and controversial. Suggested routes of infection include ascending urethral infection as a result of sexual activity, reflux of infected urine into the prostatic ducts, and haematogenous infection.

Prostatic Abscesses

Prostatic abscesses are now relatively uncommon. Most prostatic abscesses are probably complications of ABP, and there is an increased incidence in diabetic patients and patients with acquired immunodeficiency syndrome. Patients may present with acute retention, frequency and dysuria, fever, and epididymo-orchitis, and rectal examination reveals an enlarged, tender prostate with fluctuation. In the past endoscopic surgical drainage was the usual treatment, but now prostatic abscesses can be aspirated under imaging guidance using either computed tomography or transrectal ultrasound (TRUS). Antibiotics can also be introduced directly into the prostate under imaging guidance.

Chronic Bacterial Prostatitis

CBP is characterised by repeated urinary tract infection caused by the same pathogenic organism. The disease has variable clinical manifestations although some patients are diagnosed because of an incidental finding of asymptomatic bacteriuria. CBP may follow ABP, but in many patients there is no preceding attack of ABP. Most patients complain of urgency, frequency and dysuria, and pelvic and perineal pain. There are no specific findings on digital rectal examination. Microscopic examination of the expressed prostatic secretion from patients with CBP shows excess fat-laden macrophages and leukocytes, and the diagnosis is confirmed by culture of specimens of urine and prostatic secretions that localise the organism to the prostate. Multiple large prostatic calculi may be seen in men with CBP. Non-infected prostatic calculi usually cause no symptoms, but in men with bacterial prostatitis prostatic stones can become infected and serve as a source of recurrent urinary tract infection (Eykyn et al. 1974; Stamey 1981). There are no distinguishing features between those patients with CBP who have infected calculi and those without such calculi.

Non-bacterial Prostatitis

This condition is very much commoner than bacterial prostatitis. Urinary symptoms include urinary frequency and nocturia, dysuria, and pelvic, perineal and genital pain. The symptoms are similar to those of CBP, but there is no history of documented urinary tract infection. There are no specific findings on rectal examination of the prostate. As in CBP, patients with NBP have evidence of inflammation on microscopic examination of the expressed prostatic secretion, but results of culture in patients with NBP are not positive.

Tuberculous Prostatitis

This is a rare condition and in many cases is found incidentally after a transurethral resection. The route of infection is by haematogeneous spread. Rectal examination reveals a nodular non-tender prostate.

Granulomatous Prostatitis

This is an uncommon condition that mimics prostatic cancer on rectal examination. It may be idiopathic but can occur after urinary infection, transurethral prostatectomy, or needle biopsy of the prostate. The patient has a history of bladder outlet obstruction and may have a fever and arthralgia. Digital examination of the prostate reveals an enlarged gland that feels malignant. The diagnosis is confirmed by histological examination of material obtained by biopsy or transurethral resection and exclusion by culture of specific infectious causes of granulomatous prostatitis. Pathological examination demonstrates a non-caseating granulomatous inflammatory reaction which occurs in discrete foci in 20% of patients and is diffuse throughout the prostate in 80% of cases.

Ultrasonic Techniques for Examination of the Prostate

It is possible to image the prostate ultrasonically by several approaches – transabdominal, transperineal, transurethral and transrectal. The transabdominal approach uses the full bladder as an acoustic window (Fig. 1). The probe is placed in the suprapubic region, and the prostate and seminal vesicles may be visualised by tilting the probe caudally. This transabdominal approach is very acceptable to patients, but it is usually difficult to visualise the apex of the gland behind the symphysis pubis by this approach, and there may often also be difficulty in identifying small prostate glands. It is generally possible to make only a limited assessment of prostatic pathology by this route.

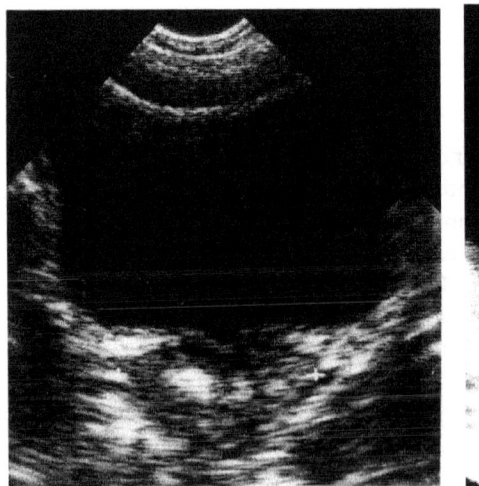 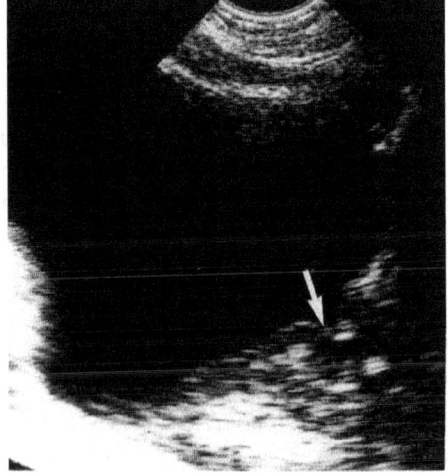

a   b

Fig. 1. Transabdominal axial (**a**) and transabdominal midline sagittal (**b**) scan of the prostate (*arrow*) visualised through the full bladder

The transperineal approach has not been widely used because of the difficulty in anatomical orientation. The apex of the gland may be clearly demonstrated by the approach, and it is a route that may be used in patients following abdominoperineal excision of the rectum.

Transurethral ultrasound images of the prostate may be obtained by using an ultrasonic probe during cystoscopy with a rigid cystoscope. Transurethral probes have been used mainly for the ultrasonic demonstration of bladder pathology, but extremely good visualisation of the transition zone and periurethral part of the prostate is possible by this route. The necessity of performing the examination in the operating room limits the widespread use of this approach.

The transrectal approach has been the most widely used route for the ultrasonic demonstration of the prostate. With modern high-frequency transducers, excellent visualisation of the internal anatomy of the prostate and seminal vesicles is possible, and a wide range of prostatic pathology may be demonstrated. Transrectal ultrasound imaging is now an established technique for the diagnosis and staging of prostatic cancer. In recent years it has been increasingly used for the diagnosis of other prostatic conditions and has been found useful in the assessment of patients with infertility, haemospermia, and prostatitis, as well as in the measurement of prostatic size in patients with benign prostatic hyperplasia.

It is often difficult to establish the diagnosis of prostatitis. Transrectal ultrasound may be considered in the investigation of patients for two reasons, firstly because of the difficulty in establishing a confident diagnosis on clinical grounds, and secondly because the findings of digital examination may suggest a diagnosis of prostatic cancer. TRUS has been used increasingly over the past decade in the diagnosis of prostatic cancer, and ultrasound examination with a high-frequency biplanar or multiplanar transducer is now an established method of demonstrating prostatic cancer. It is now accepted that the majority of cancers are hypoechoic (Griffiths et al. 1987; Lee et al. 1985), and it is a relatively simple, non-invasive process to biopsy a hypoechoic area under ultrasound guidance to achieve a histological diagnosis (Torp-Pedersen and Lee 1989). Whilst most cancers are hypoechoic, not all hypoechoic areas are cancer, and the following benign conditions may appear as hypoechoic areas within the prostate: glandular hyperplasia, prostatitis, prostatic infarcts, and smooth muscle around the ejaculatory ducts. The precise diagnosis of a hypoechoic area within the prostate can be established only by biopsy.

Method of Transrectal Ultrasound Examination of the Prostate

Equipment. A wide variety of ultrasound probes are now available for transrectal imaging. Early scans were obtained using a chair-mounted 3.5-MHz probe, but contemporary equipment uses a hand-held transducer with a frequency between 5 and 7.5 MHz. A variety of probes are available from different manufacturers with sector, linear or annular array transducers, and these may be arranged in a biplanar or multiplanar arrangement. Some probes permit the additional possibility of pulsed wave and colour Doppler imaging.

Examination Technique. The examination is usually performed with the patient lying in the left lateral decubitus position with the knees bent. It is worth ensuring that the patient is positioned with his buttock near the end of the table for optimal scanning conditions, and to achieve this it is usually necessary to support the patient's feet at the side of the table. The probe is covered with a rubber condom, and the tip lubricated with ultrasonic coupling jelly. After preliminary digital rectal examination, the probe is inserted and the balloon on the tip of the probe is inflated with 30–50 ml water.

Examination of the patient in both the transverse and longitudinal planes is necessary for a full ultrasonic examination of the gland. The gland should be scanned in the transverse plane from the base to the apex noting the overall shape and symmetry, the "capsular" integrity, and the internal echo pattern. The examination of the gland in the longitudinal plane should then be undertaken and a volume measurement of the gland obtained. The longitudinal plane provides better visualisation of the base and the apex of the gland and is the optimal imaging plane for needle insertion into the prostate and seminal vesicles for biopsy and aspiration.

Ultrasound-Guided Needle Insertion into the Prostate for Biopsy/Aspiration

It is possible to biopsy the prostate by both the transperineal and transrectal routes, and both digital examination and TRUS can be used to guide needles into suspect areas of the prostate. Transperineal biopsy of the prostate guided by axial ultrasound imaging was first described by Holm and Gammelgaard (1981), and in our own unit over 140 biopsies were performed transperineally by this route between 1985 and 1988 (Clements et al. 1990). The technique of transperineal biopsy using sagittal ultrasound images was described by Fornage et al. (1983). The transperineal route for biopsy and needle insertion has three drawbacks, however: (a) it is poorly tolerated by patients because of pain, (b) it is difficult to place needles accurately in lesions of diameter below 1 cm, and (c) it is a time-consuming procedure. It is possible to overcome these drawbacks by using the transrectal route, and needles may now be inserted transrectally under transrectal ultrasound guidance with many modern biplanar and multiplanar probes. This is now accepted as the optimal route for ultrasound-guided prostate biopsy particularly in conjunction with an automatic firing biopsy device such as the Biopty gun.

Transperineal Needle Insertion into the Prostate. For this technique the patient is placed in the lithotomy position with the legs abducted and the knees flexed. The perineal skin is cleaned with antiseptic and the region draped with sterile towels. The perineum is infiltrated with local anaesthetic. It is usually necessary to give additional intravenous sedation and an analgesic such as diazepam or pethidine for this procedure. The ultrasound probe is rotated and positioned so that the target area lies within the plane of the ultrasound image. A biopsy device is attached to the probe with needle channels corresponding to electronic markers on the ultrasound image. The needle may be inserted into the perineum and advanced into the prostate. With imaging in the longitudinal plane, the needle path may be visualised directly as it enters the gland. With the axial plane of imaging, the needle is advanced until its tip is seen as an echogenic focus on the axial image. The biopsy sample may be taken or prostatic aspiration performed once satisfactory needle placement has been confirmed ultrasonically.

Transrectal Needle Insertion into the Prostate. This technique may be performed with the patient in the left lateral position. No preliminary anaesthetic or analgesia or skin preparation is required, but the technique is usually performed under antibiotic cover. It is our practice to use 400 mg ciprofloxacin routinely 30 min before the biopsy with a further dose of 400 mg 24 h later. It should also be ascertained that the patient does not have a bleeding diathesis and is not receiving anticoagulant or aspirin therapy. Different ultrasound probes have different methods for guiding the needle into the gland; there may be an obliquely angled needle channel through the body of the ultrasound probe, or alternatively a needle guide may be attached externally to the probe. It is a particular advantage of the Bruel and Kjaer multiplanar transducer that the sector image may be obtained in both the transverse and longitudinal planes without movement of the probe. The path of needle puncture is displayed electronically on the ultrasound image on the television monitor. It is usually most satisfactory to use the longitudinal plane of imaging for transrectal biopsy, and the probe is positioned so that the target area is traversed by the puncture line. The needle may then be inserted into the target area and a biopsy sample

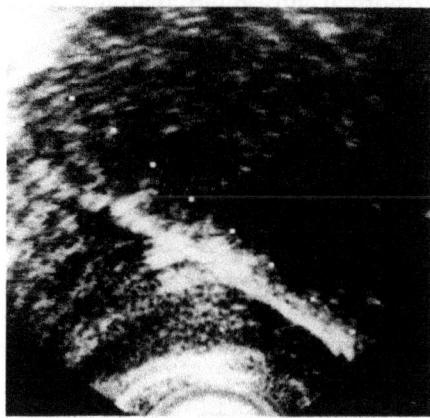

Fig. 2. Sagittal scan, showing biopsy needle passing transrectally into the prostate. *Dots*, the expected path of the biopsy needle outlined electronically on the monitor screen of the scanner

obtained (Fig. 2) or aspiration performed. This technique has been described fully by Torp-Pedersen and Lee (1989). Needle placement within the prostate by the transrectal route may be performed safely as an office procedure, but the patient should be warned of the risks of septicaemia and post-biopsy bleeding and advised of the appropriate procedures for obtaining medical advice should these complications ensue.

Normal Ultrasound Anatomy

A zonal system of anatomy of the prostate was described by McNeal (1981). In this system, the prostate is considered as three glandular zones: transition, central and peripheral, and one non-glandular region, the anterior fibromuscular stroma. These zones can be identified by transrectal ultrasound (Villers et al. 1990) and magnetic resonance imaging. In the young adult prostate, the transition zone constitutes about 5% of prostatic glandular tissue and is located on both sides of the prostatic urethra; it is in this region that benign hyperplasia develops. The central zone is relatively resistant to disease processes and constitutes about 25% of the prostatic glandular tissue in the young adult. It is situated around the base of the prostate and the ejaculatory ducts pass through central zone tissue to reach the verumontanum. The peripheral zone constitutes 70% of the glandular tissues and lies on the posterior and lateral aspect of the gland. Its ducts drain into the urethra distal to the verumontanum.

Transverse (Axial) Scans

The seminal vesicles are seen ultrasonically as paired semi-lunar structures lying posterior to the bladder above the base of the prostate with the vasa deferentia lying postero-medially (Fig. 3). The seminal vesicles may be smooth or lobulated, and within the seminal vesicles echogenic areas may be seen corresponding to the folds of the lining epithelium. The normal ultrasound anatomy of the

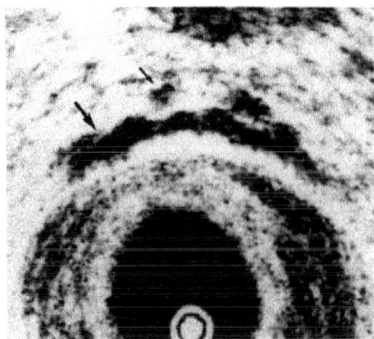

Fig. 3. Axial scan. *Small arrow*, ampulla of the vas deferens; *large arrow*, seminal vesicle

prostate is best demonstrated in young men aged 20–30 years before the onset of benign prostatic hypertrophy or focal atrophy. In the young male the prostate appears as a symmetrical semi-lunar shape triangular structure. The muscle of the preprostatic sphincter is demonstrated as a rounded echo-poor area lying anterior at the base of the prostate (Fig. 4). The zonal anatomy may be demonstrated, with the central zone being slightly more echogenic relative to the peripheral and transition zones. The ejaculatory ducts may be seen on axial scans as rounded echo-poor structures within the central zone, and the verumontanum is demonstrated as a central echogenic area which has been likened in some patients with benign hyperplasia to the Eiffel Tower (Fig. 5). The outline of the prostate is delineated by an echogenic margin caused by periprostatic adipose tissue. Within this "capsular" region the thin-walled periprostatic venous plexus lies; it is not normally visible but in some patients is seen as an echo-free band around the gland. The neurovascular bundles can be identified postero-laterally as symmetrical structures crossing this "capsular" region to enter the prostate gland. With the development of benign hyperplasia in older age in the transition zone and periurethral tissues, the remainder of the gland becomes compressed into a thin rim of surrounding tissue (Fig. 6).

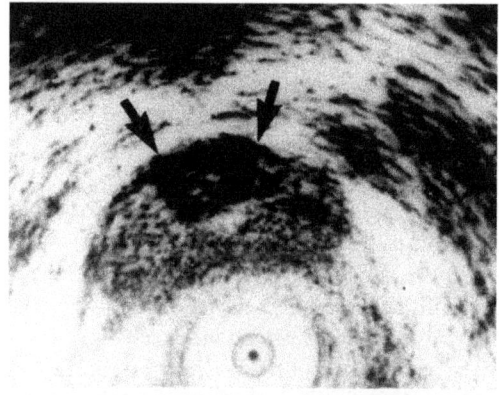

a

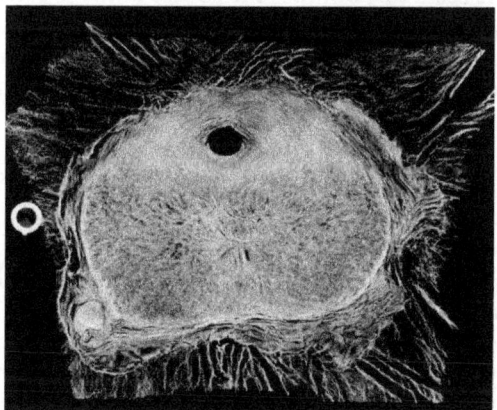

b

Fig. 4. a Preprostatic sphincter in a cadaver prostate. The sonographic scan obtained from a position near the prostatic base demonstrates an echo-poor periurethral area (*arrows*) lying in the anterior position. b Microradiograph of the cadaver prostate shown in a. The periurethral area is seen clearly as an amorphous structure surrounding the open urethra. Histological examination confirmed that this is the smooth muscle of the preprostatic sphincter. (From Griffiths et al. 1990)

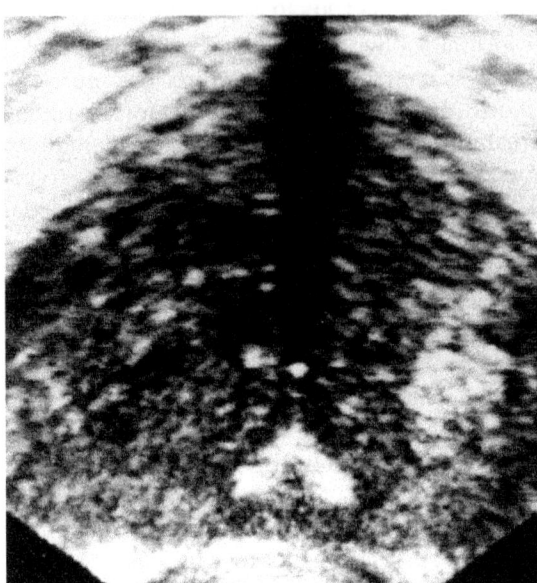

Fig. 5. Axial scan at the level of the verumontanum, which is outlined by calcification giving an "Eiffel Tower" appearance. (From Griffiths et al. 1990)

Longitudinal (Sagittal) Images

There is a 35° angulation mid-way along the prostatic urethra just proximal to the verumontanum, and this angulation divides the urethra into proximal and distal portions. The preprostatic sphincter surrounds the proximal urethra from bladder neck to the verumontanum, and the muscular tissue of the preprostatic sphincter is seen on sagittal ultrasound images as a wide echo-poor band passing from the bladder base to the verumontanum. Within this band a thin echogenic line may occasionally be seen; this outlines the course of the prostatic urethra and is caused by fine calcified deposits in submucosal glands of the proximal urethra. The zonal anatomy is well demonstrated on sagittal scans, and the ejaculatory ducts are seen as a thin echo-poor band passing through central zone towards the verumontanum (Fig. 7).

Volume Measurements

The volume of the prostate can be measured with transrectal ultrasound by several methods. With chair-mounted probes and the earliest axial scanners the volume was measured by step section planimetry. In this method the area of the gland was measured electronically on sequential scans 0.5 cm apart. The volume of the gland was computed by the scanner software from these area measure-

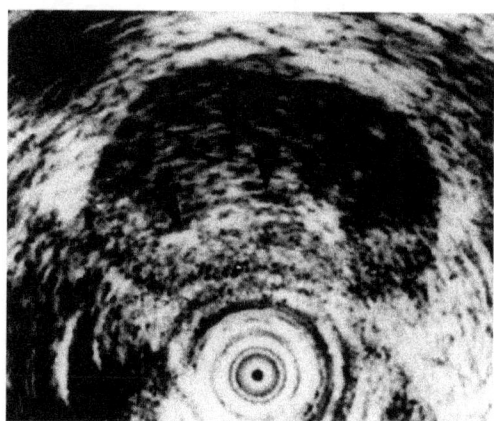

Fig. 6. a Prostatic calculi and benign prostatic hyperplasia in a cadaver prostate. The calculi are seen as echogenic areas (*arrows*) at the margin of multiple adenomata. **b** At microradiography, the adenomata are seen to be made up of multiple smaller hyperplastic nodules (*arrows*). (From Griffiths et al. 1990)

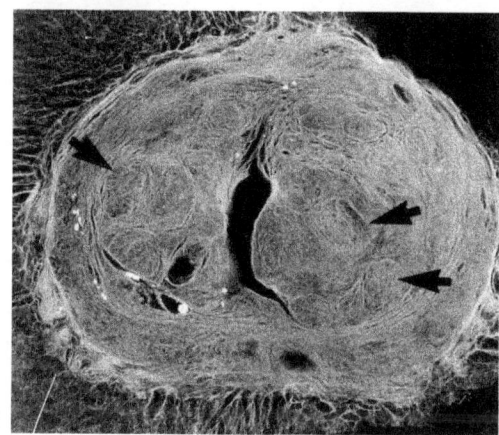

ments using the formula:

$$\text{Volume} = \sum_{i=1}^{n} \frac{1}{3}[A_i + A_{i-1} + (A_i \cdot A_{i-1})^{1/2}]h_i$$

where A_i is the area seen outlined on the ith section and h_i is the distance between the ith and $i-1$ section. Previous work by our group in cadavers demonstrated an excellent correlation between the gland volume measured by planimetry and the weight of the cadaver prostate (Clements et al. 1989).

With the introduction of hand-held probes it has been necessary to develop the use of formulae to calculate prostatic volume using measurements of the transverse gland diameter on the axial scan (width), anteroposterior gland diameter on the axial scan (height), and longitudinal diameter on the sagittal scan (length; Fig. 8). A formula that has been commonly used is the prolate ellipse formula:

$$\text{Volume} = \frac{\pi}{6} \times \text{height} \times \text{width} \times \text{length}$$

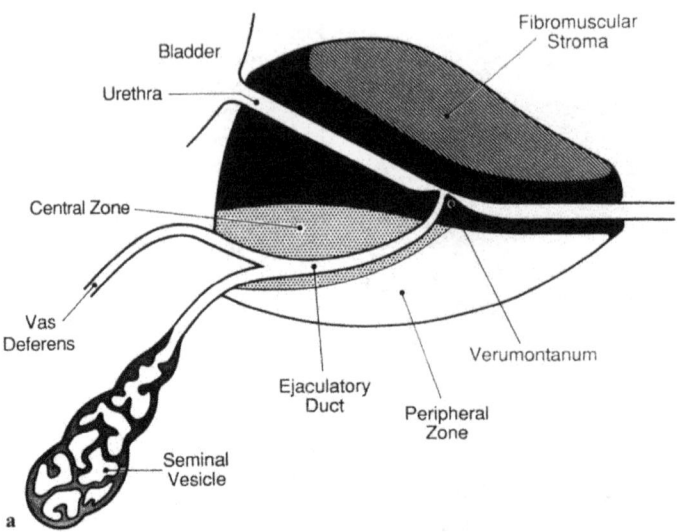

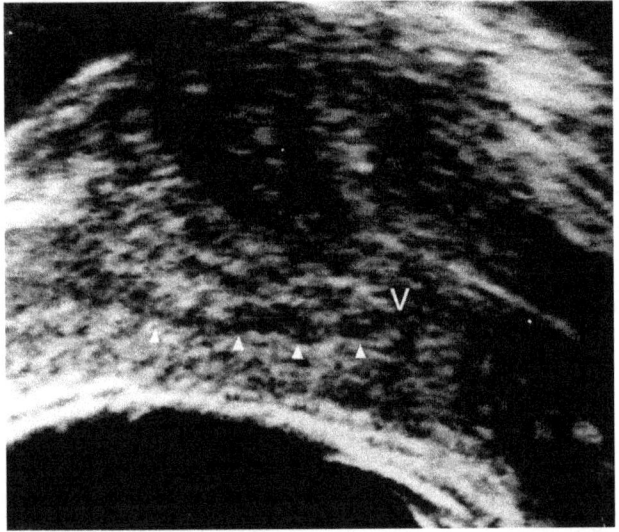

Fig. 7. a Zonal anatomy on midline sagittal scan (from Clements et al. Br. J. Radiol (1991)). **b** Midline sagittal scan. The ejaculatory duct (*arrowheads*) is outlined passing through central zone to the verumontanum (*V*)

Littrup et al. (1991) assessed prostate volume measurements with this formula and found it to be a useful practical measurement of prostatic volume. Myschetsky et al. (1991) examined 76 patients prior to radical prostatectomy and found that the following modification of the prolate ellipse to be a more reliable method of estimating gland volume than the original formula:

Volume $= 0.7 \times$ height $\times$ width $\times$ length

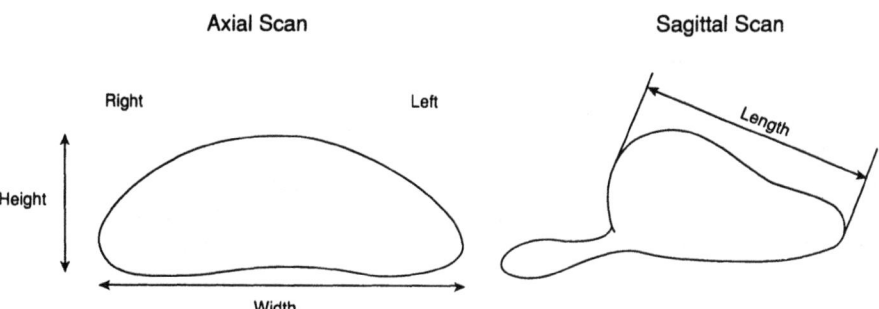

Fig. 8. Diagrammatic representation of the dimensions measured in volume calculations

There may, however, be difficulty in identifying the measuring points for the length measurement used in this formula, and this has caused other authors to explore the use of different formulae. Terris and Stamey (1991) reviewed methods of prostate volume calculation by transrectal ultrasound in 150 patients who subsequently underwent radical prostatectomy. Using multivariant regression analysis, they analysed 15 different calculations. The correlation coefficient of step-section planimetry with volume was 0.93 and the best correlation ($r = 0.94$) was obtained for the variation of the prolate spheroid formula expressed as:

$$\text{Volume} = \frac{\pi}{6} \times \text{height} \times (\text{width})^2$$

Sonographic Features of Prostatitis

A few studies have compared the transrectal ultrasound findings of prostatitis with the microscopic findings of the urine and EPS and, even more importantly, with bacterial localisation to the prostate. Griffiths et al. (1984) reported a prospective study of TRUS in prostatitis based on 40 patients with clinical symptoms and signs of prostatic inflammation. Their ages ranged from 17 to 68 years (mean 34 years). Nineteen patients had a urethral discharge and other symptoms including dysuria, perineal and testicular pain, and occasionally low back pain. Each patient underwent a full clinical examination including digital rectal examination of the prostate to assess its size, consistency, and degree of tenderness. Objective evidence of prostatic inflammation was obtained in all patients with voided, segmented, urinary stream studies, and by examination of the EPS. There was alkaline shift of the pH to above 8 in all patients. All patients were considered on the basis of these findings to have inflammation localised to the prostate and to have either a primary attack of acute prostatitis or an acute attack of relapsing chronic prostatitis. The sonographic examinations were undertaken with a chair-mounted 3.5-MHz transducer. The prostatic volume was enlarged (mean volume 38 ml). The gland was symmetrical, and in some patients the capsular margins were ill defined.

Three main sonographic features were identified: (a) An echo-poor halo was observed in the periurethral area in all cases (Fig. 9). Harada et al. (1980) noted this appearance in 50% of their cases of prostatitis but also commented that it was visualised in 69% of normal glands. (b) Multiple echo-poor areas were observed within the gland in 80% of cases, giving a heterogeneous echo pattern (Fig. 10). Histologically these areas represent areas of oedema and necrosis, and

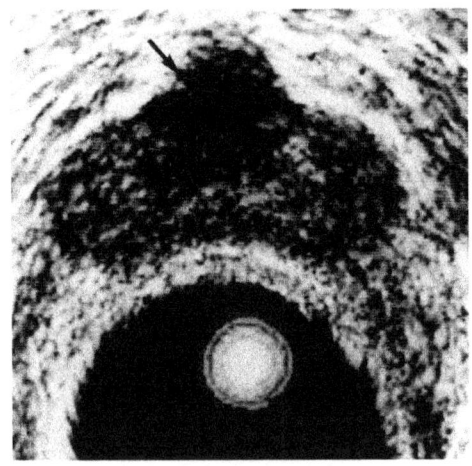

Fig. 9. Axial 4-MHz scan with echo-poor periurethral region (*arrow*) in a patient with prostatitis

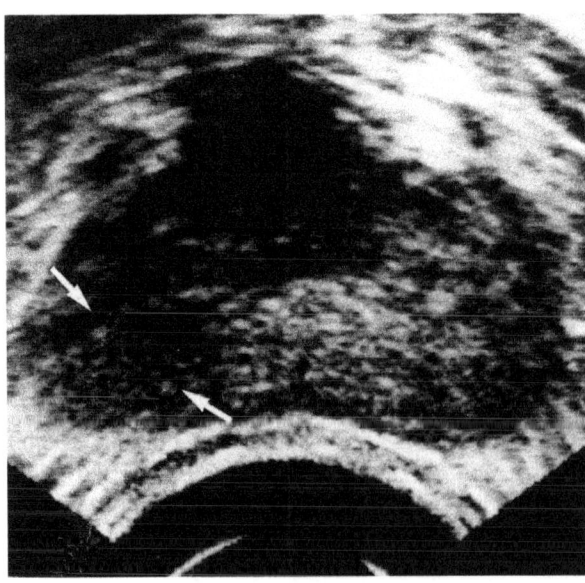

Fig. 10. Axial 7-MHz scan with echo-poor periurethral region, and an extensive echo-poor area in the right peripheral zone (*arrows*)

they were observed predominantly in the peripheral zone. (c) Enlargement of the periprostatic veins was observed in 20% of patients (Figs. 11–13). These are demonstrated sonographically as curvilinear echo free areas adjacent to the prostate.

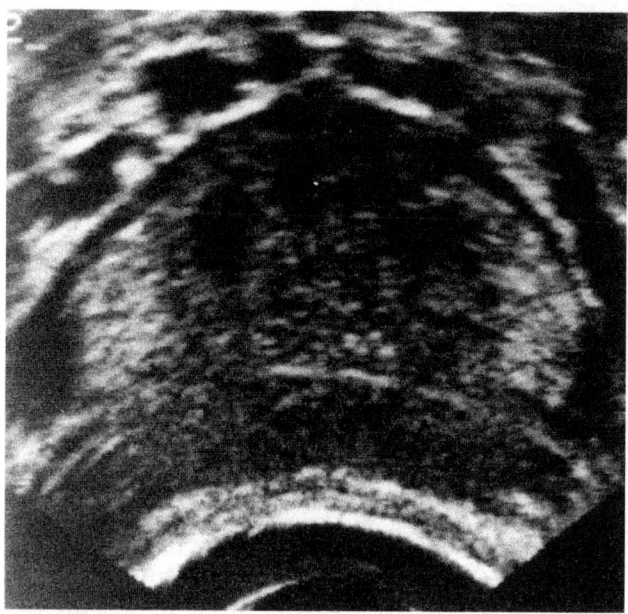

Fig. 11. Axial 7-MHz scan with marked distension of the periprostatic veins

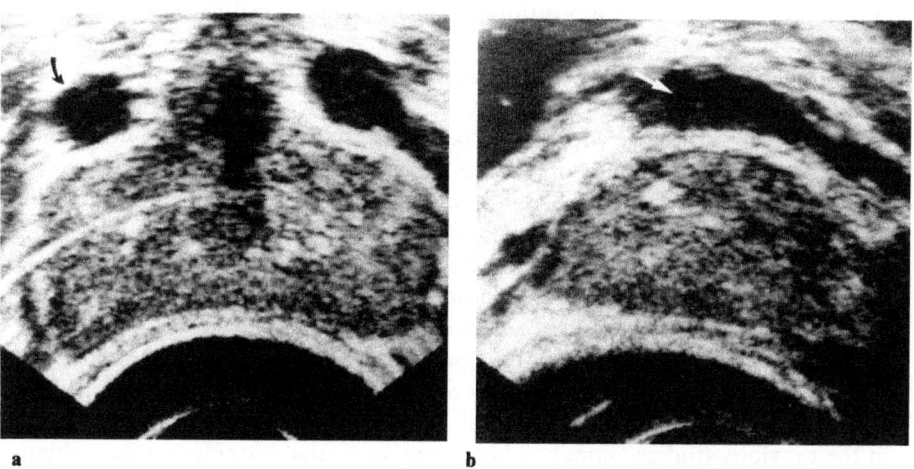

a   b

Fig. 12. Axial (a) and sagittal (b) scans showing marked distension of periprostatic veins (*arrows*) in a patient with prostatitis

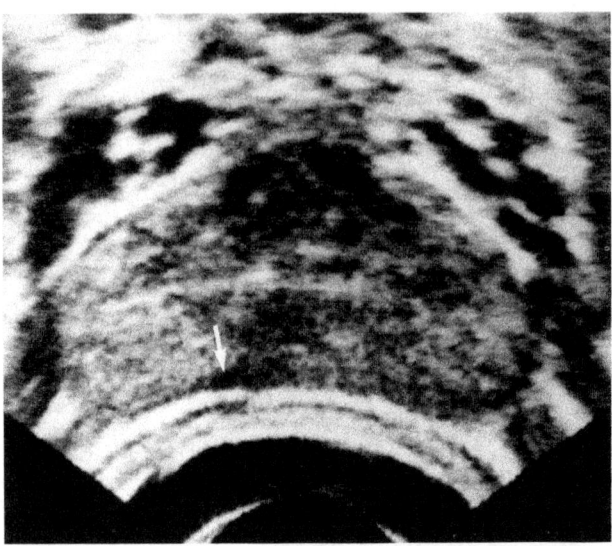

Fig. 13. Axial 7-MHz scan of a patient with prostatitis demonstrating an echo-poor periurethral region, a small echo-poor peripheral zone lesion (*arrow*), and distended periprostatic veins

Other studies have also looked at the ultrasonic features of patients with chronic prostatitis and prostatodynia. Wiegand and Weidner (1986) investigated 115 patients aged 20–78 years (mean 41 years). Chronic prostatitis was diagnosed by means of increased leukocyte numbers in prostatic secretion in 62 men, of whom 6 had chronic bacterial and 56 non-bacterial prostatitis. In another 53 patients a diagnosis of prostatodynia was established. TRUS was performed in the left lateral position with a 3.5-MHz transducer. Of the patients with chronic prostatitis 62.9% were noted to have a heterogeneous echo pattern, compared with 16.5% of patients with prostatodynia. An echo-poor periurethral region was observed in 54.9% of patients with chronic prostatitis as opposed to 17% of those with prostatodynia. Calcification was also noted to be more common in the glands of patients with chronic prostatitis than those with prostatodynia, and this increase in frequency of calcification in this study has been postulated to represent a cause of recurrent prostatitis. It is, however, the experience of our own group that calcification may be present within the gland in both malignant and benign conditions, and calcification is not a useful ultrasonic discriminant in the differential diagnosis.

Di Trapani et al. (1988) reported on the use of TRUS in 121 patients with chronic prostatitis (bacterial and non-bacterial) and prostatodynia using a 4-MHz axial probe. A similar range of abnormalities was observed to that seen in the previous studies, namely a heterogeneous prostatic echo pattern, dilatation of the periprostatic venous plexus and prostatic calcification. Although this paper gave a precise breakdown of the clinical and pathological subgroups of the 121 patients, it did not correlate the frequency of the observations to the subgroups but only described ultrasonic abnormalities in relation to the whole group of patients.

Doble and Carter (1989) reported a series of studies using TRUS in chronic prostatitis. The first study correlated sonographic abnormalities of the prostate with the leukocyte count in the expressed prostatic secretions in 60 patients with symptoms of chronic prostatitis. Ultrasound scans were performed using a 5.5-MHz transducer in the left lateral position. Eight ultrasonic features were considered: focal echogenic areas, mid-range echoes, echo-poor areas, ejaculatory duct calcification, capsular irregularity, capsular thickening, and hypoechoic periurethral zones. Sonographic abnormalities were seen more frequently in patients with borderline or definite chronic prostatitis than in prostatodynia. In a second study, the authors correlated the sonographic features of 200 men with the leukocyte count in the post-massage urine specimen (VB3). In these authors' experience, an echo-poor halo in the periurethral zone did not correlate with chronic prostatitis, and they considered it a feature of a normal gland. The other seven criteria listed above, however, correlated with the diagnosis of chronic prostatitis in this study. The authors' diagnosis of ejaculatory duct calcification in this study was based entirely on axial views, and their illustrative example of an ejaculatory duct calculus does not appear to be within the ejaculatory duct. In these circumstances the present authors doubt the validity of observations of ejaculatory duct calcification in that study. Further studies correlated pathological examination with ultrasound appearances obtained by ultrasound-guided needle biopsy. It appeared that highly echogenic areas correlate with corpora amylacea, and echo-poor areas represent areas of inflammation. Follow-up observations were also obtained. The ultrasound appearances changed in 87% of patients with prostatitis. New areas of increased echogenicity appeared in 40% of patients, whilst 47% of such areas disappeared. At follow-up 30% of echo-poor areas had disappeared. The follow-up study suggests that the development of new signs is more frequent than resolution of earlier ones in prostatitis, and there is minimal change in prostatodynia. This finding suggests that repeated scanning may increase diagnostic accuracy. The authors felt, however, that the only ultrasound feature worthy of follow-up was the echo-poor area which reflects tissue oedema. Follow-up data in prostatitis was also described by Griffiths et al. (1984), who looked at prostatic volume. Most authors consider that the gland volume increases in active prostatitis. In the study of Griffiths et al. (1984) those patients who were considered on clinical grounds to have improved in response to antibiotic treatment of prostatitis showed a mean percentage volume reduction of the prostate of 16%, whereas those with no evidence of clinical response had a mean volume increase of 13%.

Some patients with prostatitis have been treated under ultrasound guidance. Jiminez-Cruz et al. (1988) treated 51 patients with CBP using 2 ml intraprostatic amikacin 500 mg or tobramycin 100 mg weekly for 2–4 weeks. Injections were performed by the transperineal route under ultrasound guidance into the peripheral zone or echogenic areas of the prostate. Of these patients 49% were cured microbiologically, but 29% failed to respond; 43% were clinically cured, and 41% were symptomatically improved.

True prostatic calculi develop in tissues or acini of the gland. Prostatic calculi may arise spontaneously as the result of an inflammatory reaction or as a consequence of acinar obstruction. The epithelial cells of the prostatic acini undergo atrophy and degeneration and are shed to become suspended in the fluid within the acini. These hyaline masses of degenerate cells found in the prostate are called corpora amylacea. It has been suggested that prostatic calculi can be formed by consolidation and calcification of corpora amylacea (Klimas et al. 1985). Prostatic calculi vary in number from one to several hundred and can vary in size from a few millimeters to 3 cm or more. Small calculi within prostatic acini are usually associated with a chronic inflammatory infiltrate. The significance of true prostatic calculi is not known. Although the calculi may cause shedding of inflammatory cells into the prostatic fluid, they are generally considered to produce no harm. There is usually a 40%–60% failure rate following treatment of prostatitis, and it has been suggested that bacteria might persist inside stones as they do in renal calculi (Stamey 1981). It is therefore possible that calculi may be the cause of recurrent episodes of prostatitis. Prostatic calculi are readily apparent on TRUS, usually as the most strongly echogenic area within the prostate. They may be seen in benign hyperplasia and malignancy, and no specific distribution has been noted which is diagnostic of prostatitis.

Throughout the 1980s there were various developments in transducer technology, and TRUS progressed from using the original chair-mounted low-frequency probe to higher frequency hand-held radial and longitudinal biplanar and multiplanar transducers. In our department we have continued to observe with high-frequency multiplanar transducers (Fig. 13) the three signs of prostatitis observed by Griffiths et al. (1984), and we still consider them to be valid signs of an acute inflammatory process within the prostate. Engorgement of the periprostatic venous system may be particularly apparent with longitudinal imaging where the engorged veins are readily visible in the sagittal plane. These tubular periprostatic echo-free structures can be confirmed to be vascular in nature by the use of ultrasound probes which permit either pulse wave Doppler studies or colour Doppler imaging.

Colour Doppler imaging of the prostate may be of value in prostatitis although no definite study with bacteriological correlation has yet been published. Watanabe (1991) described "enhanced" Doppler signals in cases of prostatitis although he did not specify whether any intraprostatic change in Doppler flow had been demonstrated. Rifkin et al. (1991) described "diffusely abnormal flow" in 14 cases of confirmed prostatitis with a significant abnormal flow pattern to the affected area of the prostate. Lees and Rickards (1991) reported a series of 200 examinations of the prostate with colour Doppler imaging. In their experience, increases in colour Doppler imaging intensity and number of vessels were detected in both prostatic cancer and prostatitis. In prostatitis the flow increase was seen in the immediate vicinity of the urethra, and only two cases of focal flow increase in the peripheral zone were seen in patients with prostatitis.

Despite technical improvements certain sonographic features of inflammatory disease of the prostate and prostatic cancer continue to be similar, although the patient's age and clinical presentation may make the latter condition unlikely. There is a need for further studies to clarify the ultrasonic appearances of prostatitis using contemporary high-frequency multiplanar transducers and to further evaluate the possible role of colour Doppler imaging in the diagnosis of prostatitis.

Ultrasonic Appearance of Tuberculous Prostatitis

Experience with this condition is limited. In our experience, no specific ultrasonic features have been identified ultrasonically which would enable a diagnosis of tuberculous prostatitis to be made without biopsy. In one patient who presented with a left scrotal sinus, the whole of the right side of the gland appeared echo-poor (Fig. 14), and there was no calcification within the gland. In another patient there was marked calcification in the surgical capsule, but the gland texture was otherwise homogeneous.

Ultrasonic Appearance of Granulomatous Prostatitis

It has been appreciated for several years that focal granulomatous prostatitis is one of the differential diagnoses of a hypoechoic area within the prostate, yet the ultrasonic features of granulomatous prostatitis have infrequently been described

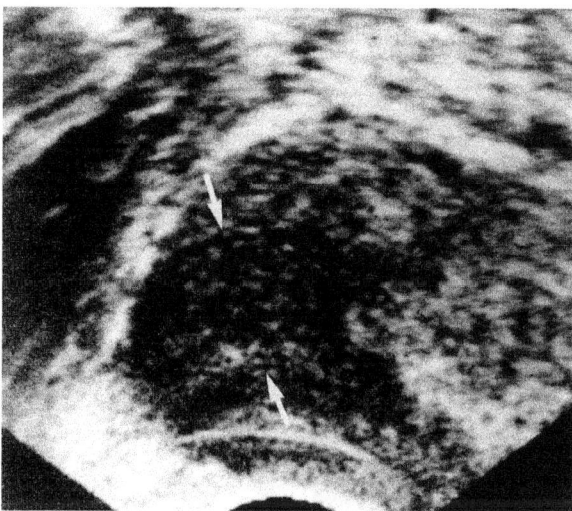

Fig. 14. Axial 7-MHz scan in a patient with tuberculous prostatitis. The whole of the right peripheral zone is echo-poor (*arrows*). Note the absence of calcification within the gland

in the literature. Bude et al. (1990) reported the ultrasonic features of six patients with granulomatous prostatitis. One patient was undergoing bacille Calmette-Guérin therapy for bladder cancer, two patients had recent urinary tract infections, and there was no known predisposing condition in the other three patients. The authors reported a focal hypoechoic lesion in one patient and multiple large and small hypoechoic areas throughout all prostatic zones in the other five. In their experience the gland was enlarged in all patients.

The ultrasonic appearances of 11 patients with granulomatous prostatitis have recently been reviewed by our group (Clements et al., 1993). The mean age was 64 years. Six patients presented with symptoms of outflow tract obstruction, four with acute retention, and one had a urinary tract infection. In all 11 patients the gland was suspicious of carcinoma on digital rectal examination. The mean serum level of prostate-specific antigen at presentation was 5.3 ng/ml. Ultrasonic examination revealed a normally sized gland in two patients, but the prostate was enlarged in nine; the mean gland volume was 41 ml. The seminal vesicles and ejaculatory ducts appeared normal in all patients. Two patients demonstrated a small calcified focus in the surgical capsule; in one patient there was extensive calcification in the surgical capsule. In all patients the periprostatic veins appeared normal. In two patients, one aged 41 years and the other 63, the periurethral area appeared abnormally hypoechoic. Focal hypoechoic areas of the peripheral zone were observed in eight patients (Fig. 15); in two of these eight patients this was accompanied by a heterogeneous texture to the central and transition zones. In three patients the gland texture was homogeneous, and no specific focal abnormality was demonstrated. In those patients with hypoechoic areas there were no special ultrasonic features that enabled a specific ultrasonic diagnosis to be established. A diagnosis of granulomatous prostatitis could be established only after histological examination of material obtained at prostatic biopsy.

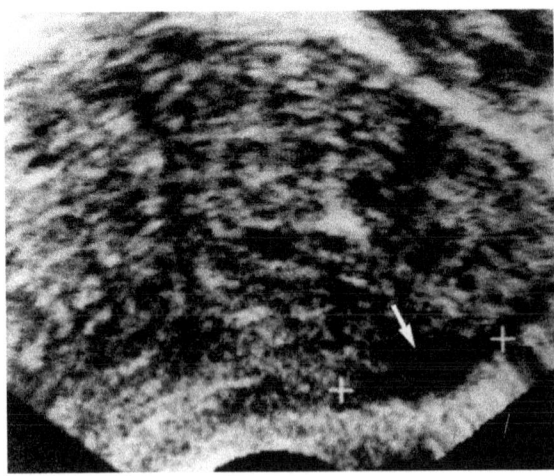

Fig. 15. Axial scan in a patient with granulomatous prostatitis. Note the echo-poor left peripheral zone (*arrow*)

Ultrasonic Appearances of Eosinophilic Prostatitis

There have been no specific reports of this condition in the ultrasonic literature. Liu et al. (1992) described three patients with eosinophilic prostatitis and referred incidentally to the TRUS findings in two of these. Both patients were reported to have hypoechoic areas in the peripheral zone. The serum level of prostate-specific antigen was considerably elevated in both patients who were considered clinically and sonographically to have prostatic cancer. No specific sonographic features of eosinophilic prostatitis were demonstrated, and, as with granulomatous prostatitis, biopsy was needed to establish the diagnosis.

Ultrasonic Appearance of Prostatic Abscess

There is considerable overlap in the clinical findings of acute prostatitis and prostatic abscess, and differentiation between the two entities may be difficult. Prostatic abscesses vary in size from microabscesses occurring in acute bacterial prostatitis to the infrequent large abscesses that need drainage. It is important to make the correct diagnosis of prostatic abscess so that drainage – whether surgical or ultrasound-guided – may be performed.

TRUS can usually be performed in patients with prostatic abscesses but may be difficult because of the markedly tender prostate. The prostate is usually

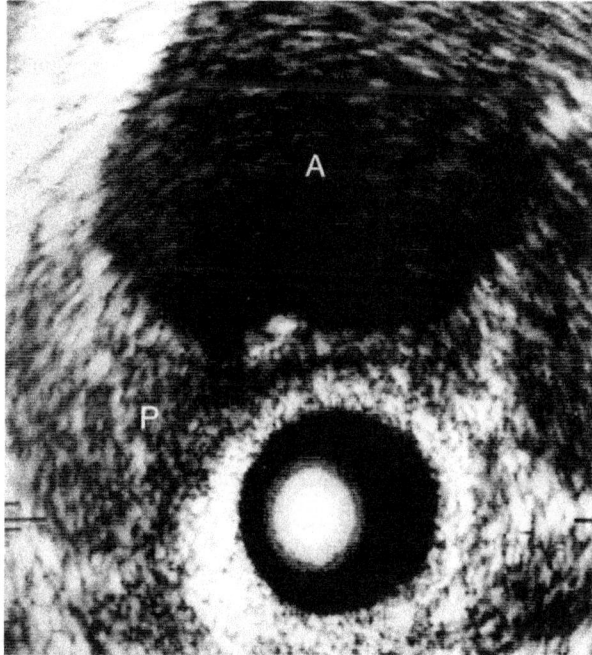

Fig. 16. Axial scan in a patient with a large abscess (A) within the prostate (P)

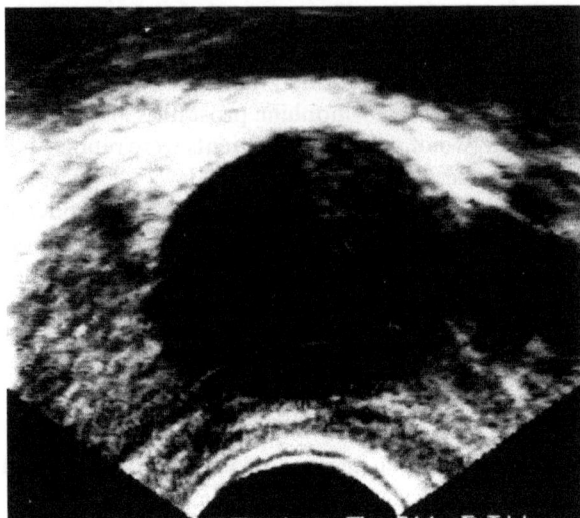

Fig. 17. Axial scan in a patient with a prostatic abscess. Note the fluid level within the abscess cavity. (Scan provided by Dr. R. Oyen, Universitaire Ziekenhuizen Leuven, Belgium)

enlarged, and the abscess cavity appears as a single or multiple localised echo-poor or echo-free area (Fig. 16). Usually some internal echoes are seen within the abscess cavity, and a fluid level may be demonstrated (Fig. 17). Acoustic enhancement may be seen. The abscess cavity is usually thick walled and may show septations. Multiple loculi may be present. The differential diagnosis of a large echo-free or echo-poor area within the prostate includes Müllerian duct cysts and seminal vesicle or ejaculatory cysts or abscesses.

Treatment of prostatic abscesses may be transurethral surgical drainage or percutaneous aspiration by the transperineal route. Both techniques may be employed successfully in a single large abscess cavity, but in complex multiloculated abscesses transurethral resection may not drain each cavity satisfactorily, and in such cases intraoperative sonography may be used to monitor whether all abscess cavities are adequately drained (Kinahan et al. 1991).

Other imaging techniques have little role in the demonstration and evaluation of prostatic inflammation, but computed tomography with intravenous contrast enhancement is able to demonstrate abscess cavities within the prostate (Thornhill et al. 1987). These may also be demonstrated by magnetic resonance imaging.

Ultrasound Appearances of Seminal Vesiculitis and Seminal Vesicle Abscesses

Seminal vesiculitis is a complication of chronic prostatitis and may either occur due to direct spread of infection from the prostate or be associated with ejaculatory duct obstruction. Along with other conditions of the seminal vesicles it is a condition that is difficult to diagnose by clinical criteria alone. The seminal vesicles can now be assessed ultrasonically in most patients undergoing a TRUS examination. Many sonographic abnormalities of the seminal vesicles appear to be non-specific and may be seen in asymptomatic men as well as in patients with chronic prostatitis and seminal vesiculitis. Specific abnormalities such as cysts or calculi may, however, be identified in the seminal vesicles and ejaculatory ducts as cause of perineal pain (Littrup et al. 1988), and these patients' symptoms might otherwise be ascribed to prostatodynia. Ultrasonic features of the seminal vesicles which have been assessed and considered by some authors to represent seminal vesiculitis include enlargement of the seminal vesicles, thickening of the septae, diffuse cystic change and increased echogenicity.

The ultrasonic features of the seminal vesicles in a group of patients with chronic NBP were assessed by Christiansen and Purvis (1991). Thirty-six men were examined, and TRUS and semen analyses were performed in each. Criteria taken as indicative of chronic inflammation of the seminal vesicles included seminal vesicle elongation and thickening of the internal septae. No clear association was noted in this series between symptom intensity and ultrasonic appearances. Because of the lack of specificity of the ultrasonic abnormalities that may be identified in the seminal vesicles, aspiration of the seminal vesicles under ultrasound guidance may be undertaken as a diagnostic procedure in patients with seminal vesiculitis. This technique has been described by Llerena and Letournean (1989). Under cover of a broad-spectrum antibiotic and using the transrectal route, a needle was inserted into the seminal vesicle. In many cases the authors found it was not easy to aspirate fluid from the seminal vesicles because of the thickness of the secretions, and in these circumstances they

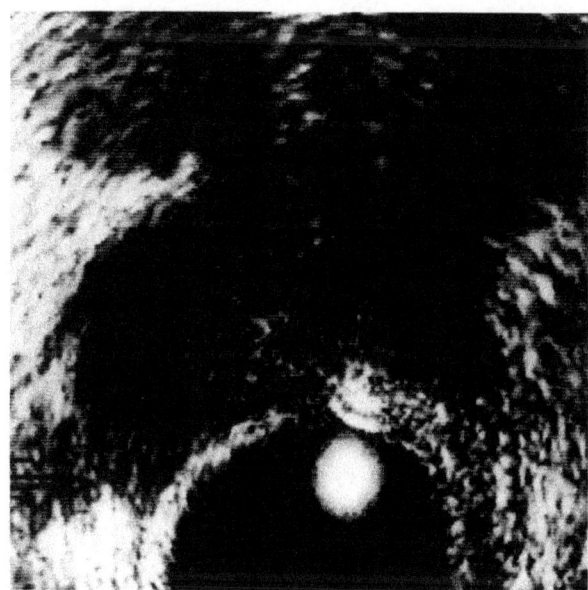

Fig. 18. Axial scan. A right seminal vesicle abscess is present

injected 1–2 ml sterile saline before attempting further aspiration. After obtaining the samples for diagnostic aspiration, each seminal vesicle was injected with 2 ml 1% lignocaine and 20–40 mg gentamicin. Temporary relief of symptoms was obtained in about 50% of patients with this procedure. A series of ultrasound-guided transperineal aspirations of the seminal vesicles was reported by Abe et al. (1989). In this series 98 patients were considered to have seminal vesiculitis on the basis of tenderness to palpation and sonographic seminal vesicle enlargement. The seminal vesicles were aspirated, and antibiotics and steroids were injected. Precise details of the treatments were not given, but clinical improvement was claimed in 61 of the 98 patients.

Seminal vesicle abscess formation may occur as a consequence of seminal vesiculitis. Seminal vesicle abscesses appear ultrasonically as thick-walled structures with a complex echo texture (Fig. 18). They may be treated successfully by aspiration under ultrasonic guidance.

Role of Transrectal Ultrasound in Clinical Management

The clinical diagnosis of prostatitis remains difficult as the history is often vague and may not be typical. Usually the diagnosis can be made by microscopy and bacteriology of divided urine samples and EPS. In these cases ultrasonography is merely a confirmatory investigation. However, some patients cannot comply with the instructions for these tests, and in some instances prostatic secretions cannot be obtained, so that bacterial confirmation is not possible. In this group ultrasonography may be critical in securing a diagnosis of prostatitis. An acute episode of prostatitis produces typical sonographic appearances which are seen consistently. Ultrasonography should still be performed in patients with confirmatory bacterial evidence of acute prostatitis to exclude the development of a prostatic abscess. TRUS is also playing an increasingly important role in the management of inflammatory prostatic disease. It is valuable in guiding precise positioning of the needle in prostatic biopsy and aspiration; the diagnosis of chronic granulomatous prostatitis can only be made histologically. TRUS is replacing surgery for aspiration of some cases of prostatic abscesses. It is still not possible to separate bacterial and non-bacterial prostatitis and prostatodynia on clinical grounds. The demonstration of a sonographically normal gland by a thorough TRUS examination of the prostate and seminal vesicles may be helpful in the management of an anxious patient with prostatodynia.

References

Abe M, Watanabe H, Kojima M, Saitoh M, Ohe H (1989) Puncture of the seminal vesicles guided by a transrectal real time linear scanner. JCU 17:173–178

Bude R, Bree RL, Adler RS, Zafar Jafri S (1990) Transrectal ultrasound appearance of granulomatous prostatitis. J Ultrasound Med 9:677–680

Christiansen E, Purvis K (1991) Diagnosis of chronic abacterial prostato-vesiculitis by rectal ultrasonography in relation to symptoms and findings. Br J Urol 67:173–176

Clements R, Griffiths GJ, Peeling WB, Edwards AM (1989) Transrectal ultrasound in monitoring response to treatment of prostate disease. Urol Clin North Am 16:735–740

Clements R, Griffiths GJ, Peeling WB, Ryan PG (1990) Experience with ultrasonically guided transperineal prostatic needle biopsy 1985–1988. Br J Urol 65:362–367

Clements R, Gower Thomas K, Griffiths GJ, Peeling WB (1993) Transrectal ultrasound appearances of granulomatous prostatitis. Clin Radiol 47:174–176

Di Trapani D, Pavone C, Serretta V, Cavallo N, Costa G, Pavone-Macaluso M (1988) Chronic prostatitis and prostatodynia: ultrasonographic alterations of the prostate, bladder neck, seminal vesicles and periprostatic venous plexus. Eur Urol 15:230–234

Doble A, Carter SSC (1989) Ultrasonographic findings in prostatitis. Urol Clin North Am 16:763–772

Eykyn S, Bultitude M, Mayo ME, Lloyd Davies RW (1974) Prostatic calculi as a source of recurrent bacteriuria in the male. Br J Urol 46:527–532

Fornage BD, Didier HT, Deglaire M, Faroux MJ, Simatos A (1983) Real-time ultrasound-guided prostatic biopsy using a new transrectal linear array probe. Radiology 146:547–548

Griffiths GJ, Crooks AJR, Roberts EE, Evans KT, Buck AC, Thomas PJ, Peeling WB (1984) Ultrasonic appearances associated with prostatic inflammation: a preliminary study. Clin Radiol 35:343–345

Griffiths GJ, Clements R, Jones DR, Roberts EE, Peeling WB, Evans KT (1987) The ultrasound appearances of prostatic cancer with histological correlation. Clin Radiol 38:219–227

Griffiths GJ, Clements R, Peeling WB (1990) Inflammatory disease and calculi. In: Resnick M (ed) Prostate ultrasonography. Decker, Philadelphia

Harada K, Tamahashi Y, Igani D, Numata I, Orikasa S (1980) Clinical evaluation of inside echo patterns in gray scale prostatic echography. J Urol 124:216–220

Holm HH, Gammelgaard J (1981) Ultrasonically guided precise needle placement in the prostate. J Urol 125:385–387

Jiminez-Cruz JF, Tormo FB, Gomez GJ (1988) Treatment of chronic prostatitis: intraprostatic antibiotic injections under echography control. J Urol 139:967–970

Kinahan TJ, Cooperberg PL, Goldenberg SL, English RA, Ajzen SA (1991) Transurethral resection of prostatic abscess under sonographic guidance. Urology 37:475–477

Klimas R, Bennett B, Gardner WA (1985) Prostatic calculi: a review. Prostate 7:91–96

Lee F, Gray JM, McLeary RD, Meadows TR, Kumasaka GH, Borlaza GS, Straub WH, Lee F Jr, Solomon MH, McHugh TA, Wolf RM (1985) Transrectal ultrasound in the diagnosis of prostatic cancer: location, echogenicity, histopathology, and staging. Prostate 7:117–129

Lees WR, Rickards D (1991) Color Doppler sonography of prostatic cancer. 77th Scientific Assembly and Annual Meeting of the Radiological Society of North America, Chicago

Littrup PJ, Lee F, McLeary RD, Wu D, Lee A, Kumasaka GH (1988) Transrectal US of the seminal vesicles and ejaculatory ducts: clinical correlation. Radiology 168:625–628

Littrup PJ, Williams CR, Egglin TK, Kane RA (1991) Determination of prostate volume with transrectal US for cancer screening II. Accuracy of in vitro and in vivo techniques. Radiology 179:49–52

Liu S, Miller PD, Holmes SAV, Christmas TJ, Kirby RS (1992) Eosinophilic prostatitis and prostatic specific antigen. Br J Urol 69:61–63

Llerena J, Letourneau JG (1989) Other prostatic interventions: seminal vesicles. Semin Intervent Radiol 6:102–107

McNeal JE (1981) The zonal anatomy of the prostate. Prostate 2:35–49

Myschetsky PS, Suburu RE, Kelly BS Jr, Wilson ML, Chen SC, Lee F (1991) Determination of prostate gland volume by transrectal ultrasound. Scand J Urol Nephrol Suppl 137:107–111

Rifkin MD, Alexander AA, Helinek TG, Merton DA (1991) Color Doppler as an adjunct to prostate ultrasound. Scand J Urol Nephrol Suppl 137:85–89

Stamey (1981) Prostatitis. J R Soc Med 74:22

Terris MK, Stamey TA (1991) Determination of prostate volume by transrectal ultrasound. J Urol 145:984–987

Thornhill BA, Morehouse HT, Coleman P, Hoffman-Tretin HC (1987) Prostatic abscess: C.T. and sonographic findings. AJR 148:899–900

Torp-Pedersen ST, Lee F (1989) Transrectal biopsy of the prostate guided by transrectal ultrasound. Urol Clin North Am 16:703–712

Villers A, Terris M, McNeal JE, Stamey T (1990) Ultrasound anatomy of the prostate: the normal gland and anatomical variations. J Urol 143:732–738

Watanabe H (1991) Transrectal sonography: a personal review and recent advances. Scand J Urol Nephrol Suppl 137:75–83

Wiegand S, Weidner W (1986) Per rectal ultrasonography of the prostate in the diagnosis of chronic prostatitis and prostatodynia. In: Therapy of Prostatitis. Zuckschwerdt, Munich, pp 177–180

Prostatitis and Male Infertility

W. Krause

Prostatitis and Parameters of Seminal Plasma, Nonsperm Cells, and Bacteria

Compounds of Seminal Plasma

As the prostate gland produces some 30% of the seminal fluid which is ejaculated (Fig. 1), it is obvious that changes in the secretory capacity of this gland due to inflammations will lead to changes in the contents of the seminal fluid. Several authors have reported on changes in the seminal plasma in relation to prostatitis. It is not proven, however, that contents of the seminal fluid besides the spermatozoa themselves are involved in the process of fertilization. This chapter discusses the changes in seminal fluid in relation to prostatitis reported in the literature and their possible role in male infertility.

Specific secretory products of the prostate in semen are citric acid, zinc, prostatic acid phosphatase, and prostate-specific antigen. The concentration of these compounds in semen is thought to be a marker for prostatic function (Table 1).

When Cooper et al. (1990) performed a biochemical analysis of specific accessory gland products in the ejaculates of 362 men suffering from various acute inflammatory diseases of the reproductive tract and 33 normozoospermic patients acting as controls, they found the concentration of citric acid to be reduced in those with prostatitis. The ejaculate content of the epididymal markers alpha-glucosidase and L-carnitine, but not glycerophosphocholine, was significantly reduced in ejaculates from men with epididymitis to about 50% and 70%, respectively. Both citric acid and alpha-glucosidase were reduced in men suffering from adnexitis, where the exact localization of the inflammation was unclear. An influence of the inflammation on seminal vesicle function, as judged from semen volumes and seminal fructose, was not obvious in these groups of patients. The results were unrelated to the microbiological flora of the semen (Fig. 2).

Grizard et al. (1985) confirmed that it is not possible with the biochemical markers used to show with any certainty a functional alteration of accessory glands in infertile men with genital tract infection. The authors assayed citric acid, acid phosphatase, and fructose in relation to sperm parameters and

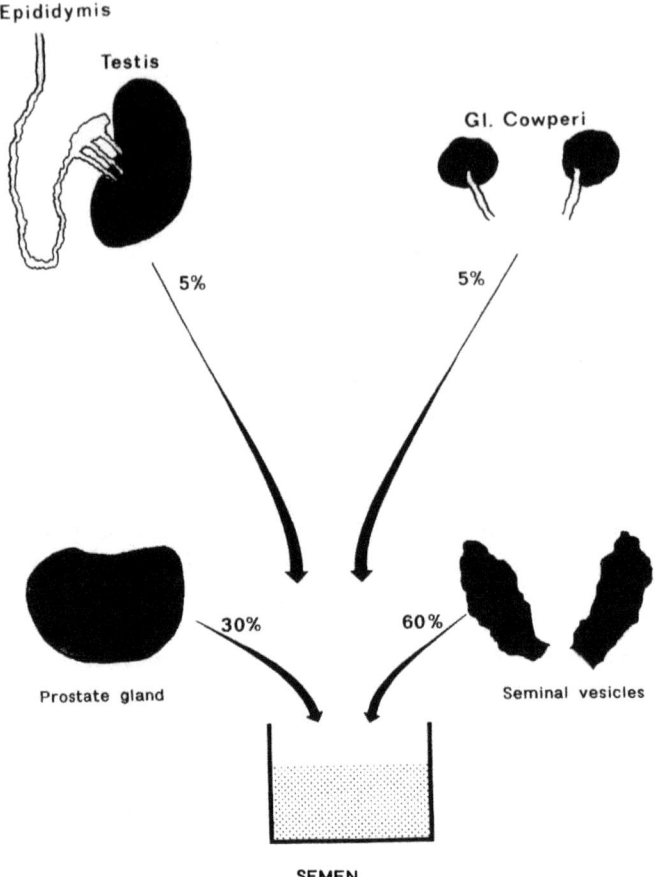

Fig. 1. Schematic representation of the components of seminal fluid

quantitative culture in three groups of men: fertile controls (donors of an insemination program) without significant bacteriospermia (group I), infertile men with significant bacteriospermia; idiopathic infertile men (group II); and infertile men with varicocele (group III). The level of significance of bacteriospermia was greater than or equal to 10^4 germs/ml ejaculate. Fructose was unaltered in the two groups of infected men. No modification of prostatic markers was observed in any groups, except in group II, where they decreased when bacteriospermia was lower than 10^5 germs/ml, and when the biological pattern of semen evoked chronic prostatitis. In men with idiopathic infertility, when bacteriospermia was higher than 10^5 germs/ml, germs were nearly always pathogenic (96%), and prostatic markers were unaltered.

The concentrations of fructose, citric acid, and zinc concentration in semen are not only useless for characterization of inflammatory intensity of prostatitis

Table 1. Specific secretory compounds of human semen

Accessory organ	Compound	Organ specificity	Inflammation specificity
Prostate	Prostatic acid phosphatase, prostate-specific antigen, zinc, citric acid	Low	Low
Seminal vesicle	Fructose	High	Absent
Epididymis	Glucosidase, carnitine, γ-glutamyl-transferase	Low	Moderate

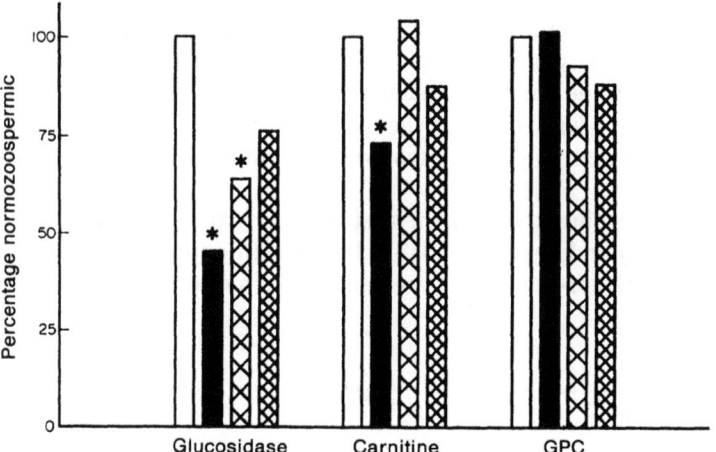

Fig. 2. Differential susceptibility of the seminal secretion of epididymal markers to inflammatory conditions. The semen content of glucosidase, carnitine, and glycerophosphocholine (*GPC*) expressed as a percentage of that in semen from normozoospermic patients in epididymitis (■), adnexitis (⊠), and prostatitis (▨). *$p < 0.05$ versus normozoospermic controls (□). (From Cooper et al. 1990)

but are also not suitable to describe therapeutic effects. Rigatti et al. (1990) studied 14 young and sexually active patients with chronic abacterial prostatitis who underwent four 60-min sessions of local prostatic hyperthermia. Biochemical patterns of seminal plasma were not significantly altered by thermotherapy, and the authors suggested preservation of the reproductive potential of these patients.

Some contradictory results are found in the study of Comhaire et al. (1989), who performed biochemical examination on semen samples from 42 infertile patients with more than 10 000 aerobic pathogens per millilitre of semen as well as 42 infertile men without signs or symptoms of infection and whose semen cultures were sterile. The authors found seminal volume to be lower and pH higher in infected than in noninfected men. The concentration of the acid phosphatase and gamma-glutamyltransferase as well as that of citric acid and fructose decreased in infected patients. When the power of the markers was evaluated for their ability to discriminate between semen of infected and noninfected infertile men by the aid of receiver-operating characteristic curves and accuracy tests, the total output of citric acid had the strongest discriminating power, followed by acid phosphatase and gamma-glutamyltransferase (Fig. 3). Measurement of the concentration of fructose was found to be non-discriminatory. Thus the method of determination (concentration versus total output) seems to influence the significance of the compound concerned.

The value of gamma-glutamyltranspeptidase (GGT) in seminal plasma as a marker of inflammation was examined in another study by the same authors (Delanghe et al. 1985). This enzyme expresses a certain heterogeneity. When the parameter was then related to the fructose concentration, acid phosphatase activity, ejaculate volume, sperm density, and number of bacteria per milliliter, multivariate regression analysis and stepwise elimination of the least fitting factors revealed that with the number of bacteria per milliliter of semen and the acid phosphatase activity with 49% of the variance of GGT-binding being explained. This result suggests that glycosylation of seminal GGT is altered by accessory gland infection.

Some studies concerning the protein distribution pattern in semen in relation to inflammatory findings are available. Disk electrophoresis of prostatic secretion proteins in polyacrylamide gel was employed in examinations of 294

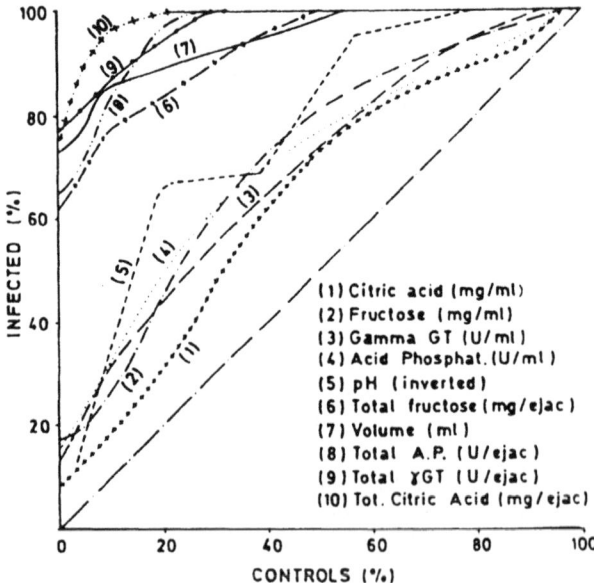

Fig. 3. Receiver-operating characteristic curves of physical and biochemical markers of semen of infected compared with noninfected fertile men. The maximal sensitivity is given by total citric acid. (From Comhaire et al. 1989)

normal subjects and sterile patients with oligo- and asthenospermia in the presence of and without chronic prostatitis by Mikhailichenko et al. (1989). Analysis of the electrophoretic picture, the microscopic examinations of prostatic secretion, and the ejaculate revealed that the progress of the inflammatory process in the prostate was associated with a drastic decrease in the concentrations of prostatic secretion proteins with a high molecular mass and an increased level of low molecular mass proteins. The authors noted that a specific electrophoretic picture is characteristic for prostatodynia, thus helping to differentiate this condition from prostatic inflammations.

Semen patterns of plasma proteins as analyzed by SDS-PAGE were found to be altered (increase in albumin concentration, decrease in prostatic markers and other anomalies) parallel to leukospermia (Colpi et al. 1988).

Seminal zinc concentration is also thought to be a specific prostatic parameter. It does not correlate with the sperm count (Krause 1991; Fig. 4). Canale et al. (1986) measured it in normospermic and infertile patients. High levels of zinc were found in semen from five patients with bilateral agenesis of the vas deferens (mean value 1411.2 μg/ml). Patients with acquired obstruction had lower levels (695.2 μg/ml). The seminal zinc level in six patients who had had a vasectomy, or who had an epididymal blockage (125.7 μg/ml) was approximately the same as in 41 controls (134.6 ± 42). The authors concluded from these values that evaluation of zinc permits merely the diagnosis of patency of the seminal pathways but does not permit identification of prostatitis.

When observing the secretion of electrolytes, the ionic composition of human prostatic fluid varies greatly among individuals, reflecting the secretory activity of the gland and the presence or absence of prostatic inflammatory disease. In normal prostatic fluid the major anion is citrate, while chloride

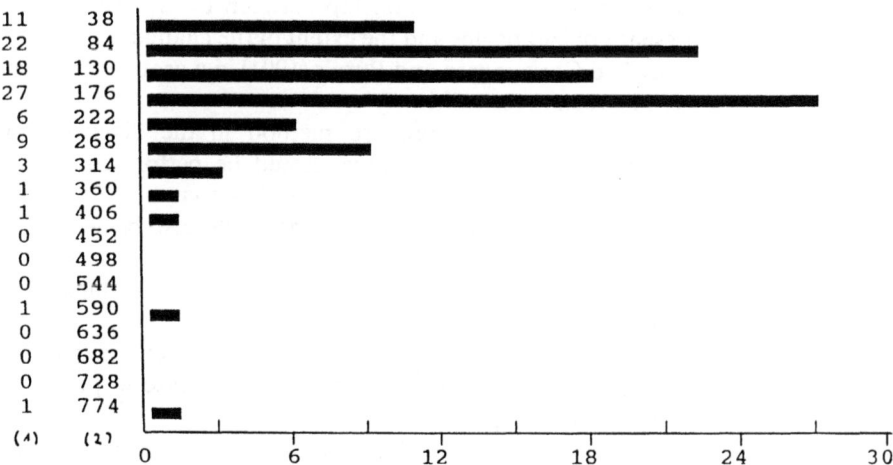

Fig. 4. Histogram of zinc concentrations in semen of randomly selected infertile men. *1*, Number of observations in each class; *2*, lower limit of classes. (From Krause 1991)

concentration is lower. Their counterions are mainly sodium and potassium, together with calcium, magnesium, and zinc (Kavanagh 1985). The author found the electrolytes to be closely correlated to each other (except for sodium, which was essentially invariant at about 145 nm). The molar changes per mole of citrate were about 0.52, potassium; -0.53, chloride; 0.17, calcium; 0.14, magnesium; and 0.09, zinc. The pH was also associated with citrate, decreasing from 8.0 to 6.2 as the citrate increased. These various ionic changes could be explained as responses to citrate secretion, without the need to propose specific transport mechanisms for the other ions measured. The marked effect of prostatic inflammation on the composition of prostatic fluid could be seen as being due mainly to decreased secretion rather than active modification.

An approach to directly measure products of inflammatory processes in addition to proteins was published by Freixia et al. (1988). These authors estimated prostaglandins of the E series (19-OH PGEs) in the seminal plasma of asthenozoospermic patients ($n = 15$) and individuals affected by prostatitis ($n = 10$) and compared to controls ($n = 13$) and secretory azoospermic patients ($n = 8$). All of them were free from infections (except individuals affected by prostatitis) or biochemical and ultrastructural problems. The results indicate that endogenous prostaglandin levels (19-OH PGEs and PGEs) bear no correlation either to motility or absence of spermatozoa. Significant increases of PGEs, however, were observed in patients with prostatitis.

Leukocytes and Erythrocytes

An important parameter of accessory gland inflammation is the presence of leukocytes in semen. A clear difference between the cell count in normal controls or patients with prostatitis is demonstrable (Fig. 5; Krause and Weidner 1983). However, there is not always a clear relationship between the severity of the symptoms or the presence of leukocytes and the extent of the changes visualized by ultrasound, as described Christiansen and Purvis (1991) in a group of 36 men with chronic abacterial prostatovesiculitis.

Ultrasonographic evaluation is a standard method in the diagnosis of prostatitis. This noninvasive imaging technique should be performed before resorting to other methods that involve manipulation (Boronat et al. 1990).

The presence of macrophages in semen (Haidl 1990) might also be helpful in diagnosing chronic unspecific genital infection and in differentiating chronic epididymal inflammation from chronic prostatitis, whereas the influence of bacteria on their presence is still controversial.

Leukospermia was significantly coupled to alterations of the seminal plasma protein composition (increase in albumin concentration, decrease in prostatic markers and other anomalies; Colpi et al. 1988).

Instead of counting leukocytes it is possible to measure the concentration of leukocyte elastase. Elastase levels over 1000 ng/ml were obtained in 14 men and positive bacterial culture in 11 men, but there was no correlation between these

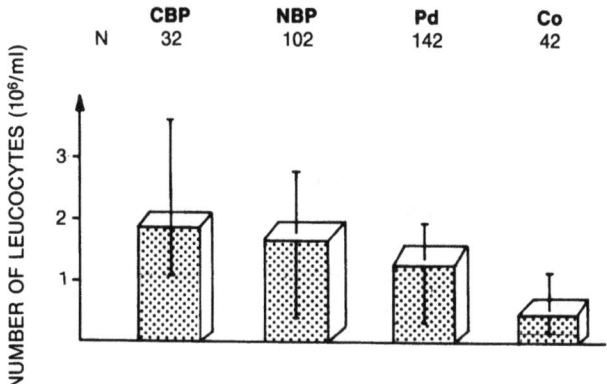

Fig. 5. Leukocyte count in semen in groups of men with different prostatic conditions. *CBP*, Chronic bacterial prostatitis; *NBP*, nonbacterial prostatitis; *Pd*, prostatodynia; *Co*, healthy control persons. (From Weidner et al. 1991a)

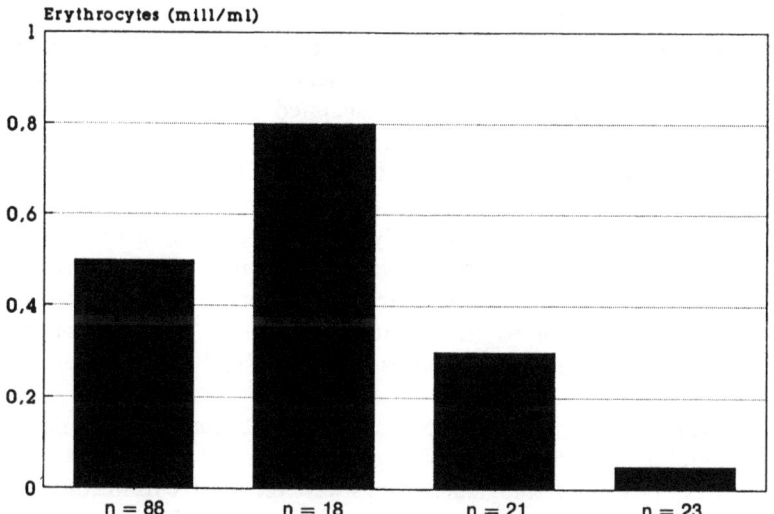

Fig. 6. Erythrocytes in seminal fluid in men with different prostatic conditions. *1*, Prostatitis without proven bacteria; *2*, bacterial prostatitis; *3*, prostatodynia; *4*, normal control persons

two sets of measurements (Cummings et al. 1990). While granulocyte elastase measurement in semen may reflect inflammation, the study suggests that it cannot be used as a simple marker of infection, particularly in a population where the prevalence of prostatitis and genital infection is low.

The admixture of erythrocytes to semen, called hemospermia, is often regarded as a sign of urogenital infection. Following routine diagnostic procedures in 72 patients this finding was ruled out in 50% of the patients examined; in 26 men chronic prostatitis was diagnosed. Additional investigation of the prostate gland and seminal vesicles by transrectal prostatic ultrasonography revealed persistent asymmetry of the latter glands as the main finding in 20 men (28%; Fig. 6; Weidner et al. 1991b).

These data were confirmed by Etherington et al. (1990), who examined the transrectal ultrasound findings in 52 patients with hemospermia. Scan abnormalities were demonstrated in 43 patients (83%). No patient was proven to have prostatic malignancy. Transrectal ultrasonography can suggest a cause of hemospermia in the majority of patients without resort to invasive investigations, and can exclude underlying prostatic malignancy. It is recommended as the first investigation in patients presenting with hemospermia.

Microbiological Agents

Ureaplasma urealyticum is considered an etiological agent in urogenital tract infections, especially prostatitis. Using the four-specimen technique, diagnosis can be based upon significant numbers of these micro-organisms. In ejaculate the critical number seems to be 10^3 cfu/ml semen to discriminate between real infection and contamination during urethral passage. In the study of Weidner et al. (1985) 46 of 412 samples (11.2%) exceeded this critical number. Most but not all patients suffering from *Ureaplasma*-associated prostatitis established by the four-specimen technique revealed significantly high ejaculate numbers, whereas all samples from patients with prostatodynia and healthy controls had lower numbers. In these cases numbers of round cells in semen, which include all leukocytes and spermatides, were significantly increased compared to prostatodynia. A significantly negative correlation was detected between the numbers of *Ureaplasma* organisms and zinc concentration in semen, and an almost identically negative correlation to the content of fructose, thus indicating secretory dysfunction of the accessory glands in ureaplasmal infections of the prostate.

It is also present in those inflammations caused by *Chlamydia trachomatis* and *Mycoplasma* (abacterial prostatitis). No pathogens at all were recordable from 31 patients. No positive cytological findings were recordable from controls (Schmidt et al. 1987, 1989).

However, one should be careful with the classification of bacteria in semen. The seminal fluid is more susceptible to contamination from urethral bacteria than the urine. This might be in part a reason for positive culture in semen of high germ numbers, suggesting a prostatic infection (Fowler and Ariano 1983).

The pattern of pathogenic bacteria in seminal alterations seems to be well characterized by the studies cited. Fowler and Ariano (1984) measured immunoglobulin A in male genital secretions with specificity for *Escherichia coli*. This was demonstrable both in seminal fluid and expressed prostatic secretions of patients with chronic bacterial prostatitis but not in fertile control patients or men from infertile marriage. This result suggests that no relation of infections with *E. coli* to male infertility exists.

Antimicrobial Drugs

The seminal fluid may also be a useful tool for demonstrating the pharma-codynamic effects of drugs used for treatment of prostatitis. For example, the study of Yasumoto and Asakawa (1988) shall be cited, in which 10 patients with prostatitis received enoxacin (ENX), and the changes in its concentration were compared, the mean ENX concentration was 3.65 $\mu g/ml$ in the group receiving 600 mg ENX and 2.60 $\mu g/ml$ in those receiving 400 mg ENX (not significantly different). When ENX was administered for 7 days, the mean ENX concentration was 3.13 $\mu g/ml$, but when it was administered for 14 days, it was 3.46 $\mu g/ml$. The concentration of ENX in the seminal fluid was higher than the minimum inhibitory concentration for the pathogens of prostatitis in every group.

Prostatitis and Sperm Parameters

Oligoasthenozoospermia is a symptom which is often thought to be connected with chronic bacterial prostatitis. In the patients reported on by Giamarellou et al. (1984), where *E. coli* and *Staphylococcus* were most commonly isolated, about 50% of the patients had symptoms and 66.7% had clinical findings; 66.5% of them had a decrease in sperm parameters.

Omer (1985) investigated 59 subfertile males to assess seminal quality, inflammatory conditions, and spermatogenic picture in relation to their sub-fertility. Defects in semen analysis were found associated with an old gonococcal infection (42.4%), schistosomiasis, (13.6%) and chronic prostatitis (5.1%).

Also, Stanislavov et al. (1990) stressed the presence of oligoasthenoterato-zoospermia in men with chronic prostatitis. In 20 cases there was a reduction in the number of spermatozoa up to $39 \times 10^6/ml$ combined with lower motility and an increased percentage of teratoforms.

Number, motility, and morphology of spermatozoa were normal in 5 patients and abnormal in 9 of 14 young and sexually active patients with chronic abacterial prostatitis in the study of Rigatti et al. (1990), who performed pretherapeutic semen analysis in patients undergoing local prostatic hyper-thermia.

The study of Grizard et al. (1985), which was cited above, reported on sperm examination, quantitative sperm culture, citric acid, acid phosphatase, and fructose assayed in three groups of men: fertile controls without significant bacteriospermia (group I), infertile men with significant bacteriospermia; idio-pathic infertile men (group II), and infertile men with varicocele (group III). In group II, motility and typical morphology percentages were lower, indepen-dently of the degree and the nature of bacteriospermia. The incidence of pathogenic bacteria was higher than in group III and linked to the degree of bacteriospermia. Thus, in the opinion of the authors, the presence of germs in ejaculate altered the motility and the typical morphology percentages of sperm.

The semen analysis of 82 patients who had signs of a chronic nonspecific genital infection showed abnormally stained flagella detected by the Shorr technique. This may be a sign of male adnexitis and might be helpful in differentiating chronic epididymal inflammation from chronic prostatitis (Haidl 1990).

A significant influence of leukocytes on sperm parameters is described by Satoh et al. (1990). Among 670 infertile men 72 were diagnosed with pyospermia by the criterion of white blood cell count (WBC) greater than or equal to 10 per high-power field (hpf) of semen. The sperm motile efficiency index, which indicates the rate of progressively motile sperm, was significantly lower in pyospermic group compared with that of nonpyospermic men (WBC less than 5/hpf semen). The mean value of granulocyte elastase in the pyospermic group was 2859.6 μg/l whereas that of nonpyospermic men was 131.6 μg/l. The authors suggested that granulocyte elastase in seminal plasma may be a cause of inhibition of sperm motility in pyospermic state.

On the other hand, Colpi et al. (1988) found conventional semen parameters not to be affected by a leukospermia itself in patients with prostatic inflammation. The seminal volume could represent an exception to this rule. However, leukospermia did significantly affect sperm viability as evaluated by the capillary tube penetration test. This is one of the first reports on possible disturbances of sperm function which does not express itself in conventional sperm parameters.

As already mentioned, zinc is secreted mainly by the prostate while vesicular, epididymal, and testicular secretions are devoid of zinc. The zinc concentration in the study of Canale et al. (1986) did not permit identification of prostatitis but only the diagnosis of patency of the seminal pathways. No correlation was found between sperm count or motility and the seminal zinc level.

A direct test of sperm viability in prostatitis was introduced by D'Agata et al. (1990) by measuring the capacity to generate reactive oxygen species (ROS), both basally and after stimulation with the calcium ionophore A23187. The authors used only the motile fraction of sperm isolated after swim-up from the semen of ten naturally fertile men and two groups of infertile patients. The latter included men with a nonbacterial inflammation of the genital tract ($n = 10$) and men unable to impregnate their partners during an intrauterine insemination programme ($n = 8$). The levels of ROS production were elevated in the sperm of some infertile men with inflammation of the genital tract compared to those found in the ten naturally fertile men. These data suggest that an excessive production of ROS by sperm may explain some cases of idiopathic male infertility.

A peculiar influence of inflammation of accessory glands on sperm function appears to be the formation of sperm autoantibodies. Witkin and Toth (1983) detected sperm antibodies in significantly more men with either culture-positive infections or a history of urethritis or prostatitis than in healthy men. The sperm antibodies belonged mostly to the IgA class. Significantly more men without sperm antibodies were fertile than those with sperm antibodies.

In a following study, Witkin and Zelikovsky (1986) evaluated 16 men immunologically with chronic prostatitis and suggested that decreased cellular immunity and enhanced humoral reactivity to sperm are common in men with chronic prostatitis. Peripheral blood mononuclear cells from 14 of 16 (88%) patients exhibited reduced or absent responses in vitro when incubated with an extract of *Candida albicans*. Sperm antibodies, evaluated by an enzyme-linked immunosorbent assay using fresh motile, homogenized spermatozoa as antigens, were found in 9 of 16 (56%) patients. Levels of IgG sperm antibodies were correlated with the degree of immunosuppression by patient sera ($p < 0.02$; Table 2).

Jarow et al. (1990) pointed to the simplicity of tests for sperm antibodies and their inexpensiveness. They noted that nonbacterial prostatitis is a risk factor for the presence of serum antisperm antibodies. They proposed performing a test for sperm antibodies in every male partner of an infertile marriage, since – in their view – studies have demonstrated a higher prevalence of antisperm antibodies among men with a history of bacterial prostatitis or urethritis. When they measured serum antisperm antibodies, using a gel agglutination assay in 28 men with chronic nonbacterial prostatitis and in age-matched control group of 69 men without a history of prostatitis, the prevalence was 25% in the test subjects and 7.2% in the healthy controls ($p < 0.05$).

In conclusion, there is no consistent evidence for an influence of prostatitis on sperm parameters except the increasing occurrence of sperm antibodies. Below we discuss whether these effects also influence male fertility.

Table 2. Antibodies to spermatozoa in men with prostatitis: patient serum/control serum (from Witkin and Toth 1983)

Patient no.	IgG	IgA	IgM
1	0.7	0.8	0.8
2	1.7*	3.8*	0.9
3	1.4	1.0	1.2
4	2.5*	3.0*	2.3*
5	1.9*	1.7*	2.9*
6	0.6	0.6	0.6
7	1.8*	0.7	0.8
8	1.4	0.6	0.6
9	1.2	1.1	0.7
10	1.2	0.6	1.0
11	1.8*	1.9*	1.0
12	2.1*	1.1	0.6
13	1.3	1.4	0.6
14	1.8*	1.3	1.1
15	1.8*	1.1	0.7
16	2.6*	1.2	1.1

*, Values at least 50% above control.

Prostatitis and Sperm Fertilization Capacity

As we know from several statistical trials, the sperm parameters which are obtained with the routine spermiogram, i.e., sperm count, motility, and morphology, are of only little value in the prediction of male fertility. The correlation of these data with the time to conception as a measure of fertility potential is poor (Fig. 7; Holland-Moritz and Krause 1992).

Most authors, however, do not consider the difference between sperm parameters and fertility and use the term infertility when they merely mean poor semen quality. Studies using the term fertility only when it is proven by statistically analyzing the conceptions are very rare. This problem must be borne in mind when considering the studies discussed in this section.

The pathophysiological mechanisms by which infection can reduce fertility in men are poorly understood. It appears not to be related to alterations in the accessory glands, even when these are demonstrated in infertile patients. In a group of 36 men examined for the diagnosis of chronic prostatovesiculitis Grizard et al. (1985) found five of them to be symptom free. They were examined firstly as part of an infertility investigation by semen analysis. While patients with prostatitis reported discomfort or pain in connection with ejaculation, the infertile patients did not claim sensations. In these patients, however, clear sonographic evidence was obtained of major inflammatory changes in both the prostate and the seminal vesicle.

The usefulness of transrectal ultrasonography is described also by Gattuccio et al. (1988). When objective clinical findings are poor or absent (such in prostatosis and prostatodynia), transrectal ultrasonography demonstrates characteristic pictures useful for diagnosis and follow-up. The urogenital inflammations may be considered as "apparatus pathology." The analysis of only inflammatory diseases of the prostate gland did not give evidence for inflammatory alterations of the rest of male genital apparatus. This inflammation did not represent the only cause of infertility, but frequently reduced the probability of male fertility.

Other evidence for the role of prostatitis in infertility is derived from the determination of IgE level in serum and semen of 92 men (Ekladios et al. 1988). Most of them (92.3%) had this in much smaller amount than that present in serum. IgE levels in serum and semen were significantly correlated to each other. Serum levels were significantly higher in men with obstructive azoospermia, especially when associated with infection. Serum levels of IgE were higher in the fertile men and in cases without infection compared with those with prostatitis although this difference was not significant.

Stanislavov et al. (1990) suggested that increased permeability of barriers of blood serum proteins might participate in the pathogenesis of the disturbed fertility. It seemed that the cause of sterility in the married couples was due to autoimmune process occurring in men with chronic nonspecific prostatitis.

IgA with specificity for antigen in the mix of common *E. coli* O-serotypes could not be detected in the seminal fluid of the fertile men or the men of infertile

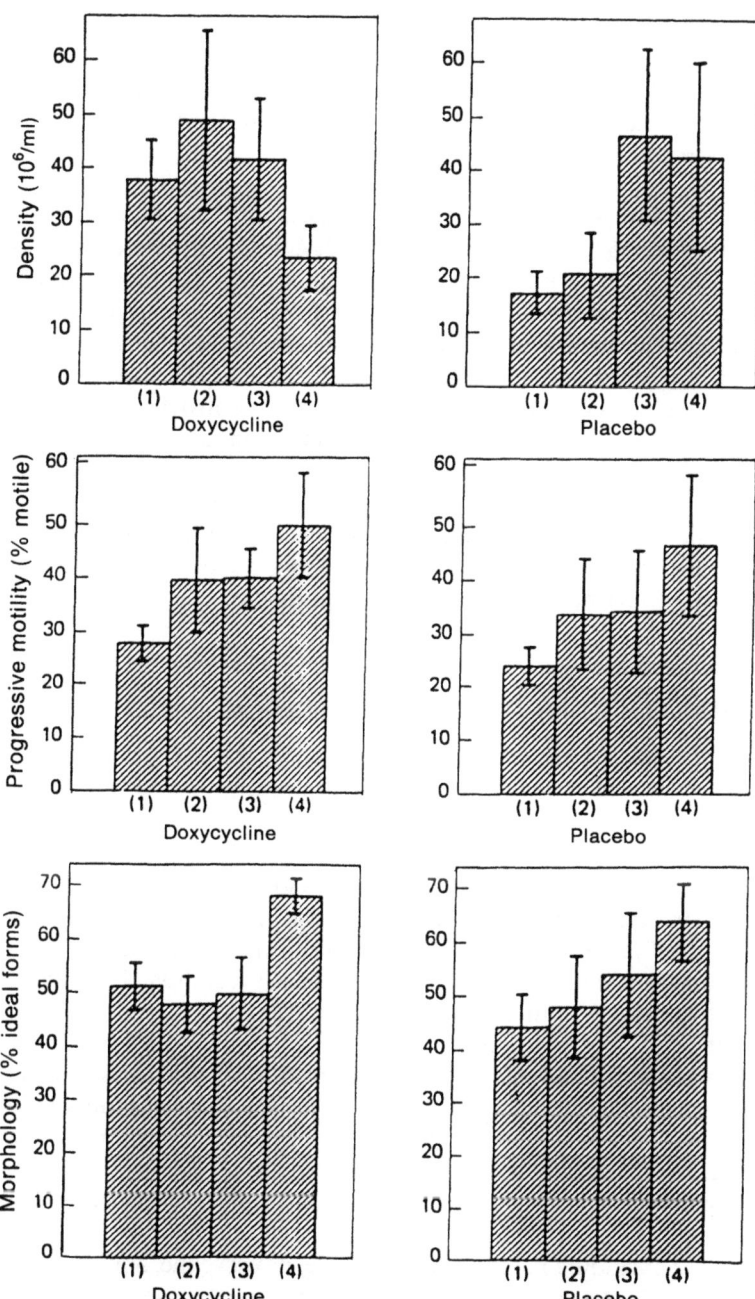

Fig. 7. Mean values for sperm density (million/ml), motility (% progressively motile sperm), and morphology (% sperm with ideal forms) in doxycycline- and placebo-treated couples. *1*, Mean value of the two semen analyses performed before initiation of treatment; *2*, value immediately after completion of treatment; *3*, value 2 months after completion of treatment; *4*, value 6 months after completion of treatment. (From Comhaire et al. 1986)

marriages. These data suggest that subclinical infection with *E. coli* are not commonly associated with infertility (Jimenez-Cruz et al. 1984).

The sperm antibodies described by Witkin and Toth (1983) belonged mostly to the IgA class. Significantly more men without sperm antibodies were fertile than those with sperm antibodies.

Suominen et al. (1983) studied 71 infertile men for the presence of seminal leukocytosis and for IgA antibodies against *C. trachomatis*. The findings were compared with those of 56 fertile men. Chlamydial IgA antibodies were found in the semen of 51.1% of infertile men with seminal leukocytosis, i.e., those defined as having asymptomatic chronic prostatitis. This frequency was significantly higher than among fertile men. The authors concluded that *C. trachomatis* might interfere with male fertility.

The role of *Ureaplasma* in male infertility is discussed controversially. Some studies describe a higher incidence of *Ureaplasma* in the genital tract of infertile couples, while others deny it. *Ureaplasma* organisms bind to human spermatozoa, and some authors have speculated on their role in abnormalities of motility and morphology of spermatozoa, thus influencing fertility. The study of Hofmann (1987) did not detect a relation of *Ureaplasma* in semen and the penetration ability of spermatozoa through cervical mucus.

Does Treatment of Prostatitis Mean Treatment of Infertility?

Antibiotics

Treatment of bacterial prostatitis (acute and chronic forms) may use antibiotic drugs which must be tested for inhibitory effects in the individual patient. Since concentration of ENX in the seminal fluid has been shown to be higher than the minimum inhibitory concentration for the pathogens of prostatitis, this may be a clinically effective drug (Yasumoto and Asakawa 1988).

Long-term treatment of chronic prostatitis with antimicrobials and their influence on semen quality and infertility were studied in 30 men (mean age of 36.7 ± 6 years) by Giamarellou et al. (1984). The infection was symptomatic in only 50% of the patients, with abnormal prostatic physical findings in 66.7%. Cardinal findings in the spermatogram were leukocytosis in 100% and oligoasthenozoospermia in 66.5% of the patients. *E. coli* and *Staphylococcus* presented the most commonly isolated bacteria in prostatic secretion cultures. Various treatment schedules, including mostly cotrimoxazole, doxycycline, and erythromycin, were given alternatively for 6–8 months. Symptoms were cured or improved in 79.7%, with elimination or improvement of abnormal physical findings in 85%, while the isolated pathogens were eradicated in all.

Consecutive treatment with doxycycline, sulfamethoxazole, and cephalexin in men with chronic prostatitis cured the subjective symptoms in 60% of the patients, and in 50% the cytological findings of the seminal parameters became normal with respect to the motility and viability of spermatozoa (Milingos et al. 1983).

In a controlled study Giorgi et al. (1989) tested the therapeutic efficacy of the second-generation quinolone ENX in patients suffering from vesicular and/or prostatic inflammations. This drug has been shown to diffuse into the prostatic fluid, achieving therapeutic concentrations either in acute or chronic pathological conditions. Thirty infertile patients referred to the Andrology Center and showing seminal signs (leukocytes, abnormal sperm forms, chemical and physical alterations, etc.) of genital tract inflammations were found to have positive sperm culture for ENX-sensitive strains. Further investigations (echotomography) showed that they were affected by prostatic and/or vesicular subacute chronic inflammations. The mean age was 32.2 years (range 20–36). The patients discontinued any previous treatment for at least 90 days. ENX was administered at a dose of 300 mg twice daily for two cycles of 10 days each, with intervals of 20 days. At the beginning and at the end of the treatment (days 0 and 60), semen analysis and culture were performed. A paired t test was employed for the statistical evaluation of data. While 26.6% of patients had an altered fluid-ification before treatment, only 10.0% of them showed this sign after treatment. A condition of hyperviscosity was present in 50% and 16.6% of patients before and after treatment, respectively. Likewise, an elevated number of leukocytes (greater than 10^6/ml) occurred in the ejaculates of 43.3% of patients and in 23.3% after ENX treatment. ENX treatment was efficacious in 89.2% of cases in the presence of either gram-positive or gram-negative bacteria.

Comhaire et al. (1986) disagreed with the suggestion that male accessory gland infection (MAGI, epididymo-prostato-vesiculitis) with abnormal semen quality is a common cause of male infertility. They presented a double-blind study of the effectiveness treating prostatitis in infertility, which is still unique. They found inflammation to be rarely the only semen abnormality in infertile couples since it occurred in no more than 1.6% of 2871 couples evaluated in seven centers over a 3-year period. Both partners of 33 infertile couples with no other demonstrable abnormality than abnormal semen and MAGI consented to participate in a double-blind trial and were treated with either doxycycline, 100 mg/day for 1 month (20 couples) or placebo (13 couples; Fig. 8). Follow-up during a total of 175 couple-months included semen analysis and the recording of pregnancy. Pregnancy occurred in two of the doxycycline-treated couples (10%) and in one of the placebo-treated couples (8%), corresponding with conception rates per month of 1.9% and 1.5%, respectively. Sperm motility and, to a lesser extent, morphology showed improvement in both groups. Evidence of infection, namely increased numbers of WBC and positive sperm culture, disappeared in both the doxycycline-treated and placebo groups. It is concluded that features of MAGI in semen may regress spontaneously and are not influenced by the doxycycline treatment. The concomitant improvement of sperm motility and morphology still does not seem to enhance the probability of conception.

In the study by Giamarellou et al. (1984), described above, spermatograms were normalized or improved in 70% of the patients, while among them nine impregnated their wives and two of them did so twice. The authors concluded that male infertility in the presence of semen leukocytosis and oligoasthenozoospermia should be investigated for underlying chronic prostatitis, while whenever proven, long-term treatment with the proper antimicrobials not only cures or improves chronic prostatitis but subsequently cures or improves male infertility.

Local treatment with antibiotic drugs was studied by Fahim et al. (1985). Seventy infertile men with chronic prostatitis were treated by prostatic massage and broad-spectrum chemotherapy as basic treatment to which intraprostatic injection of zinc or vitamin C with or without ultrasound application was added as a new line of treatment. Comparison showed no significant improvement of the additive treatment over the conventional treatment used alone. Pus cells in the expressed prostatic smear diminished significantly after treatment, which was associated with a significant increase in the percentage of motile spermatozoa and a significant decrease in abnormal forms. Bacterial flora was studied in comparison with findings in 20 cases of infertile males without prostatitis; staphylococci predominated in both patient and control groups. Despite the lack of success, this seems to be a rather heroic treatment.

Local Hyperthermia

A new method of treatment of patients with chronic prostatitis and sterility by means of ultrahigh frequency (60 W) electric field applied bitemporally has been proposed. During treatment 82% of the patients showed an increase in the number of spermatozoa in 1 ml ejaculate; the percentage of movable and morphologically normal spermatozoa was increased. Patients with chronic prostatitis and sterility showed in the prostatic secretion before treatment a predominance of B-lymphocytes over T-lymphocytes. After treatment the number of T-lymphocytes in the prostatic secretion increased, and the content of B-lymphocytes decreased. In the subpopulation of T-lymphocytes the content of T-suppressors increased, and the content of T-helpers and O-lymphocytes decreased. At the same time, patients with sterility showed an increase in blood testosterone level and a decrease in follicle-stimulating hormone. Of 67 wives of the patients with sterility 50 reported pregnancy within 6 months after beginning of the treatment (Bogolyubov et al. 1986).

Servadio and Leib (1991) treated patients with chronic prostatitis by application of rectal hyperthermia in 6-weekly, 1-h sessions of local deep microwave hyperthermia (42.5 ± 0.5°C). Since most of the patients were young and also had infertility problems, the variation of sperm analysis before and after treatment was monitored. No change for the worse was noted. On the contrary, five pregnancies followed hyperthermic treatment in this group, the result of a clear improvement in sperm analysis. The authors did not report values of semen analysis or the duration of infertility.

This treatment obviously can be safely used in patients with chronic abacterial prostatitis not responding to conventional medical therapy and desiring to preserve their reproductive potential (Rigatti et al. 1990).

Other Treatments

If conservative treatment is not successful, surgical intervention may be considered. Sometimes inflammations of male adnexes result in an obstruction of the ductus. Hamidinia (1988) found a history of epididymitis or prostatitis in four patients and a history of iatrogenic obstruction in three of five patients with obstructive azoospermia. They were evaluated by physical examination and semen analysis, including fructose studies and serum testosterone and follicle-stimulating hormone determinations. Normal spermatogenesis was shown in all patients by testicular biopsy. The patients then underwent transvasovasostomy. They had encouraging postoperative sperm counts, and fertility was demonstrated by induction of pregnancy in two cases.

References

Barsanti JA, Caudle AB, Crowell WA, Shotts EB, Brown J (1986) Effect of induced prostatic infection on semen quality in the dog. Am J Vet Res 47(4):709–712

Bogolyubov VM, Karpukhin IV, Bobkova AS, Razuvayev AV, Kozhinova EV (1986) Dynamics of spermatogenesis, hormonal and immune response of patients suffering from chronic prostatitis and sterility under bitemporal treatment with an ultra-high frequency electric field. Int Urol Nephrol 18(1):89–97

Boronat F, Broseta E, Oliver F, Vera C, Vidal J, Jimenez JF (1990) Contribution of echography to the study of the andrologic patient. Arch Esp Urol 43 Suppl 1:101–107

Canale D, Bartelloni M, Negroni A (1986) Zinc in human semen. Int J Androl 9(6):477–480

Christiansen E, Purvis K (1991) Diagnosis of chronic abacterial prostato-vesiculitis by rectal ultrasonography in relation to symptoms and findings. Br J Urol 67(2):173–176

Colpi GM, Roveda ML, Tognetti A, Balerna M (1988) Seminal tract inflammation and male infertility. Correlations between leukospermia and clinical history, prostatic cytology, conventional semen parameters, sperm viability and seminal plasma protein composition. Acta Eur Fertil 19(2):69–77

Comhaire FH, Rowe PJ, Farley TM (1986) The effect of doxycycline in infertile couples with male accessory gland infection: a double blind prospective study. Int J Androl 9(2):91–98

Comhaire FH, Vermeulen L, Pieters O (1989) Study of the accuracy of physical and biochemical markers in semen to detect infectious dysfunction of the accessory sex glands. J Androl 10(1):50–53

Cooper TG, Weidner W, Nieschlag E (1990) The influence of inflammation of the human male genital tract on secretion of the seminal markers alpha-glucosidase, glycerophosphocholine, carnitine, fructose and citric acid. Int J Androl 13(5):329–336

Cummings JA, Dawes J, Hargreave TB (1990) Granulocyte elastase levels do not correlate with anaerobic and aerobic bacterial growth in seminal plasma from infertile men. Int J Androl 13(4):273–277

D'Agata R, Vicari E, Moncada ML, Sidoti G, Calogero AE, Fornito MC, Minacapilli G, Mongioi A, Polosa P (1990) Generation of reactive oxygen species in subgroups of infertile men. Int J Androl 13(5):344–351

Delanghe J, Comhaire F, de Buyzere M, Vermeulen L (1985) Altered glycosylation of gamma-glutamyltranspeptidase (GGT) in seminal fluid from men with accessory gland infection. Int J Androl 8(3):186–192

Ekladios EM, Girgis SM, Salem D, Fahmy IM, Mostafa T, Khalil GR (1988) Immunoglobulin E in serum and semen of infertile men. Andrologia 20(6):485–491

Etherington RJ, Clements R, Griffiths GJ, Peeling WB (1990) Transrectal ultrasound in the investigation of haemospermia. Clin Radiol 41(3):175–177

Fahim MS, Ibrahim HH, Girgis SM, Essa HA, Hanafi S (1985) Value of intraprostatic injection of zinc and vitamin C and of ultrasound application in infertile men with chronic prostatitis. Arch Androl 14(1):81–87

Fowler JE, Ariano M (1983) Bacterial infection and male infertility: absence of IgA with specifity for common E coli 0-serotypes in seminal fluid of infertile men. J Urol 130:171–174

Fowler JE, Ariano M (1984) Difficulties in quantitiating the contribution of urethral bacteria to prostatic fluid and seminal fluid cultures. J Urol 132:471–473

Freixia R, Rosello J, Ramis I, Abian J, Bulbena O, Brassesco M, Gelpi E (1988) Prostaglandin levels in infertile patients affected by asthenozoospermia and prostatitis. Prostaglandins Leukot Essent Fatty Acids 31:41–44

Gattuccio F, Di Trapani D, Romano C, Turtulici B, Milici M, Pavone C, D'Alia O, Alaimo R, Latteri MA (1988) Urogenital inflammations: aetiology, diagnosis and their correlation with varicocele and male infertility. Acta Eur Fertil 19(4):201–208

Giamarellou H, Tympanidis K, Bitos NA, Leonidas E, Daikos GK (1984) Infertility and chronic prostatitis. Andrologia 16(5):417–422

Giorgi PM, Giorgi P, Canale D, Turchi P, Poggi MS, Di Coscio M, Bartelloni M, Meschini P, Andreini F, Campa M et al. (1989) Treatment of male genital infections with enoxacin. Arch Ital Urol Nefrol Androl 61(3):235–241

Grizard G, Janny L, Hermabessiere J, Sirot J, Boucher D (1985) Seminal biochemistry and sperm characteristics in infertile men with bacteria in ejaculate. Arch Androl 15(2–3):181–186

Haidl G (1990) Macrophages in semen are indicative of chronic epididymal infection. Arch Androl 25(1):5–11

Hamidinia A (1988) Transvasovasostomy – an alternative operation for obstructive azoospermia. J Urol 140(6):1545–1548

Hofmann H (1987) Genitale Mykoplasmeninfektionen – Klinik, Diagnostik und Therapie. Urologe [A]26:246–251

Holland-Moritz H, Krause W (1992) Fertility prognosis of infertile men according to semen parameters. Int J Androl 15:473–484

Jarow JP, Kirkland JA Jr, Assimos DG (1990) Association of antisperm antibodies with chronic nonbacterial prostatitis. Urology 36(2):154–156

Jimenez-Cruz JF, Martinez-Ferrer M, Allona-Almagro A, De Rafael L, Navio-Nino S, Baquero-Mochales M (1984) Prostatitis: are the gram-positive organisms pathogenic? Eur Urol 10(5):311–314

Kavanagh JP (1985) Sodium, potassium, calcium, magnesium, zinc, citrate and chloride content of human prostatic and seminal fluid. J Reprod Fertil 75(1):35–41

Krause W (1991) Die Konzentrationen von Zink im Blut und Ejakulat stehen nicht im Zusammenhang mit Spermatozoenparametern. Z Hautkr 66:1035–1037

Krause W, Weidner W (1983) Immunglobuline im Ejakulat. Aktuel Dermatol 9:91–100

Megory E, Zuckerman H, Shoham Z, Lunenfeld B (1987) Infections and male fertility. Obstet Gynecol Surv 42(5):283–290

Mikhailichenko VV, Pupkova LS, Kozlov AV (1989) Electrophoretic study of protein secretion by the prostate gland in chronic prostatitis and pathospermia. Lab Delo 1989(4):8–11

Milingos S, Creatsas G, Messinis J (1983) Treatment of chronic prostatitis by consecutive per os administration of doxycycline, sulfamethoxazole/trimethoprim, and cephlexin. In J Clin Pharmacol Ther Toxicol 21:301–305

O'Leary WM (1990) Ureaplasmas and human disease. Crit Rev Microbiol 17(3):161–168

Omer E (1985) Inflammatory conditions and semen quality among subfertile Sudanese males. Trop Doct 15(1):27–28

Rigatti P, Buonaguidi A, Grasso M, Lania C, Montorsi F, Colombo R, Galli L, Guazzoni G (1990) Morphodynamic and biochemical assessment of seminal plasma in patients who underwent local prostatic hyperthermia. Prostate 16(4):325–330

Satoh S, Satoh K, Orikasa S, Maehara I, Takahashi M, Hiramatsu M (1990) Studies on pyospermia in male infertility. Nippon Hinyokika Gakkai Zasshi 81(2):170–177

Schmidt U, Knoll B, Frille I (1987) Leukocyte detection in the semen. A contribution to the diagnosis of chronic prostatitis and silent infections of the spermatic duct. Dermatol Monatsschr 173(12):702–707

Schmidt U, Pfützner H, Hartmann M (1989) Detection of Mycoplasma hominis and Ureaplasma urealyticum in patients with leukospermia. Arch Exp Veterinarmed 43(5):801–808

Servadio C, Leib Z (1991) Chronic abacterial prostatitis and hyperthermia. A possible new treatment? Br J Urol 67(3):308–311

Stanislavov R, Tsvetkov D, Tsvetkova P (1990) Immunological studies of patients with chronic nonspecific prostatitis and infertility. Akush Ginekol (Sofiia) 29(2):57–61

Suominen J, Gronroos M, Terho P (1983) Chronic prostatitis, Chlamydia trachomatis and infertility. Int J Androl 6:405–413

Weidner W, Krause W, Schiefer HG, Brunner H, Friedrich HJ (1985) Ureaplasmal infections of the male urogenital tract, in particular prostatitis, and semen quality. Urol Int 40(1):5–9

Weidner W, Jantos C, Schiefer HG et al. (1991a) Semen parameters in men with and without proven chronic prostatitis. J Androl 26:173–183

Weidner W, Jantos C, Schumacher F, Schiefer HG, Meyhöfer W (1991b) Recurrent haemospermia – underlying urogenital anomalies and efficacy of imaging procedures. Br J Urol 67(3):317–323

Witkin SS, Toth A (1983) Relationship between genital tract infections, sperm antibodies in seminal fluid, and infertility. Fertil Steril 40:805–809

Witkin SS, Zelikovsky G (1986) Immunosuppression and sperm antibody formation in men with prostatitis. J Clin Lab Immunol 21(1):7–10

Yasumoto R, Asakawa M (1988) Enoxacin in the seminal fluid of prostatitis patients. Hinyokika Kiyo 34(6):1101–1103

Basis for Antibacterial Treatment of Prostatitis: Experimental and Clinical Pharmacokinetic Studies and Models

P.O. Madsen, P. Drescher, and T.C. Gasser

Introduction

Great effort has been invested in the treatment of chronic bacterial prostatitis, but with rather disappointing results. The best cure rates reported using trimethoprim-sulfamethoxazole and various quinolones for 4 weeks–30 months vary from 32% to 71% (Meares 1975; Andriole 1991; McGuire and Lytton 1976; Weidner et al. 1991; Paulson and DeVere White 1978). The disappointing results are probably due to poor drug penetration into the prostate (Stamey et al. 1970; Aagaard and Madsen 1991; Meares 1992). To study the principles contributing to drug penetration into the various prostatic compartments, several animal models (dogs and rats) have been used. The results should, however, be interpreted with caution before being applied clinically. Some drug penetration studies have been carried out in patients undergoing transurethral prostatic surgery, but these studies involved mainly the hypertrophied prostate, not the normal and rarely the chronically infected prostate.

This chapter evaluates the various animal and clinical models for investigation of drugs potentially useful in the treatment of infectious prostatitis.

Theoretical Considerations

Drug penetration into the prostate gland is thought to be governed by the same principles that determine drug passage across biological lipid-containing membranes in general. The original prostate studies were carried out by Stamey et al. (1970; Stamey 1972). They found that acid antibiotic drugs can be detected in prostatic secretion only in very low concentrations, even when plasma concentrations of drug were very high; in contrast, basic antibiotic drugs were found in concentrations greater than the simultaneous plasma level. This is explained by the principles that govern the passage of drugs across biological membranes, emphasizing the role of nonionic diffusion of weak acids and bases across membranes with a pH gradient. Thus drug penetration is supposedly a passive transport mechanism consisting of diffusion and concentration. Drug characteristics that determine simple diffusion and concentration and lipid solubility, degree of ionization (biological membranes do not allow the passage of charged substances), degree of protein binding, and the size and shape of the molecule (small water-soluble molecules can cross biological membranes as part of the free water diffusion). The presence of a pH gradient across a biological membrane introduces the phenomenon of ion trapping. In the dog prostate there is a pH gradient across the prostate epithelium, the pH of plasma being 7.4 and that of the prostatic secretion 6.4. Most antimicrobials are weak acids or weak bases. Therefore differences in hydrogen ion concentration in plasma and prostatic secretion are crucial to the phenomenon of ion trapping. In a stable system the uncharged fraction of a lipid-soluble drug equilibrates on the two sides of the membrane, but the charged fraction is greater on one side or the other, depending on the pH. Thus the greatest drug concentration (sum of charged and uncharged fractions) is on the side with the higher degree of ionization. A rearrangement of the Henderson-Hasselbalch equation, can be used to calculate the theoretical drug concentration ratio across a biological membrane when equilibrium is achieved (Fig. 1).

Figure 2 illustrates the situation for a base of pK_a 8.4. In dogs with a prostatic secretion of pH 6.4, weak acids (low pK_a) concentrate on the plasma

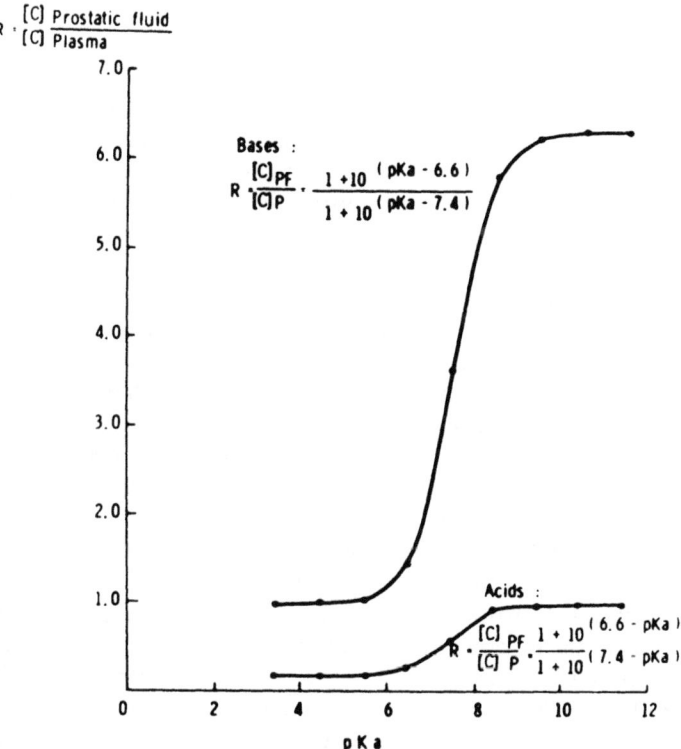

Fig. 1. Theoretical partition ratios of antibiotics between prostatic fluid and plasma

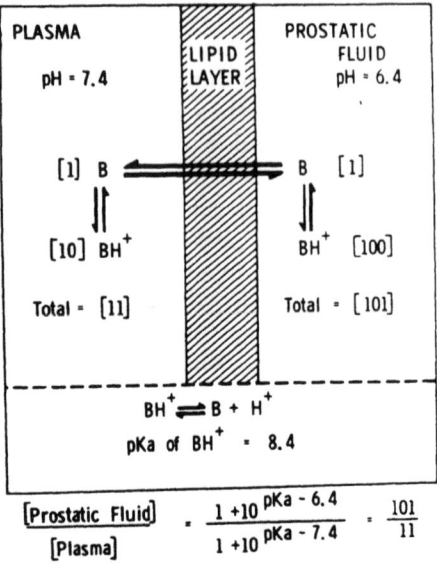

$$\frac{[\text{Prostatic Fluid}]}{[\text{Plasma}]} = \frac{1 + 10^{\text{pKa} - 6.4}}{1 + 10^{\text{pKa} - 7.4}} = \frac{101}{11}$$

Fig. 2. The ion-trapping phenomenon in a stable system across a biological membrane with a pH gradient, illustrated for a base of pK_a 8.4. Rearrangement of the Henderson-Hasselbalch equation has been used to calibrate the drug concentration ratios

side. The higher the pK_a, the higher the drug concentration is in the prostatic secretion, but never exceeding the plasma concentration. Weak bases concentrate in the prostatic secretion, and, similarly, the higher pK_a, the higher the drug concentration is. The newly developed fluoroquinolones are neither pure acids or bases but have characteristics of both (amphoteric or zwitter-ionic drugs, Gasser et al. 1986). Figure 3 shows ionization curves of an acid, a base, and an amphoteric drug, calculated using the Henderson-Hasselbalch equation. Most quinolones that are amphoteric drugs have two ionizing groups, one positively and one negatively charged, and thus two pK_a values. At one pH value, which is between the two pK_a values and is different for each amphoteric drug, the amount of charged drug is minimal (isoelectric point). At higher and lower pH values more drug is charged. Since the highest drug concentration occurs on the side with higher degree of ionization, drugs with an isoelectric point close to plasma pH should concentrate in dog prostate (but also in tissue with a pH above plasma pH). Conversely, amphoteric drugs with an isoelectric point close to prostatic secretion pH should concentrate in plasma.

The site of infection in the prostate is still under debate. In an experimental study of chronic prostatitis in dogs, the inflammatory changes were found mainly in the interstitial tissue and not in the acini as in acute prostatitis (Baumueller and Madsen 1977). Consequently, a comparison of plasma concentrations to concentrations in both prostatic secretion and prostatic interstitial fluid is of interest in evaluating the therapeutic possibilities of a given drug.

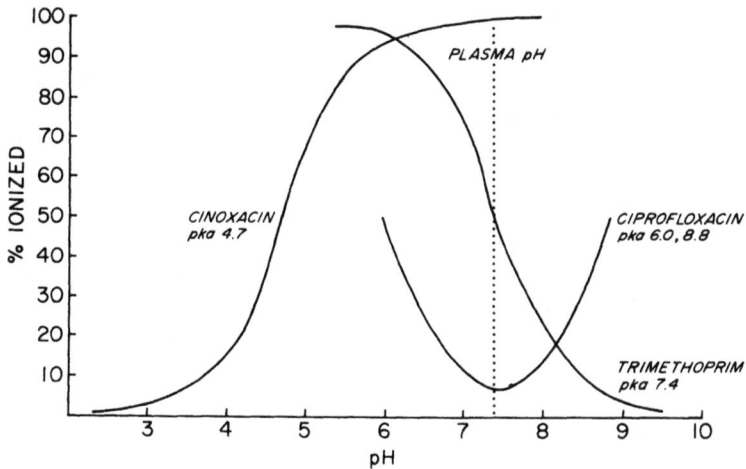

Fig. 3. Ionization curves of an acid (cinoxacin), a base (trimethoprim), and an amphoteric quinolone (ciprofloxacin) calculated by using the Henderson-Hasselbalch equation

Another interesting question is the applicability to humans of the results obtained in dog models. A basic assumption in experiments designed to study the diffusion of drugs into the prostate has been that the pH of human prostatic secretion is similar to that of the dog (about 6.5). Fair and Cordonnier (1978), however, found that the prostatic secretion of normal men is slightly alkaline, with a pH of approximately 7.3. They also found that the pH of prostatic secretion from men with prostatic infection is markedly increased (mean pH 8.34). Since the pH gradient is crucial to the ion-trapping phenomenon, one therefore cannot apply the results obtained in dogs directly to humans. Even if ion trapping should take place, it is questionable whether the trapped (and charged) fraction of a drug would have any significant antibacterial effect since it may not penetrate the bacterial wall.

Animal Studies

Dog Studies

The dog has been the most commonly used animal in experimental models for investigating diffusion of antibiotic drugs into the prostate. The dog has no functional seminal vesicles and no bulbourethral gland (Reeves and Ghilchik 1970). In other animals the secretion from these glands introduces a variable factor into the analysis of prostatic secretion. Further, the bladder of a dog is covered by peritoneum, which makes access to the prostate easier. As in humans, the dog may develop benign hyperplasia. The physiological properties of the dog prostate may therefore be somewhat similar to those of the human prostate.

In drug diffusion studies of the dog prostate, drug concentration is usually measured in prostatic secretion, plasma, and urine. Some investigators have measured the concentration in prostatic interstitial fluid as well, because studies have shown that the inflammatory changes in chronic bacterial prostatitis take place in the interstitial tissue (Baumueller and Madsen 1977). If a dog is killed at the end of a study, the concentration in the prostatic tissue is also measured.

For most drugs concentrations are several times higher in urine than in plasma, prostatic secretion, and other tissue fluids. Thus it is important to prevent urine contamination of secretions and fluids to the investigated. In 1939 Huggins et al. introduced the classical experimental dog model for quantitative studies of prostatic secretion and prevented urine contamination of prostatic secretion by transecting the bladder neck.

The experimental model of Huggins et al. (1939) has undergone several changes, as described by Mason et al. (1961). In one modification (Robb et al. 1971), a prostatostomy was performed to study the diffusion of selected sulfonamides, trimethoprim, and diaveridine into prostatic fluid of dogs.

Stamey et al. (1970) studied a large number of antimicrobial drugs, using a modification of the Huggins et al. (1939) model by ligating the bladder neck proximal to the prostate and introducing polyethylene catheters through bilateral ureterostomies. Ligation of the vas deferens permitted collection of pure prostatic secretion (Stamey 1972).

In 1977 Baumueller and Madsen developed a dog model of bacterial prostatitis, simulating the hematogenous route of infection by intra-arterially injecting a suspension of 10^6 *Escherichia coli* in 0.5 ml saline. At various intervals (1 week–2 months) after introducing the infection, they obtained prostatic secretion and finally the gland for histological examination. The acute inflammatory changes were found in the prostatic acini, and in the chronic stage the changes were seen in the interstitial tissue. The drug concentration in prostatic interstitial fluid may therefore be of importance in the treatment of chronic bacterial prostatitis.

Eickenberg et al. (1976) introduced a technique for measuring drug concentration in dog prostatic interstitial fluid. Four to five weeks prior to study they implanted in the prostatic tissue a multiperforated polypropylene capsule 1 cm in diameter with a tubing brought to the outside and buried beneath the skin. It was thus possible to collect prostatic interstitial fluid during a study by cannulating the tubings.

Our experimental dog model is a modification of this model. Approximately 4 weeks prior to study, we implant a 10×16 mm multiperforated polyethylene tissue chamber with two connecting tubings in each lateral lobe of prostate (Fig. 4). The tubings are filled with heparin, sealed, and then placed subcutaneously. At the time of study we ligate the urethra at the bladder neck and divert the urine by a cystostomy. The vasa deferentia are also ligated to prevent contamination from the testes. Prostatic secretion is obtained from a 14-F

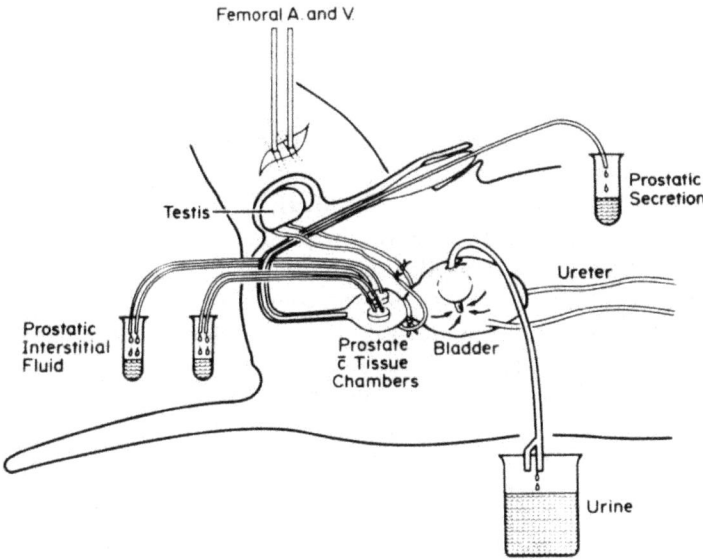

Fig. 4. Schematic drawing of dog model with implanted tissue chambers, used in our laboratory; 10 × 6 mm multiperforated tissue chambers with two connecting tubings, used for collection of prostatic interstitial fluid. This is a modification of other models (Huggins et al. 1939; Mason et al. 1961; Stamey 1972; Eickenberg et al. 1976)

urethral catheter, urine from the cystostomy, and prostatic interstitial fluid by cannulating the subcutaneously placed tubings of the tissue chambers (Fig. 4). To maintain a constant plasma drug concentration we inject intravenously a bolus of the drug followed by constant intravenous drug infusion for 4 h. To stimulate prostatic secretion, pilocarpine (0.25 mg/kg) is given intravenously initially and when needed during the study. Prostatic secretion, prostatic interstitial fluid, plasma, and urine are collected before and at 30-min intervals during a 4-h study. At the end of an experiment, the dog is killed, and tissue from various organs, including the prostate, is removed for determination of drug concentration.

Since drug diffusion into the prostate might change in the case of chronic bacterial infection, we have performed drug diffusion studies in normal prostates as well as in prostates with induced bacterial infection (Baumueller and Madsen 1977). Culture of *E. coli* from the prostatic interstitial fluid and prostatic secretion confirms the establishment of an experimental prostatitis.

Drug concentrations in tissues and various prostatic fluids are determined by bioassay using a disk diffusion method or by high-pressure liquid chromatography. To obtain enough prostatic secretion it is necessary to stimulate the secretion with pilocarpine. Plentiful thin fluid is usually obtained, but it is questionable whether this artificially induced secretion has physiological characteristics comparable to normal prostatic secretion. Further, it is questionable whether the fluid obtained from tissue chambers actually represents interstitial fluid. The presence of a tissue chamber made of polyethylene may cause a foreign body reaction in the prostate gland, and the fluid may be the result of this reaction. These elements of uncertainty should be remembered when experimental results are interpreted.

Figures 5 and 6 show typical results from drug diffusion studies. Trimethoprim (Fig. 5) is a base, and in both prostatic secretion and prostatic interstitial fluid concentrations exceed plasma levels. Ampicillin (Fig. 6) is a lipid-insoluble acid with a low pK_a and should be trapped on the plasma side and thus found only in low concentration in the prostatic secretion. Similarly, sulfonamides with concentration curves similar to ampicillin and commonly used drugs in the treatment of urinary tract infections do not gain high enough concentrations in prostatic secretion to be considered effective in the treatment of bacterial prostatitis. Table 1 shows the prostatic secretion, prostatic interstitial fluid, and

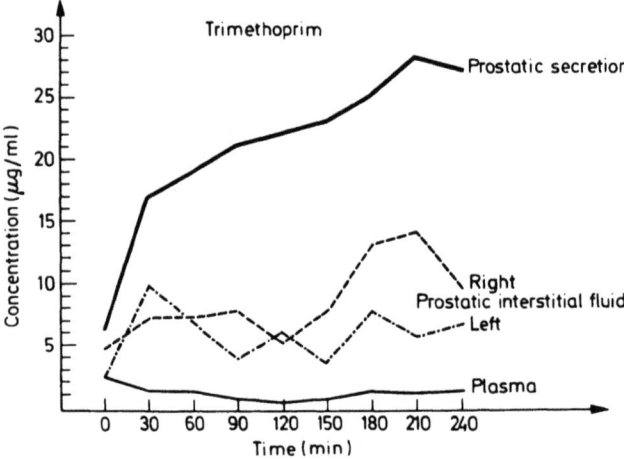

Fig. 5. Example of diffusion studies with a basic compound, trimethoprim, in dog plasma, prostatic interstitial fluid and prostatic secretion (Eickenberg et al. 1976)

Table 1. Concentrations of six quinolone derivatives in plasma, prostatic secretion and prostatic interstitial fluid during constant infusion in dogs (μg/ml; median and range)

Drug	No. of dogs	Constant infusion (mg/kg per hour)	Plasma	Prostatic secretion	Prostatic interstitial fluid
Cinoxacin	3	1	45.0 (37.0–52.0)	1.0 (0.5–2.6)	5.0 (2.4–29.6)
Norfloxacin	4	1	3.8 (2.7–11.4)	2.1 (0.7–5.1)	2.3 (1.5–4.5)
Rosoxacin	4	3	11.1 (6.0–18.0)	1.1 (0.4–2.0)	2.9 (1.5–4.5)
Ciprofloxacin	4	3	6.0 (3.6–9.9)	3.4 (1.8–7.5)	3.2 (1.6–5.4)
Amifloxacin	5	3	12.0 (9.0–9.0)	6.3 (3.6–15.0)	6.7 (4.2–20.0)
Enoxacin	5	1	2.9 (2.3–3.2)	4.2 (1.9–5.5)	3.6 (2.3–4.5)

plasma concentrations of six quinolones in dogs (Dørflinger et al. 1986). Rosoxacin and cinoxacin are acids with one pK_a and should therefore not concentrate in prostatic secretion. Amifloxacin, for instance, an amphoteric drug (pK_a1 5.8, pK_a2 7.5), has its isoelectric point close to the prostatic secretion pH and should concentrate on the plasma side, expressed as a ratio below 1. Enoxacin (pK_a1 6.0, pK_a2 8.5), ciprofloxacin (pK_a 6.0, pK_a2 8.8) and norfloxacin (pK_a1 6.3, pK_a2 8.8) have isoelectric points close to plasma pH and should concentrate in prostatic secretion, but this is true in fact only for enoxacin. Other drug characteristics, such as lipid solubility and protein binding, may account for the finding that ciprofloxacin and norfloxacin do not concentrate in prostatic secretion as predicted. However, the influence of lipid solubility and protein binding on drug diffusion are difficult to assess.

Table 2 summarizes the prostatic secretion/plasma ratios and the prostatic interstitial fluid/plasma ratios in dogs for a number of antimicrobials. Carbenicillin indanyl sodium was for many years the only antibiotic approved by the United States Food and Drug Administration for the treatment of both acute and chronic bacterial prostatitis. However, it cannot be detected in prostatic secretion and is found in the prostatic interstitial fluid in concentrations lower than the plasma level. Netilmicin, like other aminoglycosides, is a

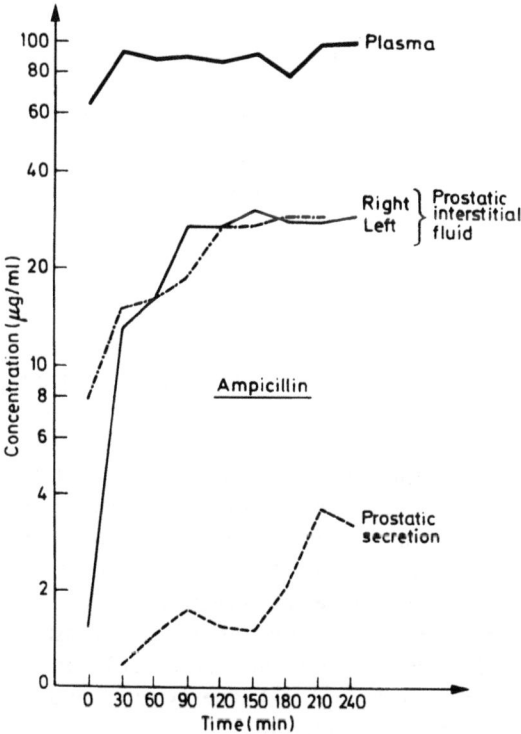

Fig. 6. Example of diffusion studies with an acid, ampicillin, in dog plasma, prostatic interstitial fluid, and prostatic secretion (Eickenberg et al. 1976)

Table 2. Prostatic secretion/plasma ratios and prostatic interstitial fluid/plasma ratios of selected representative drugs, obtained from drug diffusion studies in dogs

Drug	Chemical property	PS/p	PIF/p	Reference
Ampicillin	Acid	0.01[a]	0.34[a]	Dørflinger et al. (1986)
Amoxacillin	Acid	0.05	0.32	Dørflinger et al. (1986)
Mecillinam	Acid	0.04	0.14	Dørflinger et al. (1986)
Carbenicillin indanyl sodium	Acid	ND	0.69	Dørflinger et al. (1986)
Sulfamethoxazole	Acid	0.18	0.43	Eickenberg et al. (1976)
Sulfanilamide	Acid	0.83	–	Mason et al. (1961)
Sulfapyridine	Acid	0.50	–	Mason et al. (1961)
Doxycycline	Acid	0.59	0.72	Eickenberg et al. (1976)
Cinoxacin	Acid	0.03	0.10	Nielsen and Madsen (1988)
Rosoxacin	Acid	0.09	0.29	Frimodt-Møller et al. (1979)
Cephalothin	Acid	0.09	–	Madsen et al. (1976a)
Cephradine	Acid	0.12	–	Madsen et al. (1976a)
Netilmicin	Base	0.03	0.35	Eickenberg et al. (1976)
Erythromycin	Base	3.9	1.9	Eickenberg et al. (1976)
Oleandomycin	Base	3.25	–	Aagaard and Madsen (1991)
Trimethoprim	Base	14.8	6.7	Eickenberg et al. (1976)
Diaveridine	Base	3.10	–	Mason et al. (1961)
Rosamicin	Base	8.9	4.0	Madsen et al. (1976b)
Tetroxoprim	Base	7.9	–	Larsen et al. (1986)
Metioprim	Base	5.2	0.92	Aagaard et al. (1991)
Amifloxacin	Amphoteric	0.55	0.59	Frimodt-Møller et al. (1979)
Ciprofloxacin	Amphoteric	0.66	0.59	Frimodt-Møller et al. (1979)
Enoxacin	Amphoteric	1.51	1.32	Frimodt-Møller et al. (1979)
Norfloxacin	Amphoteric	0.43	0.49	Frimodt-Møller et al. (1979)

PS/p, Prostatic secretion/plasma ratio; PIF/p, prostatic interstitial fluid/plasma ratio; ND, not detectable.
[a] Mean.

base but does not concentrate in prostatic secretion. The reason for this surprising finding may be that netilmicin is almost totally charged at a pH of about 6.4 in prostatic secretion. The aminoglycosides, for unknown reasons, may not follow the rules of nonionic diffusion of drugs across biological membranes.

Trimethoprim is often used in combination with a sulfonamide, the optimal synergy ratio being 1:20 (Frimodt-Møller et al. 1979). As mentioned earlier, the best cure rates reported in the treatment of chronic bacterial prostatitis using trimethoprim-sulfamethoxazole range from 32% to 71%. These rather disappointing results may be caused by different degrees of penetration of the two drugs into the prostate. While trimethoprim is concentrated in the prostatic secretion, sulfamethoxazole is not. The trimethoprim-sulfamethoxazole ratio at the site of action may therefore be far from the optimal synergy ratio, and the antibacterial effect may be due to the trimethoprim alone.

On the basis of the dog experiments, trimethoprim was the drug of choice in treatment of bacterial prostatitis caused by gram-negative bacteria, and erythromycin or similar macrolide antibiotics when gram-positive organisms were considered the causative agents. These drugs concentrate well in the prostate. The new fluoroquinolones, however, with their unique pharmacokinetics and broad antibacterial spectra, now appear to be the drugs of choice. The first fluoroquinolone approved for prostatitis was ofloxacin. Other fluoroquinolones are in various stages of development.

As described above, the pH gradient across a biological membrane is of importance to the ion-trapping phenomenon. In both normal and infected dogs, the pH of prostatic secretion is approximately 6.4, as opposed to pH values of 7.3 and 8.3 in prostatic secretion of normal and infected humans (Fair and Cordonnier 1978). Results obtained in dogs must therefore be interpreted with caution.

Rat Studies

Experimental prostatitis has been induced in rats by Nielsen and Madsen (1988) and Nickel and Olsen (this volume). In the studies by Nielsen, the prostatitis in rats was induced by introducing 10^8 E. coli intravesically. Maximum infection was achieved after 4 days. In these experiments the pharmacokinetics, and also the effect on this experimental acute prostatitis by various fluoroquinolones (sparfloxacin, temafloxacin, difloxacin and ciprofloxacin), was studied. Intravenous bolus injections of these fluoroquinolones were followed by a continuous intravenous infusion adjusted according to the expected half-life of the various quinolones. Drug concentrations were determined by bioassay. All these drugs concentrated well in the prostate, reaching concentrations 2–3 times simultaneous serum concentrations. Urine concentrations exceeded serum concentrations 3–80 times. Starting on the fourth day the animals were then treated for 3 days with subcutaneous injections of the above fluoroquinolones with the dosage adjusted to the drugs' half-life and their minimal inhibitory concentration (MIC) against the E. coli strain used for the induction of the prostatitis. The best treatment results in these rats (the lowest E. coli colony counts) were found in difloxacin-treated rats, followed by temafloxacin-, sparfloxacin-, and ciprofloxacin-treated animals (Nielsen and Madsen 1988). These results of animal studies should be interpreted with caution. Clinical trials of the investigated compounds in bacterial prostatitis should also be carried out.

Studies in Humans

Drug diffusion studies in humans are difficult to carry out. Studies have been done in patients undergoing transurethral resection of the prostate for benign prostatic hyperplasia. At certain times prior to surgery, depending on the half-life of the drug to be investigated, the drug is administered orally or parenterally. Blood samples are drawn at regular intervals and prostatic tissue chips obtained

Table 3. Plasma (P) and human prostatic tissue (PT) concentrations
of norfloxacin, ciprofloxacin, enoxacin, and ofloxacin

Drug	Plasma (μg/ml)	Prostatic tissue (μg/ml)	Ratio PT/P
Norfloxacin	1.2 $\pm$ 0.6	2.2 $\pm$ 0.8	1.9
Ciprofloxacin	1.7 $\pm$ 1.0	3.3 $\pm$ 2.8	2.1
Enoxacin	2.1 $\pm$ 0.6	4.9 $\pm$ 1.7	2.5
Ofloxacin	2.9 $\pm$ 0.8	2.9 $\pm$ 1.1	1.0

at the beginning and at the end of surgery and are immediately frozen for bioassay. The drug concentration in prostatic tissue may be affected by the length of time the prostatic chips are kept in the irrigating solution at surgery. The true prostatic tissue concentration of ampicillin, for example, is assumed to be 15%–25% higher than the concentration measured in prostatic chips removed from the irrigating glycine solution after 2–5 min (Madsen et al. 1976a). In addition, it is not the diffusion of a drug into a normal or infected prostate that is studied but drug diffusion into the hyperplastic prostate gland.

Because of the high drug concentration in the urine contamination with urine is another problem in human studies. This was avoided in a study involving a 26-year-old patient with urinary diversion (cutaneous transuretero-ureterostomy because of a neurogenic bladder). On one occasion the patient received 160 mg trimethoprim and 800 mg sulfamethoxazole twice a day for 1 week before prostatic secretion was obtained by prostatic massage. The trimethoprim concentrations in prostatic secretion were found to be more than 40 times greater than those in plasma (Madsen et al. 1976b). The pH of this patient's prostatic secretion was 7, and the ratio therefore far exceeded the theoretical ratio if only passive secretion is postulated. These data imply the existence of an active concentration mechanism of trimethoprim in prostatic secretion.

The theory of an active concentration mechanism in the prostate is also supported by the findings of studies of quinolones in patients undergoing prostatectomy. Assuming a pH of the prostatic secretion close to plasma pH (i.e., no pH gradient; Fair and Cordonnier 1978), a prostatic secretion/plasma ratio of close to 1 would be expected for amphoteric drugs. However, concentration ratios considerably higher than 1 were found for several quinolones (Table 3) (Larsen et al. 1986; Aagaard et al. 1991).

Discussion

Overall, clinical application of results obtained in the laboratory has been disappointing. Several reasons must be considered, including the difference in pH of dog and human prostatic secretion (Fair and Cordonnier 1978) and the possibility of an active secretion mechanism (Madsen et al. 1976b). Despite evidence that the interstitium may be the site of infection in chronic bacterial prostatitis (Baumueller and Madsen 1977), drug concentrations in general have been measured only in prostatic secretion. In the case of marginal drug levels in plasma, the drug concentration in prostatic interstitial fluid might not exceed the MIC for a sufficient period. The existence of prostatic factor inhibiting the antibacterial effect of some drugs and thereby greatly increasing the MIC might also contribute to poor clinical results (Madsen and Whalen 1978). Thus, in spite of intensive investigation we still know little about the mechanisms that govern the transport of antibiotic drugs into the prostate, and further investigations are necessary. However, since some newer quinolones were found in human prostatic tissue in concentrations significantly higher than the MICs of most prostatitis-causing pathogens (Larsen et al. 1986), treatment of bacterial prostatitis with these compounds may become more successful.

Summary

The results of treatment of chronic bacterial prostatitis are disappointing, probably due to poor drug penetration into the prostate. The theoretical background of drug penetration into the prostate is outlined, emphasizing the phenomenon of ion-trapping and the role of nonionic diffusion of weak acids, bases and amphoteric drugs across biological membranes with a pH gradient.

Drug penetration into the prostate has been studied mainly in dogs. Some of the dog and rat models employed are described, and the pharmacokinetics of many antibiotic and chemotherapeutic agents are outlined. The results, however, are not directly applicable to humans, primarily because of the slight alkalinity of human prostatic secretion compared to the slightly acidic prostatic secretion of dogs. Some drug penetration studies have been carried out on humans undergoing prostatic surgery, but the studies involved the hyperplastic prostate, not the normal and rarely the chronically infected prostate. In spite of intensive investigations, our knowledge is still limited concerning the mechanisms that govern the transport of antibiotic drugs into the prostate and how the findings can be applied clinically.

References

Aagaard J, Madsen PO (1991) Bacterial prostatitis: new methods of treatment. Urology 37:4–8
Aagaard J, Knes J, Madsen PO (1991) Prostatic tissue levels of ofloxacin. Urology 38:380
Andriole VT (1991) Use of quinolones in treatment of prostatitis and lower urinary tract infection. Eur J Clin Microbiol Infect Dis 10(4):342–350
Baumueller A, Madsen PO (1977) Experimental bacterial prostatitis in dogs. Urol Res 5:211
Dørflinger T, Larsen EH, Gasser TC, Madsen PO (1986) The concentration of various quinolone derivatives in the dog prostate. In: Weidner W (ed) Therapy of prostatitis. Experimental and clinical data. Zuckschwerdt, Munich, pp 35–39

Eickenberg HU, Scharfenberger L, Waterman NG (1976) A new model for measuring concentration of antibiotics in prostatic interstitial fluid. Infection 4(2):108

Fair WR, Cordonnier JJ (1978) The pH of prostatic fluid: a reappraisal and therapeutic implication. J Urol 120:695

Frimodt-Møller N, Maigaard S, Madsen PO, Naber KG (1979) Co-trimazine distribution in the canine prostate. Infection 7(4):349

Gasser TC, Larsen EH, Dørflinger T, Madsen PO (1986) The influence of various body fluids and pH on E. coli MIC of quinolone derivatives. In: Weidner W (ed) Therapy of prostatitis. Experimental and clinical data. Zuckschwerdt, Munich, pp 50–53

Huggins C, Masina MH, Eichelberger L, Wharton JD (1939) Quantative studies of the prostatic secretion. I. Characteristics of the normal secretion, the influence of thyroid, suprarenal and testes extirpation and androgen substitution on the prostatic outlet. J Exp Med 70:543

Larsen EH, Gasser TC, Dørflinger T, Madsen PO (1986) The concentration of various quinolone derivatives in the human prostate. In: Weidner W (ed) Therapy of prostatitis. Experimental and clinical data. Zuckschwerdt, Munich, pp 40–44

Madsen PO, Kjaer TB, Baumueller A, Mellin H-E (1976) Antimicrobial agents in prostatic fluid and tissue. Infection 4(2):154

Madsen PO, Kjaer TB, Baumueller A (1976b) Prostatic tissue and fluid concentration of trimethoprim and sulfamethoxazole. Urology 8(2):129

Madsen PO, Whalen PR (1978) Interaction between antimicrobial agents and prostatic tissue extract and fluid. Infection 6(1):75

Mason MM, Keefe F, Boria T (1961) Specialized surgery of canine bladder and prostate gland. Isolation and collection of prostatic fluid. J Am Vet Assoc 135:1007

McGuire EJ, Lytton B (1976) Bacterial prostatitis: treatment with trimethoprim-sulfamethoxazole. Urology 7:499

Meares EM (1975) Longterm therapy of chronic bacterial prostatitis with trimethoprim-sulfamethoxazole. Can Med Assoc J Suppl 112:22s

Meares EM (1992) Prostatitis and related disorders. In: Walsh PC, Retik AB, Stamey TA et al. (eds) Campbell's urology, 6th edn. Saunders, Philadelphia, pp 807–822

Nielsen KT, Madsen PO (1988) Temafloxacin (A63004), difloxacin (A56619) and ciprofloxacin treatment of acute prostatitis. An experimental model in rats (Abstr). 2nd International Symposium on New Quinolones, Aug 25–27, Geneva

Paulson DF, DeVere White R (1978) Trimethoprim-sulfamethoxazole and minocycline-hydrochloride in the treatment of culture-proved bacterial prostatitis. J Urol 120:184

Reeves DS, Ghilchik M (1970) Secretion of the antibacterial substance trimethoprim in the prostatic fluid of dogs. Br J Urol 42:66

Robb CA, Carrol PT, Tippett LO, Landston JB (1971) The difference of selected sulfonamides, trimethoprim and diaveridine into prostatic fluid of dogs. Invest Urol 8:679

Stamey TA (1972) Urinary infection in males. In: Urinary infections. Williams and Wilkins, Baltimore, p 161

Stamey TA, Meares EM, Winningham G (1970) Chronic bacterial prostatitis and the diffusion of drugs into the prostatic fluid. J Urol 103:187

Weidner W, Schiefer HG, Brähler E (1991) Refractory chronic bacterial prostatitis: a re-evaluation of ciprofloxacin treatment after a median follow-up of 30 months. J Urol 146(2):350–352

Experimental Prostatitis

J.C. Nickel, M.E. Olson, and H. Ceri

Introduction

Prostatitis remains an enigma despite decades of clinical research (Pfau 1986; Nickel and Olson 1991). The generally held assumption in the medical community that our urologic management of this disease remains poor likely reflects our continued lack of a solid understanding of the etiology and pathogenesis of prostatitis, diagnostic systems that have been abandoned by most physicians, and clinical cure rates that are among the poorest in infectious diseases (Nickel 1992). Since not all the answers are forthcoming in our extensive clinical investigations, can experimental prostatitis offer further insight into this complex disease? In fact many of the major advances in prostate research were made possible by animal models (i.e., etiology of benign prostatic hyperplasia, androgen and antiandrogens, oncogenes, the dihydrotestosterone and 5α-reductase story etc.). In this chapter we examine a number of animal models of experimental prostatitis that have led to insights into this complex infectious disease. Animal models allow us to study the initiation and pathogenesis of disease processes in a longitudinal fashion and enable us to change experimental parameters to determine their relative influence on the progression of the disease. New diagnostic systems can be rigorously tested, and various treatments including the question of antibiotic pharmacokinetics can be explored under the various conditions.

Etiology and Pathogenesis

Experimental prostatitis can perhaps give us the greatest insight into the pathogenesis of the various prostatitis syndromes. There are remarkable similarities between the clinical prostatitis syndromes of bacterial and nonbacterial prostatitis, and many times the clinical distinction between the two is difficult. However, it is generally accepted in both acute and chronic bacterial prostatitis that the bacteria causing these conditions are similar in type and incidence to those that cause simple urinary tract infections, with aerobic gram-negative enteric bacteria (*Escherichia coli*) predominating. The role of gram-positive bacteria, such as enterococci and coagulase-negative staphylococci, anerobic bacteria and organisms such as *Chlamydia trachomatis* and *Ureaplasma urealyticum* continues to stir controversy. The development of experimental prostatitis with *E. coli* is well established in animal systems (Baumueller and Madsen 1977; Jantos et al. 1990; Neal et al. 1990; Nickel et al. 1990, 1991) and such models may be employed to test the hypothesis that other organisms, such as *C. trachomatis* (Nielsen et al. 1982), might be implicated in chronic prostatic inflammation.

While the etiologic agents in this disease remain confusing, the pathophysiology is even more so, but here experimental prostatitis has been more helpful. Maglione et al. (1986) noted that experimental surgically induced *E. coli* seminal vesiculitis in rats was occasionally complicated by *E. coli* prostatitis. However, evidence is accumulating that the pathophysiology of bacterial prostatitis is associated with retrograde bacterial ascent from the urethra, perhaps secondary to some form of intraprostatic ductal reflux. Jantos et al. (1990) inoculated the bladder of male and female *Mastomys natalensis* with *E. coli* and produced severe prostatitis. The histologic and microbiologic course of the prostatic infection resembled strongly the human disease. Chronic bacterial and nonbacterial prostatitis persisted for 6 months postinfection. Dilworth et al. (1980) used a monkey model to study the ascending route of infection in prostatitis and noted that P-fimbriae were the principle mediators of adherence to the urethral cells of the prostatic urethra. Neal et al. (1990) employed this nonhuman primate model and found that after urethral inoculation of a wild-type clinical isolate of *E. coli* the monkeys developed a prostatitis similar to that reported in humans and concluded that infection in the nonhuman primate occurs by this ascending route. They also noted histologic changes similar to that in the human disease. A reliable and consistent rat model of acute and chronic bacterial prostatitis has been developed by our research group (Nickel et al. 1991) and employed to undertake sophisticated microbial, histologic, and immunologic studies that would not be possible in a clinical patient study to further elucidate the pathogenesis of this complicated disease.

Research to date (Nickel et al. 1990, 1991; Nickel and Olson 1991) has demonstrated that once the bacteria enter the ducts and acini of the prostate gland they multiply, inducing a host response with infiltration of acute inflammatory cells into the ducts. In acute bacterial prostatitis the entire prostate gland or at least the major part of it is involved in the inflammatory process with polymorphonuclear leukocytes within and around the ducts and acini. The ducts become engorged with infiltrate made up of dead and live bacteria as well as living and dying acute inflammatory cells, desquamated epithelial cells, and cellular debris. At this point it is relatively easy to eradicate all offending organisms with appropriate antibiotic therapy for complete resolution of the inflammatory process. If bacteria persist from either acute or more likely clinically subacute inflammation, they can form small, sporadic bacterial microcolonies within the ductal system adherent to the epithelium. The bacteria produce an exopolysaccharide slime or "glycocalyx" that envelops these microcolonies, and as with other cryptic infections the micro-organisms become very quiescent, undergoing a sort of "hibernation" when the environment becomes threatening. Surrounding these focal sites of bacterial persistence are areas of lymphocytic invasion with variable infiltration of plasma cells and macrophages. Over time fibrosis occurs with subsequent permanent scarring. The pathogenesis of nonbacterial prostatitis may be similar in that intraprostatic reflux of urine, urine products, or even undetected organisms into the prostatic ducts and acini may occur (Nickel 1992).

Naslund et al. (1988) reported a study suggesting that genetic background, advancing age, and hormonal imbalance are important etiologic factors for nonbacterial prostatitis in rats. Spontaneous nonbacterial prostatitis is more common in Lewis rats than in Wistar rats and does not occur in Sprague-Dawley rats. The incidence of spontaneous prostatitis was significantly higher in older animals than in younger animals, and the administration of exogenous 17beta-estradiol increased the incidence and severity of prostatitis in old Wistar rats. Castration had a similar effect. Severe prostatitis could even be induced in young adult Wistar rats by neonatal treatment with 17beta-estradiol followed several months later in adulthood by testosterone administration. This and other studies of experimental prostatitis (Jantos et al. 1990; Nickel et al. 1990; Aronsson et al. 1988) show that nonbacterial prostatitis resulting from eradication of the bacterial agent in chronic bacterial prostatitis and chronic bacterial prostatitis with persistence of the bacterial agent are indistinguishable. In fact, prostatitis occurring in older males, discovered at time of prostate resection for obstructive and irritative symptoms, remains indistinguishable from that of bacterial prostatitis. Anecdotally, stress appears to increase the severity of the symptoms of nonbacterial prostatitis in human patients, and Gatenbeck et al. (1987) histopathologically examined rat prostate glands after a 10-day period during which the rats had been submitted to standardized stress stimuli. They demonstrated similar inflammatory histopathologic changes in the glands of all rats submitted to long-term stress stimuli that were similar to those of human males with prostatitis. In these animals there was definitely no evidence indicating a bacterial origin. Aronsson et al. (1988) confirmed this finding by subjecting rats to standardized experimental stress stimuli and again showed prostatic inflammatory changes compatible with nonbacterial prostatitis on histologic examination.

Research on the immune response to the bacterial infection in the prostate gland has led to a greater understanding of the pathogenesis of this disease and perhaps in the future may allow more precise diagnosis of the etiologic agent. In experimental chronic bacterial prostatitis we have confirmed (Nickel et al. 1990) clinical findings of increased levels of antigen-specific antibody in the prostatic secretion of animals with unresolved prostatitis as well as elevated serum antibody titers against their prostatic pathogens which return to normal with successful treatment of chronic bacterial prostatitis (Nickel et al., work in progress). We also noted deposition of antibody along the basement membranes of the prostatic ducts in the early stages of the disease with subsequent

deposition of similar antibody within the interstitium as well as the ductal
basement membrane in the later stages of the disease, which was associated with
the chronic inflammatory disruption of the normal histologic picture in the focal
area within the prostate gland (Nickel et al. 1990). The deposition of this
antibody within the prostate gland creates the chronic inflammatory state and
perhaps implicates the immune system in the pathogenesis of the disease and
possibly the resulting clinical symptoms.

Diagnosis

The history and physical examination may suggest the diagnosis, but most signs
and symptoms of bacterial prostatitis and nonbacterial prostatitis may be
indistinguishable (Nickel 1989, 1991). The necessary diagnostic routine is difficult and time consuming; however, if it is not initiated at the first presentation,
and if the patient is started on antibiotics speculatively, it becomes almost
impossible to sort out a proper diagnosis and management plan at a later date
(Nickel 1992). The technique standardized by Meares and Stamey (1968) to
differentiate the prostatitis syndromes is based on a rigid, quantitative segmented bacteriologic localization procedure that remains the gold standard for
diagnosis. However, many or most urologists do not subject their patients with
suspected prostatitis routinely to these diagnostic techniques (Nickel 1991,
1992). The identifiable shortcomings or problems with our standardized diagnostic techniques include the following. (a) Prostatic secretions cannot be
obtained from all patients all the time, and the subsequent postprostatic
specimen (VB3) is difficult to interpret. (b) Prior antibiotic therapy has in-
variably been prescribed by the primary physician without first obtaining the
proper specimens, and this may mask subsequent attempts at bacterial localization. (c) It has recently been appreciated that the bacteria are firmly adherent to
the ductal epithelium and may not be shed in significant numbers into the
expressed prostatic fluid. (d) Patients with identified bacterial prostatitis may
not respond clinically to appropriate antibiotic therapy although a so-called
"bacteriologic cure" is obtained. (e) Some patients have excessive leukocytosis in
the expressed prostatic secretion but no significant bacteria present who have
significantly benefited and even been cured by antibiotic therapy. (f) Clinical
relapses of previously proven bacterial prostatitis are not always associated with
a positive expressed prostatic secretion culture. (g) The time and expense
required to carry out these very difficult procedures is substantial, and they
consistently provide extremely low yield (Nickel 1992).

Perhaps the evaluation of experimental prostatitis may allow us to develop
more sophisticated diagnostic techniques. Ling et al. (1990) found similar
difficulties in trying to correlate cultures of ejaculate, urine, urethral swab
specimens, and biopsy cultures of the prostate from dogs with suspected
prostatitis. Our research group has demonstrated in experimental prostatitis

that has been suboptimally treated that bacteria persist in the prostate gland even when they cannot be demonstrated in the prostatic secretion (Nickel, unpublished data). We (Nickel and Costerton 1991, 1992) recently demonstrated clinical confirmation of this generally held assumption that our accepted clinical diagnostic methods are not always adequate. Patients with proven chronic bacterial prostatitis who became clinically resistant to antibiotic therapy underwent rigorous diagnostic studies 4 weeks after the therapy was discontinued. In most cases a pure culture of the initial bacterial agent was obtained from perineal prostatic biopsies even when the prostatic secretion was sterile.

Research on the immune response in both clinical and experimental prostatitis studies has led to a greater understanding of the pathogenesis of this disease, and we believe that in the future it may allow more precise diagnosis of the etiologic agent. Preliminary studies by Shortliffe and Wehner (1986) have attempted to employ the defined immunologic reaction seen in the prostate to identify the most common bacterial pathogens; however, this work has never gone beyond the initial stages primarily because it could not be validated in an adequate animal or clinical model. Our research group is presently exploiting the reliable and consistent animal model previously described (Nickel 1990) to determine whether a simple immunologic diagnostic test can differentiate nonbacterial from bacterial prostatitis (Nickel, work in progress). Once validated in an experimental animal model of prostatitis under various parameters of inflammation and before and after treatment, the results may be able to be extrapolated into the clinical situation.

Treatment

The differential diagnosis of prostatitis remains a clinical dilemma; however, the real challenge to the physician is the difficulty in treating the inflamed prostate gland. Short- and long-term therapy with what appears to be excellent antibacterial drugs that remain effective in the treatment of most urinary tract infections appear unable reliably to obtain a long-term cure of chronic prostatitis, although the organisms occasionally cultured are highly sensitive to the particular antimicrobial agents used and even remain so at the end of treatment (Aagaard and Madsen 1991; Nickel and Olson 1991). Most human pharmacokinetic studies have analyzed prostatic fluid obtained by prostatic massage or ejaculate for drug content following oral or parenteral administration of various antibiotics; however, these methods have since been disputed because of the contamination with seminal fluid or urine containing high concentrations of antibiotics. Homogenized human prostatectomy specimens have also been analyzed for drug content following preoperative antibiotic loading; however, it is apparent that this method does not measure the concentration in prostatic secretions and certainly is not an adequate measure of prostatic tissue levels, particularly in the inflamed gland.

In the late 1960s and 1970s dog models were used to investigate prostatic secretion levels of various antibiotics. The vas deferens was divided and urine diverted by ureteral cannulation or suprapubic tube. Intravenous pilocarpine was used to stimulate copious secretion of pure prostatic fluid which could be collected uncontaminated by urine at the urethral meatus. This model allowed simultaneous measurement of plasma, urine, and prostatic secretion drug levels. In 1968 Winningham et al. systematically investigated the diffusion of antibiotics from the plasma into the prostatic secretion of normal dogs employing such a model and subsequently elaborated on the pharmacokinetic basis for the observed events. They concluded that the distribution of a drug in the prostatic interstitium and prostatic secretion depends on absorption, plasma protein binding, lipid solubility, innercompartmental pH gradient, the individual antibiotic, pK_a and biotransformation. Multiple modifications of this dog model were made by Baumueller and Madsen (1977) and many others, but unfortunately no really consistent methodology has developed in the field. Sharer and Fair (1982) have reviewed the various canine models used to quantitate antimicrobial drug diffusion, and from these particular types of studies a number of antibiotics (e.g., trimethoprim, erythromycin, quinolones) have been described as the most suitable drugs for the treatment of prostatitis.

Why do antibiotics not cure chronic bacterial prostatitis more consistently? The preponderance of evidence favors incomplete sterilization of prostatic fluid probably secondary to inadequate concentration of antimicrobial agents as the most important cause for therapeutic failure. This may be due to the simple fact that the prostatic intraductal compartment is entirely different in the inflamed human prostate than in the dog (Fair et al. 1979). Also, prostatic inflammation may be a focal phenomena, and pharmacokinetics based on the entire gland may not be relevant to the sporadic infected areas. Prostatic calculi or concretions that become secondarily infected may make eradication of infection almost impossible (similar to struvite renal calculi). To attempt to answer some of their questions, Baumueller and Madsen (1977) injected *E. coli* into the prostatic arterial system 1 week prior to antibiotic treatment to create an animal model with acute bacterial prostatitis; however, inflammatory changes were mainly in the interstitial tissue and not in the acini, presumably because of the iatrogenic hematogenous route of infection. The dog studies have helped us to determine some of the factors involved in conventional antibacterial pharmacokinetics in the prostate gland, but the data obtained in these particular studies should still be interpreted with caution. Our group is presently repeating similar pharmacokinetic studies in our consistent animal model of chronic prostatitis that develops after retrograde injection of pathogens and more closely resembles the focal and intraductal nature of human disease (Nickel et al. 1991). These and other studies may help us to explain the failure of antibiotic sterilization of the prostate gland in chronic bacterial prostatitis (although our initial work shows that prostatic secretions may become sterile despite persistence of bacteria within the focal inflamed areas of the gland). Until a totally acceptable animal model can be developed, drug research will have to be guided by extrapolation of data obtained from studies already reported in the literature.

Conclusion

Animal modeling of human disease, particularly human infectious diseases, is open to scepticism, criticism, and even misinterpretation. However, in the case of chronic bacterial prostatitis, where we have not been able to find the answer to the questions of etiology, diagnosis, and even treatment in decades of clinical research, experimental prostatitis in appropriate animal models may ultimately provide the key that will unlock the mysteries of this clinical dilemma.

References

Aagaard J, Madsen PO (1991) Bacterial prostatitis: new methods of treatment. Urology Suppl 37:4–8

Aronsson A, Dahlgren S, Gatenbeck L, Stromberg L (1988) Predictive sites of inflammatory manifestation in the prostate gland: an experimental study on nonbacterial prostatitis in the rat. Prostate 13:17–24

Baumueller A, Madsen PO (1977) Experimental bacterial prostatitis in dogs. Urol Res 5:211–213

Dilworth JP, Neal DE, Fussell EN, Roberts JA (1980) Experimental prostatitis in nonhuman primates. I. Bacterial adherence to the urethra. Prostate 17:227–231

Fair WR, Crane DB, Schiller N, Heston WDW (1979) Reappraisal of treatment in chronic bacterial prostatitis. J Urol 121:437–441

Gatenbeck L, Aronsson A, Dahlgran S, Johansson B, Stromberg L (1987) Stress stimuli-induced histopathological changes in the prostate: an experimental study in the rat. Prostate 11:69–76

Jantos C, Altmannsberger M, Weidner W, Schiefer HG (1990) Acute and chronic bacterial prostatitis due to E. coli: description of an animal model. Urol Res 18:207–211

Ling GV, Nyland TG, Kennedy PC, Hager DA, Johnson DL (1990) Comparison of two sample collection methods for quantitative bacteriologic culture of canine prostatic fluid. J Am Vet Med Assoc 196:1479–1482

Maglione W, Nardi A, Cranz C, Clavert A, Bollack C (1986) Acute vesiculitis and its prostatic complications caused by E. coli. Urol Res 14:265–266

Meares EM Jr, Stamey TA (1968) Bacteriologic localization patterns in bacterial prostatitis and urethritis. Invest Urol 5:492–518

Naslund MJ, Strandberg JD, Coffey DS (1988) The role of androgens and estrogens in the pathogenesis of experimental nonbacterial prostatitis. J Urol 140:1049–1053

Neal DE, Dilworth P, Kaack MB, Didier P, Roberts JA (1990) Experimental prostatitis in nonhuman primates. II. Ascending acute prostatitis. Prostate 17:233–239

Nickel JC (1989) Evaluation and management of the many syndromes of prostatitis. Can J Diagn 6:19–28

Nickel JC (1991) The prostatitis syndromes. A continuing enigma for the family physician. Can Fam Physician 37:921–928

Nickel JC (1992) New concepts in the pathogenesis and treatment of prostatitis. Curr Opin Urol 2:37–43

Nickel JC, Costerton JW (1991) Bacterial localization in antibiotic resistant bacterial prostatitis. J Urol 145:236A

Nickel JC, Costerton JW (1992) Coagulase-negative staphylococcus in chronic prostatitis. J Urol 147:398–401

Nickel JC, Olson ME (1991) Prostatitis: the enigma continues. Contemp Urol [Can] 1(4):4–12

Nickel JC, Olson ME, Barabas A, Benediktsson H, Dasgupta MK, Costerton JW (1990) Pathogenesis of chronic bacterial prostatitis in an animal model. Br J Urol 66:47–54

Nickel JC, Olson ME, Costerton JW (1991) Rat model of experimental bacterial prostatitis. Infection 19 Suppl 3:126–130

Nielsen DS, Golubjatnikov R, Dodge R, Madsen PO (1982) Chlamydial prostatitis in dogs: an experimental study. Urol Res 10:45–49

Pfau A (1986) Prostatitis: a continuing enigma. Urol Clin North Am 13:695–715

Sharer WCV, Fair WR (1982) The pharmacokinetics of antibiotic diffusion in chronic bacterial prostatitis. Prostate 3:139–148

Shortliffe LMD, Wehner N (1986) The characterization of bacterial and non-bacterial prostatitis by prostatic immunoglobulins. Medicine (Battimore) 65:399–414

Winningham DG, Nemoy NJ, Stamey TA (1968) Diffusion of antibiotics from plasma into prostatitic fluid. Nature 219–139

III. Acute Bacterial Prostatitis

Acute Prostatitis and Prostatic Abscess

W. Vahlensieck, Jr., and A.G. Hofstetter

According to the 1978 classification by Drach et al., the prostatic exprimation in acute bacterial prostatitis (ABP) shows an abundant amount of white cells (WBC) and bacterial culture shows typical pathogens. The prostate gland is very tender on palpation (Drach et al. 1978).

Prostatic abscess (PA) shows the same symptoms and findings. Fluctuation of the gland is quite often palpable. Demonstration of liquid areas within the gland by imaging procedures confirms the diagnosis.

Epidemiology

ABP accounts for 4% and PA for 3% of all cytologically confirmed inflammatory diseases of the prostate gland (Leistenschneider and Nagel 1978). Since the beginning of the antibiotic era, prostatic abscess formation has been rare because of declining gonococcal urethritis and associated stricture disease (Brawer 1992; Brawer and Stamey 1987; Dajani and O'Flynn 1968; Mariani et al. 1983; Meares 1986; Trapnell and Roberts 1970). Although microabscesses often develop early in the course of ABP, the appropriate use of modern antimicrobial agents generally eliminates the infection and prevents abscess formation (Meares 1986). Today the incidence of PA ranges between 0.5% and 2.5% of all patients admitted to hospital for prostatic disease and accounts for approximately 0.02% of urologic outpatients (Dajani and O'Flynn 1968; Pai and Bhat 1972; Trapnell and Roberts 1970). The incidence for the whole population is about 0.007‰ (Trapnell and Roberts 1970).

We have found 46 articles dealing with PA in the English literature since 1970, many reporting only one case. Although prostatic abscess may occur in patients of any age, men 50 years and older are predisposed for prostatic abscess (Meares 1986; Trapnell and Roberts 1970). In an analysis of 36 well-documented patients with PA since 1970 the average age was 56.25 years (Bartlett et al. 1978; Bergner et al. 1981; Brawer and Stamey 1987; Chia et al. 1986; Cytron et al. 1988; Dennis and Donohue 1985; Inoshita et al. 1983; Kadmon et al. 1986; Learmonth and Philp 1988; Lentino et al. 1984; Marans et al. 1991; Mariani et al. 1983; Mitchell and Blake 1972; Morrison et al. 1988; Papanicolaou et al. 1987; Rorvik and Daehlin 1989; Sohlberg et al. 1991; Sugao et al. 1986; Vaccaro et al. 1986;

Washecka and Rumancik 1985; Weinberg et al. 1985; Woo et al. 1987). Patients with PA in the antibiotic era were 20–30 years older than patients in the preantibiotic era (Cytron et al. 1988, Pai and Bhat 1972). The youngest patient reported in the literature was a 46-day-old infant with metastatic PA (Heyman and Lombardo 1962).

Etiology and Pathogenesis

Since gonococcal infections are rare today, most authors report gramnegative bacteria, especially *Escherichia coli*, as the most frequent cause of ABP, followed by staphylococci (Dajani and O'Flynn 1968; Kadmon et al. 1986; Meares 1980). Drach and Kohnen (1977) however found more gram-positive cocci than gram-negative organisms in ABP. ABP may also be caused by *Chlamydia trachomatis* (Bruce and Reid 1989). Systemic fungi and anaerobes are sporadically found in PA but not in ABP (Table 1) (Bartlett et al. 1978; Brawer and Stamey 1987; Dajani and O'Flynn 1968; Kadmon et al. 1986; Trapnell and Roberts 1970; Vahlensieck 1987; Youngen et al. 1967).

In 1931 Sargent and Irwin reported a 75% incidence of *Neisseria gonor-rhoeae* in 42 cases of PA. In the reviewed literature since 1970 only Pai and Bhat have reported a case of gonococcal PA (Pai and Bhat 1972). About 75% of the abscesses today are caused by coliform gramnegative organisms, mainly strains of *Escherichia coli*, followed by grampositive bacteria, mainly staphylococci (Kadmon et al. 1986; Meares 1986). Anaerobic organisms, especially *Bacteroides fragilis*, alone or in combination with coliforms or *Pseudomonas aeruginosa* and fungi have been implicated sporadically (Bartlett et al. 1986; Bergner et al. 1981; Inoshita et al. 1983; Kadmon et al. 1986; Meares 1986; Schwarz 1982; Vahlen-

Table 1. Bacterial spectrum in prostatic abscess ($n = 36$)

	n	%
Escherichia coli	19	53
Other Enterobacteriaceae	7	19
Gram positive/negative bacteria (systemic infection)	7	19
Anaerobia	6	17
Fungus	4	11
Mycobacterium tuberculosis	1	3
Neisseria gonorrhoeae	0	0

Numbers exceed 100% and $n = 36$ because of multiple reportings. From: Bartlett et al. (1978), Bergner et al. (1981), Brawer and Stamey (1987), Chia et al. (1986), Cytron et al. (1988), Dennis and Donohue (1985), Inoshita et al. (1983), Kadmon et al. (1986), Learmonth and Philp (1988), Lentino et al. (1984), Marans et al. (1991), Mariani et al. (1983), Mitchell and Blake (1972), Morrison et al. (1988), Papanicolaou et al. (1987), Rorvik and Daehlin (1989), Sohlberg et al. (1991), Sugao et al. (1986), Vaccaro et al. (1986), Washecka and Rumancik (1985), Weinberg et al. (1985), Woo et al. (1987)

sieck 1987). In 1987 Brawer and Stamey reported 15 cases of anaerobic prostatic abscess. Systemic mycosis caused by *Cryptococcus neoformans, Blastomyces dermatitidis, Coccidioides immitis,* or *Histoplasma capsulatum* can involve the prostate gland and cause PA (Bergner et al. 1981; Inoshita et al. 1983; Marans et al. 1991; Schwarz 1982; Vahlensieck 1987). *Candida albicans* may infect the prostate gland by ascending hematogenous route and rarely cause PA (Lentino et al. 1984; Vahlensieck 1987).

The route of infection in most cases is canalicular ascending with influx of infected urine into the prostatic ducts (Brawer and Stamey 1987; Kirby et al. 1982; Meares 1980, 1986; Trapnell and Roberts 1970). This is promoted especially in older patients by bladder outlet obstruction caused, for example, by neurogenic bladder, urolithiasis, carcinoma of the prostate and benign prostatic hyperplasia, urinary tract infection, adnexitis, or transurethral instrumentation including previous prostatectomy, prostate needle biopsy, or indwelling catheter (Bartlett et al. 1986; Bergner et al. 1981; Brawer and Stamey 1987; Chia et al. 1986; Cytron et al. 1988; Dennis and Donohue 1985; Inoshita et al. 1983; Kadmon et al. 1986; Learmonth and Philp 1988; Lentino et al. 1984; Marans et al. 1991; Mariani et al. 1983; Mitchell and Blake 1972; Morrison et al.1988; Pai and Bhat 1972; Papanicolaou et al. 1987; Rorvik and Daehlin 1989; Sohlberg et al. 1991; Steinhardt 1988; Sugao et al. 1986; Trapnell and Roberts 1970; Vaccaro et al. 1986; Trapnell and Roberts 1970; Vaccaro et al. 1986; Washecka and Rumancik 1985; Weinberg et al. 1985; Woo et al. 1987). At least

Table 2. Predisposing factors in prostatic abscess ($n = 127$)

	n	%
Urologic		
Bladder outlet obstruction	18	14
Urinary tract infection	16	13
Urethritis, prostatitis	6	5
Transurethral instrumentation, prostatic biospy	6	5
Urinary catheter	6	5
None	76	60
General		
Diabetes mellitus	32	25
Other immunosuppressive therapy or disease	6	5
Infectious focus	3	2
None	89	70

Numbers exceed 100% and $n = 127$ because of multiple reportings. From: Bartlett et al. (1978), Bergner et al. (1981), Brawer and Stamey (1987), Chia et al. (1986), Cytron et al. (1988), Dennis and Donohue (1985), Inoshita et al. (1983), Kadmon et al. (1986), Learmonth and Philp (1988), Lentino et al. (1984), Marans et al. (1991), Mariani et al. (1983), Mitchell and Blake (1972), Morrison et al. (1988), Pai and Bhat (1972), Papanicolaou et al. (1987), Rorvik and Daehlin (1989), Sohlberg et al. (1991), Steinhardt (1988), Sugao et al. (1986), Trapnell and Roberts (1970), Vaccaro et al. (1986), Washecka and Rumancik (1985), Weinberg et al. (1985), Woo et al. (1987)

50% of reported PA cases are a result of instrumentation or indwelling catheters (Meares 1980, 1986, 1991).

Gramnegative Enterobacteriaceae are the most common organisms involved in this entity (Brawer and Stamey 1987; Kadmon et al. 1986; Thornhill et al. 1987). In 8%–27%, metastatic hematogenous or lymphogenous spread or direct bacterial inoculation by transrectal biopsy or inflammatory disease of the rectum are causes of ABP or abscess formation (Brawer and Stamey 1987; Drach and Kohnen 1977; Hofstetter 1983; Kohnen and Drach 1979; Learmonth and Philp 1988; Meares 1980, 1986; Pai and Bhat 1972; Trapnell and Roberts 1970). Primary foci may be general infectious diseases such as melioidosis, typhus, salmonellosis, or systemic mycosis (Bergner et al. 1981; Heyman and Lombardo 1962; Inoshita et al. 1983; Learmonth and Philp 1988; Marans et al. 1991; Morrison et al. 1988; Pai and Bhat 1972; Schwarz 1982; Trapnell and Roberts 1970; Vahlensieck 1987; Woo et al. 1987). On the other hand, bacteria may spread from infected eye sockets, skin abscesses, or other localized foci (Trapnell and Roberts 1970). In these cases grampositive cocci such as staphylococci are found predominantly (Brawer 1992; Kadmon et al. 1986; Meares 1986; Youngen et al. 1967). Diabetes mellitus and other immunocompromising factors including end stage renal insufficiency, immunosuppressive therapy, recent antibiotic exposure, alcohol abuse, intravenous drug abuse, and hospitalization predispose for ABP and PA formation (Brawer 1992; Kadmon et al. 1986; Marans et al. 1991; Meares 1986; Pai and Bhat 1972; Thornhill et al. 1986; Youngen et al. 1967).

Pathology

In ABP within ducts, acini, and adjacent stroma neutrophilic granulocytes in variable numbers and debris are found. The ductal and acinar lining epithelium cells are necrotic (Leistenschneider and Nagel 1978; Petersen 1986). Most commonly small, localized microabscesses with destruction of prostatic glands and stroma are found (Drach and Kohnen 1977; Meares 1980; Petersen 1986). Less commonly, confluence of microabscesses is observed, forming PA (Petersen 1986). In PA, besides larger amounts of pus, multiple leukocytes are seen. Epithelial cell groups are small and exhibit unclear cell borders (Leistenschneider and Nagel 1978). Otherwise PA looks very similar to ABP (Leistenschneider and Nagel 1978). Prostatic fragments of benign nodular prostatic hyperplasia obtained by transurethral resection in 3.7% of cases contain areas with signs of ABP (Kohnen and Drach 1979). Further study is required to learn more about the etiology and clinical significance of such incidentally found foci of acute inflammation (Kohnen and Drach 1979; Petersen 1986).

PA may be unilocular or multilocular and may be limited only to the prostate gland. The dense capsule of the prostate may contain the abscess and favor spontaneous transurethral drainage (5% of cases) (Bartlett et al. 1986;

Bergner et al. 1981; Brawer and Stamey 1987; Chia et al. 1986; Cytron et al. 1988; Dennis and Donohue 1985; Inoshita et al. 1983; Kadmon et al. 1986; Learmonth and Philp 1988; Lentino et al. 1984; Marans et al. 1991; Mariani et al. 1983; Mitchell and Blake 1972; Morrison et al. 1988; Pai and Bhat 1972; Papanicolaou et al. 1987; Rorvik and Daehlin 1989; Sohlberg et al. 1991; Sugao et al. 1986; Trapnell and Roberts 1970; Vaccaro et al. 1986; Washecka and Rumancik 1985; Weinberg et al. 1985; Woo et al. 1987). The PA may, however, in 2–3% of cases extend out of the prostate into soft tissues of the pelvis. When it is confined, pus may collect around the seminal vesicles above the prostate in the subperitoneal space (Trapnell and Roberts 1970; Washecka and Rumancik 1985). Direct peritoneal invasion and subsequent peritonitis are unusual (Mitchell and Blake 1972). The anterior urogenital diaphragm usually prevents the infection from reaching the anterior perineum. However, the inflammation may extend along the pubovesical ligaments and spread to the prevesical fascia and invade the rectum. It may then extend to the posterior perineum by dissecting around the anus. If the infection invades the levator ani muscle, it may spread into the ischiorectal fossa. Thus, the sequelae of a prostatic abscess may be of such severity as to obscure the very origin of the abscess as well as impede an accurate and timely diagnosis (Washecka and Rumancik 1985). Perforation into the rectum occurs in 2% of cases (Bartlett et al. 1986; Bergner et al. 1981; Brawer and Stamey 1987; Chia et al. 1986; Cytron et al. 1988; Dennis and Donohue 1985; Inoshita et al. 1983; Kadmon et al. 1986; Learmonth and Philp 1988; Lentino et al. 1984; Marans et al. 1991; Mariani et al. 1983; Mitchell and Blake 1972; Morrison et al. 1988; Pai and Bhat 1972; Papanicolaou et al. 1987; Rorvik and Daehlin 1989; Sohlberg et al. 1991; Sugao et al. 1986; Trapnell and Roberts 1970; Vaccaro et al. 1986; Washecka and Rumancik 1985; Weinberg et al. 1985; Woo et al. 1987).

Symptoms

Symptoms of ABP and PA include (Hofstetter 1983; Hofstetter and Eisenberger 1986; Meares 1980, 1991; Rorvik and Daehlin 1989):

Pain
    Low back, suprapubic or infrapubic
    Perineal
Obstructive voiding symptoms
    Dysuria, urinary retention
Irritative voiding symptoms
    Frequency (diuria, nocturia), alguria
    Urgency, urge incontinence
Hematuria, urethral discharge

Epididymitis, hemospermia
Rectal tenesmi
Painful bowel movements
Fever, prostration, myalgia
Chills, arthralgia, malaise

Patients with ABP complain of sudden chills, fever often over 39°C, low back and perineal pain, painful bowel movements, urethral discharge, and hematuria plus irritative and obstructive voiding symptoms or complete urinary retention.

In some recent series fever has been found in only about 50% and rectal discomfort in only about 20% of cases (Meares 1986). Generalized malaise, prostration, arthralgias, and myalgias are also observed (Hofstetter 1983, 1987; Hofstetter and Eisenberger 1986; Meares 1986, 1991). The symptoms often recur or persist even after adequate antibiotic treatment of an infectious episode, indicating relapse (Dajani and O'Flynn 1968; Vaccaro et al. 1986; Weinberg et al. 1985). PA should be suspected after persisting or recurring symptoms in spite of appropriate antibiotic treatment of urinary tract infection or prostatitis (Dajani and O'Flynn 1968). The symptoms in prostatic abscess are very similar to those in ABP and therefore clinical differentiation very difficult (Dajani and O'Flynn 1968; Rorvik and Daehlin 1989). Today the clinical presentation is less dramatic (Cytron et al. 1988; Mitchell and Blake 1972; Sugao et al. 1986; Washecka and Rumancik 1985). Spontaneous rupture of the abscess into the perineum (2%–3%), rectum (2%), or urethra (5%) occurs only rarely in the antibiotic era (Cytron et al. 1988; Mitchell and Blake 1972; Sugao et al. 1986; Washecka and Rumancik 1985). Up to one-third of PA cases are accompanied by adenocarcinoma (Washecka and Rumancik 1985).

Findings

On rectal examination in ABP the gland characteristically is tender, warm, and swollen with partly or total indurations (Meares 1991). In this stage of disease prostatic massage and also endourologic procedures are contraindicated. This could lead to even more severe pain and possibly bacteremia (Brawer and Stamey 1987; Brawer 1992; Hofstetter and Eisenberger 1986; Hofstetter 1983; Meares 1991). In the asymptomatic form of ABP palpable indurations lead to a diagnostic biopsy or cytology and incidental finding of ABP.

PA, besides the findings mentioned in ABP shows a fluctuation during palpation in 21%–88% of cases (Brawer and Stamey 1987; Brawer 1992; Mariani et al. 1983; Pai and Bhat 1972; Trapnell and Roberts 1970; Youngen et al. 1967). In 36 well-documented patients since 1970 a fluctuation was reported in 53% of cases (Bartlett et al. 1986; Bergner et al. 1981; Brawer and Stamey 1987; Chia et al. 1986; Cytron et al. 1988; Dennis and Donohue 1985; Inoshita et al. 1983, Kadmon et al. 1986; Learmonth and Philp 1988; Lentino et al. 1984; Marans et al. 1991; Mariani et al. 1983; Mitchell and Blake 1972; Morrison et al. 1988; Papanicolaou et al. 1987; Rorvik and Daehlin 1989; Sohlberg et al. 1991; Sugao et al. 1986; Vaccaro et al. 1986; Washecka and Rumancik 1985; Weinberg et al. 1985; Woo et al. 1987). The gland is enlarged in 75% of the cases (Weinberg et al. 1985). Abscess encapsulation after a longer time may lead only to palpable tender nodes without fluctuation and to biopsy for differentiation of cancer. Prostatic abscess might also be an incidental finding in asymptomatic patients. Pus is expressed into the urethra on rectal examination in 3% of cases (Bergner et al. 1981; Cytron et al. 1988; Papanicolaou et al. 1987).

Besides the urologic findings the patient's cardiovascular, pulmonary, immunologic, and renal status should be ascertained to judge the patient's ability to deal with the ABP and PA and its sequelae (Brawer and Stamey 1987).

When prostatic secretions are obtained in ABP or PA, numerous white blood cells and fat-laden macrophages are seen microscopically. In most cases the causative organism is also found in the primary or midstream urine culture (Brawer 1992; Hofstetter 1983; Meares 1991). Also, pyuria and microhematuria are observed (Hofstetter 1983, 1987). Before the initiation of antimicrobial therapy some authors recommend blood cultures for both anaerobic and aerobic bacteria (Brawer 1992). In encapsulated PA the urinary findings may be normal.

When a diagnostic perineal puncture is performed to ascertain a prostatic abscess and its bacteriology, appropriate antimicrobial treatment should be started first to avoid septicemia (Brawer and Stamey 1987). Transrectal aspiration material might be contaminated by rectal bacterial flora (Brawer and Stamey 1987).

Serum parameters show nonspecific signs of inflammation such as leukocytosis, with a shift to the left in the complete blood cell count and rapid blood sedimentation rate (Brawer 1992; Hofstetter and Eisenberger 1986; Hofstetter 1983). Electrolyte values, blood urea nitrogen, creatinine, and serum glucose levels should be determined to evaluate the patient's general condition and possible risk factors (Brawer 1992).

A flat-plate X-ray film of the abdomen rules out radiopaque infectious calculi, having followed former generalized urinary tract infection episodes, and renal ultrasound concomitant hydroureteronephrosis (Brawer 1992). An intravenous pyelogram may also demonstrate ureteropyelectasis and elevation of the bladder base (Dajani and O'Flynn 1968; Mariani et al. 1983). An influx into the prostate gland during retrograde urethrocystography confirms preexisting inflammatory changes of the gland (Dennis and Donohue 1985). This examination should not be performed in the acute stage of the disease unless antibiotic treatment has been started.

If PA or ABP are suspected, endoscopy should be performed only after initiation of appropriate antibiotic treatment. Urethrocystoscopy does not give specific information of diagnostic value in PA (Cytron et al. 1988; Kadmon et al. 1986; Rorvik and Daehlin 1989) unless the abscess perforates during the examination (2% of cases) (Bartlett et al. 1978; Dennis and Donohue 1985). A diffuse inflammation of the urethral epithelial cells in the prostatic urethra may be seen.

Whenever prostatic abscess is suspected, the prostate gland should be examined by imaging procedures. The clinical diagnosis before the sonography and computed tomography era was made preoperatively in only 21%–88% of cases (Pai and Bhat 1972; Trapnell and Roberts 1970; Youngen et al. 1967). Computed tomography and magnetic resonance imaging are expensive and not universally available but reveal excellent results especially in prostatic abscess (Brawer 1992; Dennis and Donohue 1985; Kadmon et al. 1986; Marans et al. 1991; Meares et al. 1986; Vaccaro et al. 1986; Washecka and Rumancik 1985). On computed tomography, prostatic abscess shows well-defined areas of low attenuation after administration of intravenous contrast medium (− 19 to 26 HE) (Dennis and Donohue 1985; Rorvik and Daehlin 1989; Thornhill et al. 1987). The appearance may be singular or multiple (Thornhill et al. 1987). All lobes can be affected (Thornhill et al. 1987). Enhancing rims around the abscess are seen in 40%, prostatic calcifications in 20% (Thornhill et al. 1987). All PAs were identified correctly on computed tomography performed on ten patients (Brawer and Stamey 1987; Dennis and Donohue 1985; Kadmon et al. 1986; Lentino et al. 1984; Marans et al. 1991; Rorvik and Daehlin 1991; Vaccaro et al. 1986; Washecka and Rumancik 1985). On magnetic resonance imaging of PA the lesions display low signal intensity on short TE (T1) images, with increased signal intensity on long TE images (T2) (Papanicolaou et al. 1987).

Transrectal ultrasound is the method of choice in patients presenting with clinical signs of urinary tract or prostatic infection and having poor or partial response to antibiotic therapy (Cytron et al. 1988; Griffiths et al. 1984; Lee et al. 1986; Rorvik and Daehlin 1989). Well-documented signs in chronic clinical prostatitis are varying gland echogenicity, echolucent zones, capsular irregularity and thickening, ejaculatory duct echoes, calcifications, and periurethral irregularity (Doble and Carter 1989; Griffiths et al. 1984). In acute prostatitis less information is available. The gland appears enlarged, with increased antero-posterior diameter, a more rounded configuration and a symmetric capsule. Hypoechogenic areas due to edema and swelling may be seen, mainly in the peripheral zone. After effective treatment these changes may resolve (Brawer 1992; Doble and Carter 1989; Greenberg et al. 1981; Peeling and Griffiths 1984; Spirnack and Resnick 1984). With abscess formation focal anechoic or hypo-echoic zones with irregular internal echoes, septations, thickened wall, and indistinct borders with the surrounding parenchyma are typical patterns (Brawer 1992; Cytron et al. 1988; Greenberg et al. 1981; Papanicolaou et al. 1987; Sugao et al. 1986). There are two types of abscess, a distinct one and a more diffuse form (Chia et al. 1986; Sugao et al. 1986). Müllerian duct cyst, prostatic utricle cyst, cystic degeneration in benign prostatic hyperplasia, prostatic retention cyst, cavitary prostatitis, seminal vesicle or ejaculatory duct cysts, and necrotic or mucinous carcinoma may have similar sonographic features (Chia et al. 1986; Papanicolaou et al. 1987). All PAs were identified correctly on TRUS in

15 patients (Cytron et al. 1988; Papanicolaou et al. 1987; Rorvik and Daehlin 1989; Sohlberg et al. 1991; Sugao et al. 1986; Weinberg et al. 1985).

In ABP and PA there is marked accumulation on gallium-67 scan in the prostate gland. After micturition and bowel movements a barium enema and combined anterior and posterior views of the pelvic region may help to differentiate the accumulation in the prostate gland from bladder or bowel accumulation (Mariani et al. 1983; Sullivan et al. 1984). Only two reports on this subject have been published (Mariani et al. 1983; Sullivan et al. 1984).

Follow-up examinations every 2nd or 3rd day are required when imaging procedures are normal but clinical findings still suggest prostatic abscess (Brawer and Stamey 1987).

Differential Diagnosis

Prostatic congestion (prostatodynia) fails to show findings of acute inflammatory disease; there may also be perineal and low back pain and a tender prostate gland (Hofstetter 1983; Vahlensieck and Dworak 1988). The complaints in acute pyelonephritis are more directed towards the flanks, and the prostate is not tender on palpation (Hofstetter and Eisenberger 1986; Hofstetter 1983). Prostatic infarction, bladder outlet obstruction secondary to vesical calculi, benign prostatic hyperplasia or carcinoma with secondary bacterial cystitis, and acute perirectal abscess may have similar signs (Brawer and Stamey 1987; Brawer 1992; Pai and Bhat 1972; Youngen et al. 1967). Also urethritis, inflammation of the Cowper glands, and spermatocystitis must be ruled out (Brawer 1992; Brawer and Stamey 1987; Pai and Bhat 1972; Youngen et al. 1967). The differential diagnosis between acute prostatitis with sepsis and bladder outlet obstruction, and prostatic abscess is always difficult (Kadmon et al. 1986; Weinberg et al. 1985).

Medication Therapy: General Measures

The intense inflammation of the gland in ABP allows good penetration of antimicrobial drugs into the prostatic tissue even by those drugs which normally diffuse poorly into prostatic tissue and secretions (Table 3) (Hofstetter 1983, 1987; Madsen et al. 1993; Meares 1991; Stamey 1980). Following urine and blood cultures therapy with a fluoroquinolone, benzylpyrimidine/sulfonamide combination such as cotrimoxazole or especially in septic cases with an aminoglycoside/beta-lactam-antibiotic combination (preferably gentamicin or tobramycin/ampicillin or third-generation cephalosporins) should be started. Within 48 h after the fever subsides, patients who initially received intravenous

Table 3. Selection of antimicrobial therapy for acute bacterial prostatitis and prostatic abscess

Substance	Dose	Number of daily doses
Cotrimoxazole	960 mg	2
Trimethoprim	8–10 mg/kg	2–4
Ampicillin/gentamicin	2 g/1–5 mg/kg	4/3
Norfloxacin	400 mg	2
Ciprofloxacin	500 mg	2
Ofloxacin	200 mg	2

From: Meares (1991)

medication can usually be converted to oral preparation (Meares 1991). Following the acute treatment, oral long-term antibiotics should be used for a total duration of antibiotic therapy of 30–90 days to prevent relapse or chronic bacterial prostatitis (Brawer 1992; Cytron et al. 1988). Since anaerobic bacteria may be causative in PA in about 15% of the cases metronidazole, clindamycin, or chloramphenicol should be added whenever PA is suspected and primary therapy is not effective (Mariani et al. 1983).

Urethral catheter or transurethral instrumentation is contraindicated during the early treatment because of compromised prostatic gland drainage. All patients with urinary retention should have a punch suprapubic cystostomy under local anesthesia (Brawer and Stamey 1987; Hofstetter 1983; Hofstetter and Eisenberger 1986; Meares 1991). As auxiliary measures intravenous fluids, analgesics, antipyretics, spasmolytics, stool softeners, bed rest, sitz baths, and increased fluid intake (2–3 1/day) are recommended (Brawer 1992; Brawer and Stamey 1987; Hofstetter 1983, 1987; Hofstetter and Eisenberger 1986; Meares 1991). The number of patients with ABP who must be hospitalized because of possible sepsis and shock varies from author to author depending on the urinary retention or for need of parenterally administered antimicrobial therapy (Brawer and Stamey 1987; Hofstetter 1983; Hofstetter and Eisenberger 1986; Meares 1991). Patients with PA should be hospitalized in most cases (Weinberg et al. 1985).

Operative Therapy

ABP does not require operative therapy. Only if PA or chronic bacterial prostatitis as complications occur, one of the following procedures is indicated (Table 4). PA rarely is cured by antimicrobial therapy and other auxiliary measures mentioned for treatment of ABP (Meares 1991). Definitive abscess

Table 4. Drainage methods in prostatic abscess ($n = 60$)

	n	%
Transurethral unroofing	10	17
Transurethral resection	6	10
Transperineal aspiration	15	25
Finger guidance	4	27
Ultrasound guidance	11	73
With catheter drainage	2	13
With 1% neomycin irrigation	4	27
Transrectal incision	2	3
Transperineal incision	30	50

Numbers exceed 100% and $n = 60$ because of multiple reportings:
From: Bartlett et al. (1978), Bergner et al. (1981), Brawer and Stamey
(1987), Chia et al. (1986), Cytron et al. (1988), Dennis and Donohue
(1985), Inoshita et al. (1983), Kadmon et al. (1986), Learmonth and
Philp (1988), Lentino et al. (1984), Marans et al. (1991), Mariani et al.
(1983), Mitchell and Blake (1972), Morrison et al. (1988), Pai and Bhat
(1972), Papanicolaou et al. (1987), Rorvik and Daehlin (1989), Sohlberg et al. (1991), Sugao et al. (1986), Vaccaro et al. (1986), Washecka
and Rumancik (1985), Weinberg et al. (1985), Woo et al. (1987)

drainage is mandatory (Brawer 1992). The abscess should be treated operatively
by either transurethral unroofing with drainage of the abcess or formal resection
as introduced by Timberlake in 1938 (Brawer 1992; Hofstetter and Eisenberger
1986; Kadmon et al. 1986; Marans et al. 1991; Rorvik and Daehlin 1989;
Timberlake 1938; Trapnell and Roberts 1970; Vaccaro et al. 1986). A formal
resection may lead to bacteremia via the open venous sinus (Vaccaro
et al. 1986). Therefore transurethral unroofing seems to be the method of choice
(Kadmon et al. 1986; Trapnell and Roberts 1970). Computed tomography may
aid in planning the exact cut to unroof the abscess (Vaccaro et al. 1986). In 72
well-documented cases of PA ten (16.7%) underwent transurethral unroofing
and six (10.0%) formal transurethral resection of the prostate without evidence
of recurrence (Bartlett et al. 1986; Bergner et al. 1981; Brawer and Stamey 1987;
Chia et al. 1986; Cytron et al. 1988; Dennis and Donohue 1985; Inoshita et al.
1983; Kadmon et al. 1986; Learmonth and Philp 1988; Lentino et al.
1984; Marans et al. 1991; Mariani et al. 1983; Mitchell and Blake 1972; Morrison
et al. 1988; Pai and Bhat 1972; Papanicolaou et al. 1987; Rorvik and Daehlin
1989; Sohlberg et al. 1991; Sugao et al. 1986; Vaccaro et al. 1986; Washecka and
Rumancik 1985; Weinberg et al. 1985; Woo et al. 1987).

Perineal abscess puncture under digital or ultrasonic guidance with or
without pigtail catheter drainage and/or antibiotic irrigation is also possible
(Brawer and Stamey 1987; Hofstetter and Eisenberger 1986; Hofstetter 1983;
Kadmon et al. 1986; Marans et al. 1991; Rorvik and Dachlin 1989; Trapnell and

Roberts 1970; Vaccaro et al. 1986) after initiation of appropriate antibiotic therapy. In perineal abscess puncture, the patient's perineum is infiltrated with a 0.5% lidocaine solution. Then an 18-G spinal needle or a renal puncture needle is placed into the abscess under digital or ultrasonic guidance. After aspiration of all pus the abscess cavity may be filled with contrast medium. A J-tip guide wire is then passed into the abscess cavity and the needle is withdrawn. An 8.3-F pigtail catheter may finally be placed into the abscess cavity and left in place until all drainage ceases. The catheter is secured with a nonabsorbable stitch to the perineal skin (Kadmon et al. 1986). Percutaneous drainage has the advantages of being simple, and needing only local anesthesia. Especially in moribund patients not tolerating anesthesia for transurethral resection or anuric patients, it provides dependent drainage without urethral manipulation and indwelling catheter (Kadmon et al. 1986). Disadvantages are a small catheter lumen which might be obstructed by pus and possible damage to the perineal nerves by the procedure itself or by spreading infectious material.

In 72 well-documented cases of PA 15 patients (25.0%) underwent transperineal abscess aspiration (Bartlett et al. 1986; Bergner et al. 1981; Brawer and Stamey 1987; Chia et al. 1986; Cytron et al. 1988; Dennis and Donohue 1985; Inoshita et al. 1983; Kadmon et al. 1986; Learmonth and Philp 1988; Lentino et al. 1984; Marans et al. 1991; Mariani et al. 1983; Mitchell and Blake 1972; Morrison et al. 1988; Pai and Bhat 1972; Papanicolaou et al. 1987; Rorvik and Daehlin 1989; Sohlberg et al. 1991; Sugao et al. 1986; Vaccaro et al. 1986; Washecka and Rumancik 1985; Weinberg et al. 1985; Woo et al. 1987). Three patients (20%) needed a second aspiration, five (33.3%) another second procedure (two transurethral resection, two open perineal abscess incision, one spontaneous rectal perforation after transperineal abscess aspiration) because of failure. Transrectal abscess incision or aspiration was used in only two of 60 cases (3.3%) (Weinberg et al. 1985). Because of possible contamination by the rectal bacterial flora the transrectal route should be used only in perirectally perforated PA which might be difficult to drain completely transurethrally or perineally (Weinberg et al. 1985). Formal immediate perineal incision with abscess drainage, originally proposed as the method of choice and used in 50% (30/60) of patients, should be performed only in desperate cases because of possible damage to the neurovascular bundle leading to erectile impotence (Bartlett et al. 1986; Bergner et al. 1981; Brawer and Stamey 1988; Chia et al. 1986; Cytron et al. 1988; Dennis and Donohue 1985; Inoshita et al. 1983; Kadmon et al. 1986; Learmonth and Philp 1988; Lentino et al. 1984; Marans et al. 1991; Mariani et al. 1983; Mitchell and Blake 1972; Morrison et al. 1988; Pai and Bhat 1972; Papanicolaou et al. 1987; Rorvik and Daehlin 1989; Sohlberg et al. 1991; Sugao et al. 1986; Vaccaro et al. 1986; Washecka and Rumancik 1985; Weinberg et al. 1985; Woo et al. 1987). Four of 30 patients (13%) after perineal PA drainage needed a second procedure for definitive cure (Pai and Bhat 1972).

In conclusion, transurethral unroofing of PA is the method of choice in PA limited to the prostate gland. In poor risk patients or anuric patients transperineal aspiration with ultrasound guidance should be performed. In perforated abscesses or recurrence open abscess drainage is mandatory.

Complications

With sufficient therapy chronic bacterial prostatitis can be prevented in most cases of ABP (Brawer and Stamey 1987; Meares 1991). ABP may otherwise also lead to urinary retention, cystitis, pyelonephritis, urosepticemia, epididymoorchitis, and prostatic abscess, especially in non-compliant patients (Dajani and O'Flynn 1968; Fowler 1987; Meares 1986, 1991; Trapnell and Roberts 1970).

PA may perforate spontaneously into the rectum, urethra, or the perineal region (Hofstetter 1983). In a literature review Mitchell and Blake, including mostly patients of the preantibiotic era, reported an incidence of spontaneous rupture of PA to the urethra in 19% (30/162) of the cases, to the rectum in 3% (5/162), and into the perineum in 2% (4/162) (Mitchell and Blake 1972). They reported only two cases with peritonitis, indicating extension of the PA through the tough fascia of Denonvilliers; both patients died (Mitchell and Blake 1972). Trapnell and Roberts (1970) reported on a 3% incidence of abscess penetration to the ischiorectal fossa and a 1% incidence of concomitant scrotal abscess. Pai and Bhat reported a fatal case of development of an epidural abscess with bacterial spreading to the epidural space via Batson's system of veins (Pai and Bhat 1972). When not treated adequately, total urinary incontinence caused by necrosis of the complete prostate gland and internal sphincter and distorsion of the external sphincter by scars as a late sequela may occur (Duvie 1988).

In the preantibiotic era mortality in PA ranged from 6 to 30% (Woo et al. 1987). The mortality from prostatic abscess has decreased following the introduction of antibiotic therapy to 3 to 16% (Cytron et al. 1988; Dajani and O'Flynn 1968; Pai and Bhat 1972; Trapnell and Roberts 1970; Youngen et al. 1967). Prostatic abscess may recur if definitive treatment after diagnostic puncture is delayed (see "Operative therapy") (Lentino et al. 1984; Mariani et al. 1983).

Follow-up

One week after ending antibiotic treatment a check-up according to Meares and Stamey should determine cessation of the bacterial prostatitis (Meares and Stamey 1968; Stamey 1980). If bacteria are still found another antibiotic course for 6 weeks is indicated (Brawer and Stamey 1987). After surgical drainage of PA symptomatic improvement occurs within 24–48 h (Weinberg et al. 1985). Success of prostatic abscess drainage should be followed by long-term transrectal ultrasound and culture check-up (Brawer 1992; Brawer and Stamey 1987; Cytron et al. 1988). A formal resection of the prostate is not mandatory in all cases after transurethral abscess unroofing (Vaccaro et al. 1986). It seems reasonable to give low-dose, long-term antibiotic prophylaxis after surgical PA drainage for about 3 months. This is mandatory if *Pseudomonas pseudomallei* is the causative agent (Woo et al. 1987).

References

Bartlett JG, Weinstein WM, Gorbach SL (1978) Prostatic abscesses involving anaerobic bacteria. Arch Intern Med 138:1369–1371

Bergner DM, Kraus SD, Duck GB, Lewis R (1981) Systemic blastomycosis presenting with acute prostatic abscess. J Urol 126:132–133

Brawer MK (1992) Acute prostatitis and prostatic abscess. In: Drach GW (ed) Common problems in infections and stones. Mosby, Baltimore, pp 99–105

Brawer MK, Stamey TA (1987) Prostatic abscess owing to anaerobic bacteria. J Urol 138:1254–1255

Bruce AW, Reid G (1989) Prostatitis associated with Chlamydia trachomatis in 6 patients. J Urol 142:1006–1007

Chia JK, Longfield RN, Cook DH, Flax BL (1986) Computed axial tomography in the early diagnosis of prostatic abscess. Am J Med 81:942–944

Cytron S, Weinberger M, Pitlik SD, Servadio C (1988) Value of transrectal ultrasonography for diagnosis and treatment of prostatic abscess. Urology 32:454–458

Dajani AM, O'Flynn JD (1968) Prostatic abscess. A report of 25 cases. Br J Urol 40:736–739

Dennis MA, Donohue RE (1985) Computed tomography of prostatic abscess. J Comput Assist Tomogr 9:201–202

Doble A, Carter S (1989) Ultrasonographic findings in prostatitis. Urol Clin North Am 16:763–772

Drach GW, Kohnen PW (1977) Prostatitis. In: Tannenbaum M (ed) Urologic pathology: the prostate. Lea and Febiger, Philadelphia, p 157

Drach GW, Meares EM, Fair WR, Stamey TA (1978) Classification of benign diseases associated with prostatic pain: prostatitis or prostatodynia? J Urol 120:266

Duvie SO (1988) Bacterial prostatitis: an unusual cause of total urinary incontinence and its surgical management. J Urol 139:139–141

Fowler JE (1987) Prostatitis. In: Gillenwater JY, Grayhack JT, Howard SS (eds) Adult and pediatric urology. Year Book Medical Publishers, Chicago, pp 1220–1244

Greenberg M, Neiman HL, Brandt TD, Falkowski W, Carter M (1981) Ultrasound of the prostate. Radiology 141:757–762

Griffiths CJ, Crooks AJR, Buck AC, Roberts EE, Evans KT, Thomas PJ, Peeling WB (1984) The ultrasonic appearance of prostatic infection. Clin Radiol 35:343–345

Heyman A, Lombardo LJ Jr (1962) Metastatic prostatic abscess with report of a case in a newborn infant. J Urol 87:174–177

Hofstetter AG (1983) Urethro-Adnexitis des Mannes: Urethritis, Prostatitis und Vesikulitis. In: Stille W, Schilling A (eds) Infektionen des Harntraktes. Zuckschwerdt, Munich, pp 79–88

Hofstetter AG (1987) Therapie der Urethro-Adnexitis. Fortschr Antimikrob Antineoplast Chemother 6–10:2219–2221

Hofstetter AG, Eisenberger F (1986) Urologie für die Praxis. Bergmann, Munich, pp 109, 116

Inoshita T, Youngberg GA, Boelen LJ, Langston J (1983) Blastomycosis presenting with prostatic involvement: report of 2 cases and review of the literature. J Urol 130:160–162

Kadmon D, Ling D, Lee JKT (1986) Percutaneous drainage of prostatic abscesses. J Urol 135:1259–1260

Kirby RS, Lowe D, Bultitude MI, Shuttleworth KED (1982) Intraprostatic urinary reflux: an aetiological factor in abacterial prostatitis. Br J Urol 54:729–731

Kohnen PW, Drach GW (1979) Patterns of inflammation in prostatic hyperplasia: a histologic and bacteriologic study. J Urol 121:755–760

Learmonth DJ, Philp NH (1988) Salmonella prostatic abscess. Br J Urol 61:163

Lee F Jr, Lee F, Solomon H, Straub WH, McLeary RD (1986) Sonographic demonstration of prostatic abscess. J Ultrasound Med 5:101–102

Leistenschneider W, Nagel R (1978) Zytologische Diagnose und Klassifizierung entzündlicher Prostataerkrankungen. Aktuel Urol 9:185–193

Lentino JR, Zielinski A, Stachowski M, Cummings JE, Maliwan N, Reid RW (1984) Prostatic abscess due to Candida albicans. J Infect Dis 149:282

Madsen PO, Drescher P, Gasser TC (1993) Experimental and clinical pharmacokinetic studies and models. Basis for antibacterial treatment. In: Weidner W, Schiefer HG, Madsen PO (eds) Prostatitis. Springer Berlin Heidelberg New York, pp 110–122

Marans HY, Mandell W, Kislak JW, Starrett B, Moussouris HF (1991) Prostatic abscess due to Histoplasma capsulatum in the acquired immunodeficiency syndrome. J Urol 145:1275–1276

Mariani AJ, Jacobs LD, Clapp PR, Hariharan A, Stams UK, Hodges CV (1983) Emphysematous prostatic abscess: diagnosis and treatment. J Urol 129:385–386

Meares EM Jr (1980) Prostatitis syndromes: new perspectives about old woes. J Urol 123:141

Meares EM Jr (1986) Prostatic abscess. J Urol 136:1281–1282

Meares EM Jr (1991) Prostatitis. Med Clin North Am 75:405–424

Meares EM, Stamey TA (1968) Bacteriologic localization patterns in bacterial prostatitis and urethritis. Invest Urol 5:492–518

Mitchell RJ, Blake JRS (1972) Spontaneous perforation of prostatic abscess with peritonitis. J Urol 107:622–623

Morrison RE, Lamb AS, Craig DB, Johnson WM (1988) Melioidosis: a reminder. Am J Med 84:965–967

Pai MG, Bhat HS (1972) Prostatic abscess. J Urol 108:599–600

Papanicolaou N, Pfister RC, Stafford SA, Parkhurst EC (1987) Prostatic abscess: imaging with transrectal sonography and MR. AJR 149:981–982

Peeling WB, Griffiths GJ (1984) Imaging of the prostate by ultrasound. J Urol 132:217–224

Petersen RO (1986) Urologic pathology. Lippincott, Philadelphia, pp 600–601

Rorvik J, Daehlin L (1989) Prostatic abscess: imaging with transrectal ultrasound. Scand J Urol Nephrol 23:307–308

Sargent JC, Irwin R (1931) Prostatic abscess: clinical study of 42 cases. Am J Surg 11:334–337

Schwarz J (1982) Mycotic prostatitis. Urology 19:1–5

Sohlberg OE, Chetner M, Ploch N, Brawer MK (1991) Prostatic abscess after transrectal ultrasound guided biopsy. J Urol 146:420–422

Spirnack JP, Resnick MI (1984) Transrectal ultrasonography. Urology 23:461–467

Stamey TA (1980) Pathogenesis and treatment of urinary tract infections. Williams and Wilkins, Baltimore

Steinhardt GF (1988) Prostatic suppuration and destruction in patients with myelodysplasia: a newly recognized entity. J Urol 140:1002–1006

Sugao H, Takiuchi H, Sakurai T (1986) Transrectal longitudinal ultrasonography of prostatic abscess. J Urol 136:1316–1317

Sullivan WT, Rosen PR, Weiland FL, Ritchey ML (1984) Prostatic uptake of Ga-67. Radiology 152:537

Thornhill BA, Morehouse HT, Coleman P, Hoffman-Tretin JC (1987) Prostatic abscess: CT and sonographic findings. AJR 148:899–900

Timberlake G (1938) An electro-prostatome; relief of prostatic abscesses and acute obstructive prostatitis by transurethral prostatomy. J Urol 40:343–345

Trapnell J, Roberts M (1970) Prostatic abscess. Br J Surg 57:565–569

Vaccaro JA, Belville WD, Kiesling VJ, Davis R (1986) Prostatic abscess: computerized tomography scanning as an aid to diagnosis and treatment. J Urol 136:1318–1319

Vahlensieck W Jr (1987) Mykosen des Urogenitaltraktes. Urologe [B] 27:151–156

Vahlensieck W, Dworak O (1988) Abgrenzung der rezidivierenden Prostatakongestion von der chronischen Prostatitis. Helv chir Acta 55:293–296

Washecka R, Rumancik WM (1985) Prostatic abscess evaluated by serial computed tomography. Urol Radiol 7:54

Weinberg M, Pitlik SD, Rabinovitz M, Morduchowicz G, Rosenfeld JB, Cytron S, Servadio C (1985) Per-rectal ultrasonography for diagnosis of and guide to drainage of prostatic abscess. Lancet 2:772

Woo ML, Chan PSF, French GL (1987) A case of melioidosis presenting with prostatic abscess in Hong Kong. J Urol 137:120–121

Youngen R, Mahoney SA, Persky L (1967) Prostatic abscess. Surg Gynec & Obst 124:1043–1046

IV. Chronic Bacterial Prostatitis

Etiology, Pathogenesis, and Inflammatory Reactions in Chronic Bacterial Prostatitis

A.J. Schaeffer

Prostatitis is one of the commonly encountered inflammatory diseases in urologic practice. Inflammation of the prostate gland may be due to bacterial or nonbacterial causes. Healthy patients show a minimal amount of inflammation in prostatic secretions. Evaluation of a patient with prostatitis requires actual determination of the number of white blood cells in the prostatic fluid so that patients with elevated numbers of white cell counts, that is, with prostatitis, can be separated from those without prostatitis.

Definition of Prostatitis

The definition of prostatitis is based on determination of the degree of inflammation that is found in normal prostatic fluid. This is done by microscopic examination of expressed prostatic fluid and by counting the number of white blood cells per high-power field. It is important to obtain prostatic fluid carefully because white blood cells from the foreskin or urethra can contaminate the expressed prostatic fluid and give a false impression of inflammation. Therefore, prior to collecting fluid the foreskin should be retracted and the area carefully washed. The patient should then be asked to urinate and the urethral specimen, that is, the first 10 ml urine, collected for urinalysis. If there is any evidence of inflammation in the first 10 ml voided urine, the patient has urethritis, and assessment of prostatic fluid inflammation is not valid. Similarly, the patient's midstream urine specimen should be analyzed. Evidence of cystitis, as determined by white blood cells in the midstream urine specimen, invalidates any assessment of prostatic fluid for inflammation. If a patient does have urethritis or cystitis, he must be treated with appropriate antimicrobial therapy, and a sufficient time must be allowed to wait for the inflammatory reaction to subside.

Collection of Specimen

After examination of the urine, the prostate gland should be massaged gently and expressed prostatic secretions collected on a slide as they emerge from the urethral meatus. A cover slip should then be placed on top of the expressed prostatic secretions and microscopic examination of the expressed prostatic fluid performed to determine the number of white blood cells per high-power field. Available data suggest that white blood cells are rarely present in normal prostatic fluid. We studied 119 consecutive patients with no history, symptoms, or physical findings (excluding prostatic fluid evaluation) of urinary tract inflammation, normal prostate glands by digital examination, and fewer than two white blood cells per high-power field in the first 10 ml voided urine and no or insignificant growth on urine culture (Schaeffer et al. 1981) (Fig. 1). Of these patients, 31 were judged to have no urologic disease, and they had prostatic fluid containing 0.7 ± 0.41 white blood cells per high-power field, and 88, with a variety of noninflammatory urologic diseases, had 3.8 ± 0.83 white blood cells per high-power field in the prostatic fluid. There were two white blood cells or fewer per high-power field observed in 97% of the patients with no urologic disease and in 75% with noninflammatory urologic disease and normal prostatic glands by digital examination. Only 13 of the 119 patients in these two groups had 10 white blood cells or more per high-power field. Similar results have been reported (Blacklock 1969; Anderson and Weller 1969). It therefore appears that clinically significant inflammation is present when prostatic fluid contains 10 or more white blood cells per high-power field.

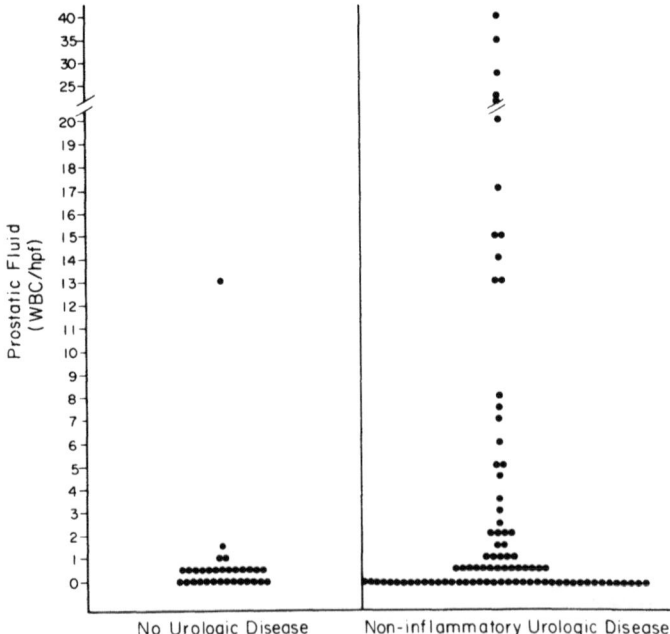

Fig. 1. White blood cell count per high-power field (*WBC/hpf*) in prostatic fluid in patients with no urologic disease (*n* = 31) and in patients with noninflammatory urologic diseases (*n* = 88). (From Schaeffer et al. 1981)

Prostatic inflammation also can be assessed by identifying changes in biochemical indicators of epithelial cellular damage. Lactate dehydrogenase (LDH) is an enzyme that reversibly catalyzes the reduction of pyruvate to lactate in the presence of nicotinamide adenine dinucleotide. Electrophoretic separation and semiquantitation of LDH have identified isoenzyme fractions 1 through 5. One of the characteristics of LDH is a shift to predominantly LDH-5 in the presence of malignancy or inflammation (Goldman et al. 1964; Carjaval et al. 1975). Previous studies have shown that ratios of LDH-5/LDH-1 in prostatic fluid are above 2 in 80% of patients with identifiable prostatic malignancy, in more than 10% of patients with benign prostatic hyperplasia, and in many patients with prostatitis (Hein et al. 1975; Grayhack et al. 1977a, b).

We have assessed the degree of inflammation in consecutive prostatic fluid specimens from patients without urinary tract disease and from those with symptoms or findings of infectious or noninfectious urologic abnormalities. The data suggest that white blood cells and high LDH-5/LDH-1 ratios are frequently associated with clinically significant disorders, indicating that cellular damage from noninfectious agents or conditions can cause or be associated with prostatitis.

Causes of Elevated White Blood Cell Count

The causes of elevated white blood cell count may be transient or permanent. Transient causes include ejaculation, urethritis, or acute cystitis or prostatitis. Chronic or long-standing inflammation is due to chronic bacterial prostatitis or so-called nonbacterial prostatitis, which may be due to as yet unrecognized infectious diseases or other conditions that could cause increased white cell counts, for example, infertility.

Etiology and Pathogenesis of Bacterial Prostatitis

Bacterial prostatitis is caused by the same bacteria that cause acute urinary tract infection and include *Escherichia coli, Klebsiella, Enterobacter*, and other *Enterobacteriaceae*. Gram-positive organisms, such as *Enterococcus faecalis* and *Staphylococcus epidermidis* are uncommon causes of acute bacterial prostatitis. *Pseudomonas* and other nosocomial strains should be suspected if the patient has recently had instrumentation, particularly in a hospital setting. The pathogenesis of bacterial prostatitis is unknown. Presumably ascending urethral infection, after a vaginal or rectal inoculation of the urinary meatus during sexual intercourse, plays an important role. Direct extension or lymphatic spread of fecal micro-organisms, as well as hematogenous spread, are also possible routes of infection. Some investigators have postulated that reflux of urine into the prostate ducts can cause prostatic calculi because the stones contain constituents commonly found in the urine but foreign to prostatic secretions. These stones are very prevalent in men over the age of 50 and usually produce no symptoms. However, if bacteria become entrapped with the stones, they may act as a nidus for bacteria, protecting them from the action of the antimicrobial drug.

Chronic Bacterial Prostatitis

This is a subtle disease characterized by a relatively asymptomatic period between episodes of recurrent bacteriuria. It is impossible to diagnose by physical examination. It is caused by small numbers of bacteria in the prostatic fluid and may be difficult to eradicate with antimicrobial therapy. Most patients are asymptomatic until they have recurrent urinary tract infections, a hallmark of this condition. Bacterial lower urinary tract localizations are a prerequisite for antimicrobial therapy.

The prostatic fluid shows increased numbers of white blood cells, and frequently large oval brown bodies (macrophages) are also identified. The inflammatory response may persist independent of bacteriologic response. Patients can be cured of the bacterial element of the chronic bacterial prostatitis and continue to have white blood cells in their prostatic fluid. Conversely, the white blood cell count may diminish despite persistence of bacteria in the prostate gland.

Treatment of chronic bacterial prostatitis with trimethoprim introduce: sulfamethoxazole or the fluoroquinolones can achieve cure rates in the range of 30%–70%. If antimicrobial therapy is not effective in curing the patient, long-term suppressant antimicrobial therapy must be utilized to prevent symptomatic urinary tract infections. Alternatively, the infected tissue may be resected transurethrally or, if cancer is present, a prostatectomy performed to achieve a cure.

Nonbacterial Prostatitis

Nonbacterial prostatitis, by definition, is not due to the common uropathogens. It is the most common form of prostatitis syndrome, approximately eight times more common than bacterial prostatitis. Usually the symptoms, physical findings, and microscopic appearance of the prostatic expressates in nonbacterial prostatitis and chronic bacterial prostatitis are indistinguishable. However, in patients with nonbacterial prostatitis, typically there is no history of urinary tract infection, and results of localization cultures are negative. The patient with nonbacterial prostatitis can be characterized by obstructive voiding symptoms, pain in the perineum or urethra, pelvis or scrotum, or low back area. However, approximately one-third of all patients with nonbacterial prostatitis are asymptomatic.

The possibility that *Chlamydia, Ureaplasma,* or *Mycoplasma* play a role in the etiology of nonbacterial prostatitis is controversial. Most investigators have found that *Mycoplasma* and *Ureaplasma* are not causative agents in nonbacterial prostatitis (Berger et al. 1989; Mårdh and Colleen 1975; Mårdh et al. 1978; Meares 1973). In 1983, however, Brunner et al. found a tenfold, or greater, increase in quantitative counts of *Ureaplasma urealyticum* in prostatic cultures compared with urethral cultures in 82 (13.7%) of 597 patients who appeared to have nonbacterial prostatitis. Most of these patients were said to respond favorably to tetracycline. Until culture results are substantiated by demonstration of antigen-specific immune response in the prostatic secretions, however, *Ureaplasma urealyticum* remains an unconfirmed pathogen in prostatitis.

Chlamydia trachomatis is also a controversial cause of this condition. Berger et al. (1989) and Mårdh and Colleen (1975) studied 50 or more patients with nonbacterial prostatitis and found little or no evidence that *C. trachomatis* is an etiologic agent. Poletti et al. (1985), however, performed transrectal aspiration biopsies of the prostate in 30 men with nonbacterial prostatitis and reported isolating *C. trachomatis* in tissue cultures from 10 (33%). In an accompanying editorial Schachter (1985) expressed concern about the authors' methods of identifying *Chlamydia* and the observation that all 30 men had positive urethral cultures for *Chlamydia*. He raised the questions about specimen contamination. Shortliffe and Wehner (1986) and Shortliffe et al. (1985) detected insignificant antigen-specific antibody elevations against *Chlamydia* in the prostatic secretion of patients with nonbacterial prostatitis. No unequivocal evidence therefore exists to support the etiologic role of *Chlamydia* for nonbacterial prostatitis. *Chlamydia* therefore, must play an insignificant role in this condition.

The possibility exists that urine refluxing into the prostatic ducts, particularly if it contains strong antimicrobials such as the fluoroquinolones or tetracycline, could conceivably lead to inflammation of the prostate; however, this has not been demonstrated scientifically. Many patients do have prostatic calculi with inflammation and are asymptomatic. Others have prostatic calculi without inflammation. The interaction is asymptomatic. The interaction is probably complex and warrants further study.

Prostatodynia (Pelviperineal Pain)

It should be clear from the above that prostatic fluid does not normally contain white blood cells. Even in the presence of white blood cells the patient may or may not be symptomatic. Therefore the relationship of pain in and around the prostate and inflammation is unclear. Attempts to implicate the prostate as the cause of the vague complex of symptoms associated with prostatodynia is appealing but may be misleading. Particularly in the absence of inflammation, it is unwise to assume that the prostate is the cause of the patient's symptoms. Other systems, such as musculoskeletal or gastrointestinal, may cause these symptoms. Careful evaluation of these structures is indicated.

Summary

Prostatic inflammation is rarely found in healthy individuals. Care must be taken to collect specimens to prevent contamination of prostatic fluid. Acute causes of inflammation, such as urethritis or intercourse, should be recognized and the diagnosis of prostatitis not applied to these patients, unless these factors are eliminated. Chronic inflammation, due to bacterial infections or commonly to nonbacterial causes, may be difficult to treat. If bacterial infections are present, long-term antimicrobial therapy is recommended and is effective in approximately 70% of patients. In the absence of infection, antimicrobial therapy should not be utilized and, in fact, may cause some inflammation and symptoms. Supportive therapy, including analgesics and anti-inflammatory drugs, is recommended and has varying results.

References

Anderson RU, Weller C (1979) Prostatic secretion leukocyte studies in nonbacterial prostatitis (prostatosis). J Urol 121:292–294
Berger RE, Krieger JN, Kessler D, Ireton RC, Close C, Holmes KK, Roberts PL (1989) Case–control study of men with suspected chronic idiopathic prostatitis. J Urol 141:328–331
Blacklock NJ (1969) Some observations on prostatitis. In: Williams DC, Briggs MH, Stanford M (eds) Advances in the study of the prostate. Heinemann, London, pp 37–55
Brunner H, Weidner W, Schiefer HG (1983) Studies on the role of Ureaplasma urealyticum and Mycoplasma hominis in prostatitis. J Infect Dis 147:807–813
Carvajal HF, Passey RB, Berger M, Travis LB, Lorentz WB (1975) Urinary lactic dehydrogenase isoenzyme 5 in the differential diagnosis of kidney and bladder infections. Kidney Int 8(3):176
Goldman RD, Kaplan NO, Hall TC (1964) Lactic dehydrogenase in human neoplastic tissue. Cancer Res 24:389
Grayhack JT, Wendel EF, Lee C, Oliver L (1977a) Analysis of prostatic fluid in prostatic disease. Cancer Treat Rep 61:205
Grayhack JT, Wendel EF, Lee C, Oliver L, Cohen E (1977b) Lactate dehydrogenase isoenzymes in human prostatic fluid: an aid in recognition of malignancy? J Urol 118:204
Hein RC, Grayhack JT, Goldberg E (1975) Prostatic fluid lactic dehydrogenase isoenzyme patterns of prostatic cancer and hyperplasia. J Urol 113:511
Mårdh P-A, Colleen S (1975) Search for uro-genital tract infections in patients with symptoms of prostatitis. Studies on aerobic and strictly anaerobic bacteria, mycoplasma, fungi, trichomonads and viruses. Scand J Urol Nephrol 9:8–16
Mårdh P-A, Ripa KT, Colleen S et al. (1978) Role of Chlamydia trachomatis in non-acute prostatitis. Br J Vener Dis 54:330–334

Meares EM Jr (1973) Bacterial prostatitis versus "prostatosis": a clinical and bacteriological study. JAMA 224:1372–1375

Poletti F, Medici MC, Menozzi MG, Sacchini P, Stagni G, Toni M (1985) Isolation of Chlamydia trachomatis from the prostatic cells in patients affected by nonacute abacterial prostatitis. J Urol 134:691–693

Schachter J (1985) Is Chlamydia trachomatis a cause of prostatitis (Editorial)? J Urol 134:711

Schaeffer AJ, Wendel AJ, Dunn JK, Grayhack JT (1981) Prevalence and significance of prostatic inflammation. J Urol 125:215–219

Shortliffe LMD, Wehner N (1986) The characterization of bacterial and nonbacterial prostatitis by prostatic immunoglobulins. Medicine (Baltimore) 65:399–414

Shortliffe LMD, Elliott KM, Sellers RG et al. (1985) Measurement of chlamydial and ureaplasma antibodies in serum and prostatic fluid of men with nonbacterial prostatitis (Abstr). J Urol 133 (42):276A

The Treatment of Chronic Bacterial Prostatitis: Principles and Management

A. Pfau

Introduction

Chronic bacterial prostatitis (CBP) is a subtle disease, often insidious in its onset, that challenges the acumen as well as the patience and determination of every urologist, when it comes to cure this disease. However, CBP is a clinical entity accurately defined by two basic features: recurrent urinary tract infections (UTIs) and persistence of gram-negative enterobacteria, mainly *Escherichia coli*, in the prostatic secretion. CBP is probably the most common cause of recurrent UTIs in the male patient because the bacterial pathogen often persists unaltered in the prostatic secretion during antibacterial therapy, frequently insufficient and inadequate, and eventually reinfects the urine after treatment is withdrawn. CBP is mainly a bacteriologic diagnosis and, therefore, sequential bacteriologic localization cultures of the initially voided urine, the midstream urine, and the expressed prostatic secretion (EPS) are essential in reaching the right diagnosis and cannot be replaced by any other method. Demonstration of gram-negative bacteria in the EPS in the presence of sterile initial and midstream urine cultures are highly diagnostic for CBP. Alternatively, a significantly higher bacterial level (of a log or more) in the EPS compared to the initial urethral specimen is also considered diagnostic of CBP.

CBP is a clinical entity difficult to treat and cure, a fact already recognized in the early 1970s. The main difficulty derived from the fact that the majority of the antibacterial drugs available on the market and so effective in the treatment of UTIs were not effective in the treatment of CBP because they were unable to penetrate the electrically charged lipid membrane of the prostatic epithelium and achieve effective therapeutic levels within the prostatic acini (Winningham et al. 1968).

This was beautifully demonstrated by the experimental studies on diffusion kinetics of a large number of antibacterial drugs from plasma into the prostatic fluid in the normal dog by Stamey et al. (1970), which showed that in order to penetrate the lipid membrane of the prostatic epithelium a drug must first be lipid soluble and minimally bound to the plasma proteins and, then, have a favorable dissociation constant (pK_a) which enables the drug to achieve a high fraction of uncharged (un-ionized) molecules in the plasma; only these un-charged molecules are free to cross the prostatic epithelium and diffuse into the prostatic fluid, where they become ionized, and then are thus unable to cross back into the plasma (phenomenon of ion trapping) to finally accumulate to effective therapeutic levels within the prostate. Furthermore, under the presumption that the pH of the prostatic fluid in the normal dog, which is acidic at about 6.4, is similar to that of the prostatic fluid in man with CBP and in the presence then of a pH gradient of 7.4 to 6.4 between the plasma and prostatic fluid, it was concluded that a weak base would be the ideal drug for treatment of CBP.

According to the above criteria, the adequate antibacterial considered in the early 1970s to meet all the requirements for adequate diffusion and concentration in the prostatic fluid was trimethoprim, a lipid-soluble weak base with a favorable pK_a of 7.3 (meaning that more than 50% of its molecules in the plasma are available in the uncharged form for diffusion into the prostate) and a protein binding of about 45%, that was bactericidal against gram-negative organisms. In the prostatic fluid of the uninflamed prostate in the dog (Reeves and Ghilchik 1970; Robb et al. 1971; Granato et al. 1973; Stamey et al. 1973) as well as the uninflamed prostatic tissue and prostatic fluid in man (Oosterlinck et al. 1975; Madsen et al. 1976; Wright et al. 1982) trimethoprim reached 2–10 times as high concentrations as in the plasma, more than adequate to reach the minimal inhibitory concentration (0.5–1.5 µg/ml) versus gram-negative enterobacteria in CBP (Carroll et al. 1971); in one patient with a urinary diversion a 20–40 times prostatic fluid to plasma ratio of trimethoprim was found in the presence of a prostatic fluid pH of 6.9 (Madsen et al. 1976). These investigations also showed that the combination of trimethoprim with sulfamethoxazole potentiates the activity of trimethoprim by appreciably reducing its minimal bactericidal concentration and even lowering it below its minimal inhibitory concentration for gram-negative enterobacteria when used alone (Carroll et al. 1971).

Treatment with Cotrimoxazole-Trimethoprim

Following the studies in normal dog and human and assuming that the physicochemical conditions in the normal prostate are similar to those in CBP, cotrimoxazole and in the later stages trimethoprim alone, were heralded as the ideal drugs in the treatment of CBP. The optimistic expectations of this treatment, however, were only partially fulfilled. Short-term treatment for 1 or a number of weeks with cotrimoxazole did not cure at all (Pfau and Sacks 1976) or only a very limited number of cases of CBP (Meares 1975). Long-term treatment of 3–5 months with cotrimoxazole (160 mg trimethoprim + 800 mg sulfamethoxazole 2 × daily) or pure trimethoprim (100 mg 3 × daily) cured only 30%–40% of the patients with CBP (McGuire and Lytton 1976; Stamey 1980; Meares 1982; Pfau 1986; Table 6) in spite of the fact that the pathogens in the prostate remained sensitive to trimethoprim or cotrimoxazole during the treatment in the majority of the cases. In view of the appreciable difficulty to cure

A. Pfau

CBP and the significant number of relapses, sterilization of the urine and prostatic secretion during and a short time following treatment are by no means a definite sign of cure. *Only repeated sterile urine and prostatic secretion cultures for at least 12 months following completion of treatment are able to assure the cure of CBP.*

Case Study

Table 1 summarizes the cure of an *E. coli* CBP cured by long-term treatment with cotrimoxazole. A 56-year-old man was first seen at the Hadassah Medical Center Outpatient Clinic in January 1975 because of recurrent *E. coli* UTIs, sometimes accompanied by high fever and chills, for the past 30 years in spite of repeated antibacterial treatment. Antibacterial therapy was usually effective,

Table 1. Management of a 56-year-old man with chronic bacterial prostatitis cured by long-term cotrimoxazole

Date	Days on (+) or off (−) drug	Drug	Colonies per milliliter[a]			Organism
			First-voided	Midstream	EPS	
27/ 1/75				100 000		*E. coli*
10/ 2/75	+ 13	Ampi	0	0	1 900	*E. coli*
20/ 2/75	− 8	Ampi	0	0	30 000	*E. coli*
28/ 2/75	− 14	Ampi	100 000	100 000	100 000	*E. coli*
	(Cystoscopy and localization)					
				CB 100 000		*E. coli*
				WB 1 200		*E. coli*
			RK1 0	LK1 100 000		*E. coli*
			RK2 0	LK2 50 000		*E. coli*
			RK3 0	LK3 50 000		*E. coli*
24/ 3/75	+ 3	Kana	0	0	0	
18/ 4/75	− 15	Kana	0	0	0	
23/ 5/75	− 50	Kana	0	0	1 000	*E. coli*
6/ 6/75	+ 8	TMP-SMX	0	0	0	
17/10/75	+ 140	TMP-SMX	0	0	0	
9/ 1/76	− 84	TMP-SMX	0	0	0	
24/12/76	− 433	TMP-SMX	0	0	0	
9/12/77	− 754	TMP-SMX	0	0	0	
5/12/78	− 1115	TMP-SMX	0	0	0	
29/11/82	− 2568	TMP-SMX	0	0	0	

[a] Low counts of gram-positive organisms (staphylococci, streptococci, diphtheroids) not included. EPS, expressed prostatic secretion; Ampi, ampicillin (500 mg q.i.d.); Kana, kanamycin (1000 mg b.i.d. for 3 days + 500 mg b.i.d. for 11 days i.m.); TMP-SMX, cotrimoxazole (trimethoprim 160 mg + sulfamethoxazole 800 mg); CB; catheterized bladder urine; WB, washed bladder (after 3000 ml sterile water irrigation); RK1–RK3, serial catheterized right kidney urines; LK1–LK3, serial catheterized left kidney urines.

and the symptoms disappeared within a few days. In recent years the *E. coli* UTIs occurred 4–5 times a year.

According to the history the patient underwent in 1936, at the age of 17, a transurethral ureteral meatotomy because of a left ureterocele. A recent excretory urogram revealed a normal hypertrophied right kidney (14.7 × 8 cm), whereas the small left kidney (9.4 × 6.3 cm) showed irregular borders, deformed calices, and delayed secretion of the contrast medium. A cystogram revealed left vesicoureteral reflux into the dilated lower third of the ureter. Several urologists had advised the patient to have a left nephroureterectomy, as they considered the left contracted kidney as the source of the recurrent UTIs. Physical examination revealed a slightly enlarged, smooth and nontender prostate. The urine grew more than 10^5 colonies per milliliter of *E. coli*.

As the patient experienced high fever on his first visit, he was subjected to a 2-week ampicillin treatment (500 mg 4 × daily). During and following the treatment repeated sequential localization cultures of the urine and EPS clearly revealed the presence of *E. coli* CBP (Table 1). Two weeks after completion of the ampicillin treatment, which sterilized his urine, the patient was again infected with *E. coli*. Differential ureteral bacteriologic studies (Stamey and Pfau 1963) revealed a sterile right kidney but an infected left kidney with *E. coli*. The patient was now given a 14-day treatment with kanamycin which quickly sterilized his urine and EPS. The patient felt well, but 50 days following completion of the kanamycin treatment his follow-up EPS cultures grew again *E. coli* (Table 1). This time the patient was subjected to a 5-month cotrimoxazole treatment, which sterilized his EPS cultures and definitely cured his *E. coli* CBP after 30 years of recurrent *E. coli* UTIs. The urine and EPS cultures remained sterile for the next 7 years following completion of the cotrimoxazole treatment, with the exception of an asymptomatic *Staphylococcus epidermidis* and enterococcal bacteriuria of urethral origin which was treated successfully with ampicillin and kanamycin.

This case illustrates well that in a male patient with a nonobstructed urinary tract and in the absence of renal calculi an upper UTI most probably originates in the prostate.

Case Study

Table 2 summarizes the cure of an *E. coli* CBP cured by long-term treatment with pure trimethoprim. A 45-year-old patient was seen at the Hadassah Medical Center Outpatient Clinic in December 1979 because of three recurrent attacks of high fever up to 39°C and chills accompanied by frequency, urgency, dysuria, and terminal hematuria during the past 5 months in spite of repeated 10-day antibacterial treatment with cotrimoxazole or nitrofurantoin and temporary symptomatic improvement. During the last attack the patient also developed a right epididymitis. The urine cultures grew *E. coli* every time during these attacks. Physical examination revealed a normal nontender prostate. The

Table 2. Management of a 45-year-old man with chronic bacterial prostatitis cured by long-term trimethoprim

Date	Days on (+) or off (−) drug	Drug	Colonies per milliliter[a]			Organism	EPS	
			First-voided	Midstream	EPS		White blood cell count (mm³)[b]	pH
7/12/79			200	0	100 000	E. coli	15 000	7.7
14/12/79	+ 3	TMP	0	0	70	E. coli		8.2
11/ 4/80	+ 122	TMP	0	0	0			
2/ 7/80	− 80	TMP	0	0	0		10 000	6.8
14/ 1/81	− 276	TMP	0	0	0			7.4
16/12/81	− 613	TMP	0	0	0			
30/ 1/84	− 1388	TMP	0	0	0		14 000	6.5
8/ 8/84	− 1578	TMP	0	0	0		3 100	6.5
10/12/91	− 4262	TMP	0	0	0			

EPS, expressed prostatic secretion; TMP, trimethoprim (100 mg t.i.d.).
[a] Low counts of gram-positive organisms (staphylococci, streptococci, diphtheroids) not included.
[b] According to Anderson and Weller (1979).

excretory urogram was normal. Sequential localization cultures of the urine and prostatic secretion clearly revealed the prostate as the source of the relapsing *E. coli* infections (Table 2). The patient was subjected to a 4-month trimethoprim treatment (100 mg 3 × daily) which quickly sterilized his prostate. Repeated follow-up cultures of the urine and EPS for the next 11 years remained sterile while the patient felt well.

Treatment with Kanamycin

In view of the fact that cotrimoxazole or trimethoprim were able to cure only one-third of the patients with CBP, there was an urgent need for additional antibacterials able to penetrate the prostatic epithelial barrier and achieve adequate concentrations in the prostate. A report by Meares and Stamey in 1968 of a single case of CBP cured by a 5-day treatment of intramuscular kanamycin drew our attention to this antibacterial. We then subjected in the mid-1970s three patients with CBP, who did not respond to long-term treatment with cotrimoxazole, to a modified 14-day intramuscular kanamycin treatment (1000 mg 2 × daily for the fist 3 days + 500 mg 2 × daily for the next 11 days); all these patients were cured (Pfau and Sacks 1976). On the basis of this initial success we decided to subject every new patient with CBP first to a short-term intramuscular kanamycin treatment and, if unsuccessful, to continue with long-term cotrimoxazole or trimethoprim treatment. In the following years kanamycin revealed itself as an effective antibacterial, curing another one-third of our patients (Pfau 1986, 1991; Table 6). Kanamycin, like trimethoprim, is a weak base with a favorable pK_a of 7.2, is not at all bound to the plasma proteins, achieves high serum levels of 35–40 μg/ml, and is an effective antibacterial against gram-negative bacteria; it is, however, lipid insoluble and should therefore have been incapable of crossing the lipid membrane of the prostatic epithelium. The fact that kanamycin still achieved an appreciable success in curing one-third of our patients with CBP means that in spite of its lipid insolubility, kanamycin is able to cross the prostatic epithelium, probably because of altered conditions occurring in the presence of CBP, and achieve a sufficient concentration to eradicate the pathogenic bacteria within the prostate in some patients.

Case Study

Table 3 summarizes the cure of a *Citrobacter diversus* CBP by a short-term kanamycin treatment. A 46-year-old man was seen at our Outpatient Clinic in December 1984 because of a 2-month history of recurrent *E. coli* UTIs accompanied by high fever up to 39°C and chills, which did not respond to repeated antibacterial treatment with cotrimoxazole or nitrofurantoin. The patient was

Table 3. Management of a 46-year-old man with chronic bacterial prostatitis cured by short-term kanamycin

Date	Days on (+) or off (−) drug	Drug	Colonies per milliliter[a]			Organism	EPS	
			First-voided	Midstream	EPS		White blood cell count (mm³)[b]	pH
16/12/84				100 000	100 000	E. coli	24 000	
24/12/84	+6	Nitro	0	0	100 000	E. coli	37 500	
31/12/84	−3	Nitro	100 000	100 000	50 000	Cit. div.		
5/ 1/85								
	(Patient starts kanamycin treatment)							
7/ 1/85	+2	Kana	0	0	2 100	Cit. div.	38 500	
16/ 1/85	+11	Kana	0	0	0		1 300	8.5
13/ 2/85	−25	Kana	0	0	0		300	8.0
22/ 4/85	−93	Kana	0	0	0		9 700	8.2
15/ 7/85	−177	Kana	0	0	0		1 700	8.2
13/ 1/86	−359	Kana	0	0	0		12 500	7.9
22/12/86	−702	Kana	0	0	0		7 000	7.0
27/ 4/87	−828	Kana	0	0	0		11 000	
9/ 5/88	−1206	Kana	0	0	0		3 100	
3/ 7/89	−1626	Kana	0	0	0		4 300	
18/ 9/91	−2221	Kana	0	0	0			

Nitro, nitrofurantoin (100 mg q.i.d.); Kana, kanamycin (1000 mg b.i.d. for 3 days + 500 mg b.i.d. for 11 days i.m.); Cit. div., Citrobacter diversus.

[a] Low counts of gram-positive organisms (staphylococci, streptococci, diphtheroids) not included.

[b] According to Anderson and Weller (1979).

sensitive to cotrimoxazole as he developed a generalized rash on his body. Following the second UTI, he developed difficulties in micturition and subsequently acute urine retention, which necessitated a temporary indwelling catheter. The patient was relieved of the catheter after 1 week and had a normal micturition subsequently.

When seen by us, the patient felt relatively well but the urine culture grew more than 10^5 colonies per milliliter of *E. coli*. Physical examination revealed a small, smooth, and nontender prostate. Following pretreatment with nitrofurantoin macrocrystals (100 mg 4 × daily) for a number of days, sequential localization cultures clearly revealed the prostate as the source of the *E. coli* infections (Table 3). After nitrofurantoin was stopped, the patient quickly developed a new urinary tract infection, this time with *Citrobacter diversus*. Sequential localization cultures again revealed the prostate as the source of the new infection. The patient was started on a 14-day intramuscular kanamycin treatment which quickly sterilized the cultures, including the EPS. During the next 6 years the patient remained symptomless, and the urine and EPS cultures remained sterile.

The failure of trimethoprim, as well as kanamycin, to cure only two-thirds of the patients with CBP in spite of the fact that the gram-negative pathogens remained sensitive to these antibacterials throughout the whole treatment, demanded further explanation. Additional investigations revealed that the prostatic fluid underwent profound physicochemical alterations in CBP, such as a steep rise to an alkaline pH of 8–8.4 from a pH of 6.3–7.3 in normal conditions (a difference of almost 2 pH units), thus contradicting the original concept of similarity of conditions in the uninflamed canine or human prostate and the inflamed human prostate in CBP (Anderson and Fair 1976; Pfau et al. 1978; Fair et al. 1979).

Consequently the formerly supposed pH gradient of 7.4/6.4 between plasma and prostatic fluid was abolished and reversed to a pH gradient of 8.4/7.4 in favor of the prostatic fluid in the presence of CBP. In these new conditions the total amount of any antibacterial base such as trimethoprim or kanamycin is higher in the plasma than in the prostatic fluid. Therefore, the concentration of trimethoprim or kanamycin in the prostatic fluid of patients with CBP at a pH of 8.4 is approximately half the simultaneously measured plasma level. In view of these new findings, we should be careful not to draw definite conclusions as to the concentration and activity of an antibacterial in the alkaline prostatic secretion of a patient with CBP from the data obtained in the acidic prostatic secretion of the uninflamed canine or human prostate. In fact, it now became clear that a better experimental model for predicting concentrations of antibacterial drugs in the prostatic fluid of men with CBP would probably be the level achieved in the alkaline salivary fluid and not the acidic prostatic fluid in the normal dog because the pH of the salivary fluid between 8 and 9 correlates better with the pH of the prostatic fluid of men with CBP (Granato et al. 1973).

These new facts explained why the biologic fraction of a weak base such as trimethoprim or kanamycin, concentrating at a pH above 8 in the inflamed prostate, was often inadequate to eradicate many of the gram-negative pathogens. On the other hand, however, the fact that these drugs still cured some of the patients with CBP meant that even low prostatic fluid levels of these antibacterials, inferior to those in the plasma but maintained for long periods of time, were sufficient enough to eradicate some of the gram-negative pathogens within the prostate (Pfau et al. 1978; Fair et al. 1979). Thus, a reappraisal of the former treatment was required, and weak acids, not weak bases, preferably with a high pK_a, meaning a high fraction of uncharged molecules in the plasma, should be looked for in the presence of CBP. Theoretically, at least, weak acids should reach higher concentrations in the prostatic fluid than in the plasma in the presence of an 8.4/7.4 pH gradient in favor of the prostatic secretion.

Treatment with Fluoroquinolones (Ciprofloxacin, Norfloxacin)

Around the mid-1980s we were able to cure about two-thirds of our patients with CBP using kanamycin, cotrimoxazole, or trimethoprim. At the same time a new group of antibacterial agents, revealing a potent bactericidal activity against gram-negative pathogens causing CBP, the fluoroquinolones, became available. Some of them, such as ciprofloxacin or norfloxacin, were described as achieving therapeutic concentrations in the prostate and, therefore, adequate in CBP. Both ciprofloxacin and norfloxacin are lipid-soluble weak acids of a zwitterionic nature ($pK_{a1} = 6.0$–6.4, $pK_{a2} = 8.8$–8.9), and have a low protein binding of 13%–36%, qualities which should enable them to cross the prostatic epithelium and achieve, at least theoretically, higher concentrations in the prostatic fluid than in the plasma in the presence of an alkaline prostatic pH of 8–8.4 as happens in CBP.

The data available from measurements obtained again only from the uninflamed prostate of dog and man is, however, not uniform. Whereas the ratios of ciprofloxacin or norfloxacin concentrations between prostatic tissue, as well as prostatic interstitial fluid or prostatic secretion, and plasma were less than 1 in some investigations (Frimodt-Møller et al. 1984; Dan et al. 1986), they were equal to 1 (Bologna et al. 1983; Sabbay et al. 1986) or higher than 1 in others (Dalhoff and Weidner 1984; Bergeron et al. 1985; Larsen et al. 1986; Gombert et al. 1987). A recent study by Naber et al. (1989) demonstrated lower ciprofloxacin concentrations in the prostatic secretion of the uninflamed human prostates than in plasma and attributed the higher concentrations in some of the previous studies to the contamination of the prostatic secretion by the high ciprofloxacin concentrations in the urine expelled prior to collection of the prostatic secretion. Still, the concentrations of cipro- or norfloxacin reached in the prostatic tissue or secretion of the uninflamed prostate proved to be above the minimal inhibitory concentration for most of the gram-negative pathogens causing CBP. Furthermore, recent reports revealed significant cure rates by cipro- or norfloxacin in patients with well-documented CBP (Pfau 1991;

Schaeffer and Darras 1990; Weidner et al. 1991). The data on the effectiveness of ofloxacin in CBP is still insufficient (Cox 1989; Naber 1989).

In our hands the 3- to 5-month treatment with ciprofloxacin (500 mg, 2 × daily) cured about 70% of the patients with CBP subjected to this treatment; some of these patients had already received repeated short- and long-term antibacterial treatment without any appreciable result.

Case Study

Table 4 summarizes the cure of a patient with *E. coli* CBP by long-term treatment with ciprofloxacin. A 30-year-old man was first seen at the Hadassah Medical Center Urologic Clinic in July 1989, 1 week after an attack of high fever up to 39°C and chills, accompanied by frequency, urgency, dysuria and macroscopic hematuria as well as a flu-like sensation of myalgia along his extremities. A urine culture grew 50 000 colonies per milliliter of *E. coli*. The patient first received amoxicillin (500 mg 3 × daily) and then cephalexin (500 mg 3 × daily) for the next 10 days. The patient's general condition improved although he continued to complain of frequency.

Physical examination revealed a normal nontender prostate. The excretory urogram was within normal limits. Urine cytology was normal. Repeated sequential localization cultures of the urine and prostatic secretion revealed the prostate as the source of the previous *E. coli* UTI (Table 4). In the presence of an *E. coli* CBP, we first started with a 14-day amikacin treatment (500 mg 3 × daily the first 3 days + 500 mg 2 × daily the next 11 days), as kanamycin was not available. The prostatic secretion, however, again grew small numbers of *E. coli* 14 days following completion of the amikacin treatment. We then assigned the patient to a 5-month ciprofloxacin treatment (500 mg 2 × daily). Except a one-time minimal *E. coli* urethral infection (Table 4), which was treated with a 5-day nitrofurantoin macrocrystals treatment (100 mg 4 × daily), repeated urine and prostatic secretion cultures following completion of the ciprofloxacin treatment remained sterile for the next 2 years and the patient symptomless.

Two of our patients with an *E. coli* CBP initially reacted well to different long-term antibacterial treatments, including a 3-month ciprofloxacin treatment, but one became reinfected with an *E. coli* whereas the second one with *Enterobacter aeroqenes* and *Pseudomonas aeruginosa*. Both these patients were subsequently subjected to a 5-month treatment with norfloxacin (400 mg 2 × daily) following which they were cured, as they are symptomless, and repeated urine and EPS cultures remained sterile for about 3 years following completion of the treatment (Table 6).

The few patients with CBP who do not respond to any of the above antibacterial regimens are maintained symptomless by daily low-dose suppressive antibacterial treatment such as 40 mg trimethoprim + 200 mg sulfamethoxazole or 50 mg nitrofurantoin macrocrystals.

Table 4. Management of a 30-year-old man with chronic bacterial prostatitis cured by long-term ciprofloxacin

Date	Days on (+) or off (−) drug	Drug	Colonies per milliliter[a]			Organism	EPS
			First-voided	Midstream	EPS		White blood cell count (mm)[b]
28/ 6/89				50000		E. coli	10000
6/ 8/89	− 25	Ceph	0	0	1 200	E. coli	10000
20/ 8/89	− 39	Ceph	100	0	50000	E. coli	24000
24/ 9/89	− 14	Amika	0	0	310	E. coli	700
1/ 1/90	+ 67	Cipro	0	0	0		9 100
2/ 4/90	− 14	Cipro	0	0	0		4 400
16/ 9/90	− 166	Cipro	0	0	0		3 900
17/12/90	− 257	Cipro	0	0	0		
7/ 4/91	− 369	Cipro	300	0	400	E. coli	5 700
18/11/91	− 594	Cipro	0	0	-0		2 000
12/ 4/92	− 740	Cipro	0	0	0		1 500

Ceph, cephalexin (500 mg t.i.d.); Amika, amikacin (500 mg t.i.d. for 3 days + 500 mg b.i.d. for 11 days); Cipro, ciprofloxacin (500 mg b.i.d. for 5 months).
[a] Low counts of gram-positive organisms (staphylococci, streptococci, diphtheroids) not included.
[b] According to Anderson and Weller (1979).

We would like to emphasize that in our experience repeated trials with a 1-month minocycline, doxycycline, or carbenicillin indanyl sodium treatment, a 3-month treatment with rifampicin + cotrimoxazole or repeated local transperineal intraprostatic injections with gentamicin or cefazolin were unsuccessful in curing even a single case of CBP (Pfau 1986).

Lastly, it should be mentioned that, whereas sterilization of the urine and the EPS occurs almost immediately following adequate antibacterial treatment in CBP, the accompanying high white blood cell counts and the high pH values of the EPS return to normal values very slowly, sometimes years after completion of the treatment (Tables 2–4; Pfau et al. 1978).

Surgery in the Treatment of CBP

Surgery is the last resort in the treatment of CBP and should be reserved only to patients over the age of 50 years with an associated pathology such as benign hyperplasia of prostate or infected prostatic calculi in whom repeated adequate antibacterial treatment did not sterilize the prostate. However, it is our feeling that in view of the great advances in the effective cure of CBP by antibacterial treatment in the past 10 years, prostatectomy should become less necessary even in selected cases.

It should be emphasized that prostatectomy (transurethral, supra- or retropubic) met only with partial success in the cure of CBP (Stamey 1980). This could be explained by McNeal's studies in 1968 which showed greater susceptibility to inflammation of the peripheral zone of the true prostate than the periurethral glands. Following this assessment and using a radical transurethral prostatectomy, Meares (1986) cured ten patients with CBP who did not respond to previous antibacterial therapy.

To increase the effectiveness of the surgical intervention in the cure of CBP, we have modified the routine retropubic prostatectomy by adding the following three steps: (a) removal of all the calculi, if present, following adenomectomy; (b) careful excision of the posterior capsule of the prostate together with the bladder neck as far as possible laterally and distally to the vicinity of the verumontanum; and (c) repeated washing of the operative area with 1% neomycin solution and injection of the residual posterior as well as the anterior prostatic capsule with a solution of 1000 mg kanamycin dissolved in 10 ml water.

Applying these principles, three patients over the age of 50 were cured who had documented CBP and benign hyperplasia of prostate, and who did not respond to repeated antibacterial treatment before the era of the fluoroquinolones and underwent a modified retropubic prostatectomy.

Case Study

Table 5 illustrates the cure of a patient with CBP by a modified retropubic prostatectomy. A 53-year-old man was referred in November 1979 to

Table 5. Management of a 53-year-old man with chronic bacterial prostatitis cured by a modified retropubic prostatectomy

Date	Days on (+) or off (−) drug	Drug	Colonies per milliliter[a]			Organism
			First-voided	Midstream	EPS	
3/12/79	− 14	TMP-SMX		100 000		E. coli
9/12/79	+ 3	Nitro	0	0	2 000	E. coli
12/12/79	+ 6	Nitro	0	0	300	E. coli
24/12/79	− 8	Nitro	100 000	100 000	100 000	E. coli
27/12/79	(Patient starts pure trimethoprim treatment)					
23/ 1/80	+ 28	TMP	0	0	0	
25/ 4/80	+ 121	TMP	0	0	20	Ps. aer.
2/ 6/80	− 38	TMP	100 000			E. coli
12/ 6/80	+ 10	Kana	0	0	0	
5/ 9/80	− 86	Kana	100	0	100 000	Kle. pn.
						Ps. aer.
6/10/80	− 117	Kana	0	0	100 000	E. coli
8/ 4/81	− 301	Kana	100 000	100 000		Str. faec
					30	E. coli
					30	Ent. cl.
	(Patient starts amoxicillin treatment)					
13/ 7/81	− 56	Amoxi	0	0	200	Kle. pn.
					80	Aeromonas
					300	E. coli
24/ 8/81	+ 34	TMP-SMX	0	0	1 000	E. coli
14/ 9/81	+ 55	TMP-SMX		100 000		E. coli
16/10/81	+ 7	Nitro	50 000	50 000	100 000	E. coli
25/11/81	+ 47	Nitro	5 000	0	100 000	E. coli
17/ 2/82	+ 18	Mino	0	0	100 000	E. coli
10/ 1/83	+ 12	Carb	15 000	100	100 000	Kle. pn
7/ 1/83	+ 19	Carb		100 000		Kle. pn
13/ 2/85			100 000	100 000	70 000	Str. faec
					20 000	Ps. aer
					1 000	E. coli
21/ 3/85	(Modified retropubic prostatectomy)					
17/ 5/85	− 58	RPP		0		
17/ 5/85	− 58	RPP		0		
14/ 4/86	− 390	RPP		0		
6/ 4/87	− 747	RPP		0		
8/ 8/88	− 1237	RPP		0		
28/ 3/90	− 1834	RPP		0		
17/ 9/90	− 2007	RPP		0		
17/ 2/92	− 2554	RPP		0		

Nitro, nitrofurantoin (100 mg q.i.d.); TMP, pure trimethoprim (200 mg b.i.d. for 2 weeks + 100 mg t.i.d. for 3.5 months); Kana, kanamycin (1000 mg b.i.d. for 3 days + 500 mg b.i.d. for 11 days); Amoxi, amoxicillin (250 mg q.i.d. for 10 days); TMP-SMX, cotrimoxazole (160 mg trimethoprim + 800 mg sulfamethoxazole); Mino, minocycline (200 mg b.i.d. for 2 days + 100 mg b.i.d. for 28 days); Carb, carbenicillin indanyl sodium (764 mg q.i.d.); RPP, retropubic prostatectomy. *Ps. aer.*, *Pseudomonas aeruginosa*; *Kle. pn.*, *Klebsiella pneumoniae*; *Str. faec.*, *Streptococcus faecalis*; *Ent. cl.*, *Enterobacter cloacae*.
[a] Low counts of gram-positive organisms (staphylococci, streptococci, diphtheroids) not included.

the Hadassah Medical Center Outpatient Clinic because of recurrent UTIs over the past year in spite of repeated antibacterial treatment. During the last year the patient experienced frequency and urgency, moderate difficulties in micturition accompanied in the last days by fever up to 39.5°C and a urethral discharge. Physical examination revealed a moderately enlarged prostate but otherwise nontender and normal in consistency. The urine, which was extremely foul smelling, showed frank pyuria, and the culture grew more than 10^5 colonies per milliliter of *E. coli*. The excretory urogram was normal, but the bladder emptied with a residual urine of about 50 ml.

The patient was started on nitrofurantoin macrocrystals, and after the fever disappeared, repeated localization cultures of the urine and EPS were carried out; the cultures clearly revealed the prostate as the source of the recurrent *E. coli* UTIs (Table 5).

During the years 1979–1985 the patient received repeated treatments with pure trimethoprim, kanamycin, minocycline, doxycycline, cotrimoxazole, nitrofurantoin macrocrystals, amoxicillin, carbenicillin indanyl sodium, and low-dose nalidixic acid. In spite of careful follow-up the patient developed recurrent UTIs mainly with *E. coli* and sometimes with *Streptococcus faecalis* or *Klebsiella pneumoniae*, often accompanied by high fever, for which the patient was repeatedly hospitalized. The EPS cultures were infected practically all the time and grew besides *E. coli*, *P. aeruginosa*, *Aeromonas*, *Citrobacter freundii*, *K. pneumoniae*, *Enterobacter cloacae*, *Proteus mirabilis*, or *Proteus vulgaris*.

In view of the fact that we were not able to sterilize the prostate in this patient in spite of almost continuous antibacterial treatment and in view of the presence of an enlarged prostate, which caused difficulties in micturition, the patient was subjected to a modified retropubic prostatectomy in 1985. During the operation multiple small calculi were removed from the area between the prostatic adenoma and the prostatic capsule as well as from the bladder. Following an uneventful recovery, the patient became symptomless and remained with a sterile urine for the next 6 years.

Conclusion

Chronic bacterial prostatitis, the most common cause of recurrent UTIs in the male patient, is a well-defined clinical entity but one difficult to cure because the majority of antibacterials available on the market are not able to penetrate the prostatic epithelium and concentrate within the prostate; moreover, even the antibacterials which penetrate the prostatic epithelium cure only some of the patients with CBP. In view of our experience of 20 years and a cure rate of 90% (Table 6), we recommend today starting every patient with well-documented CBP on a 14-day intramuscular treatment of kanamycin (Table 7). Only those patients who do not respond to short-term kanamycin treatment should receive a 5-month treatment of either cotrimoxazole, trimethoprim, or one of the two

Table 6. Treatment results in 45 men with chronic bacterial prostatitis caused by gram-negative bacteria

Drug or procedure	Patients		Age (years)		Status	Follow-up (days)	
	n	%	Median	Range		Median	Range
Cotrimoxazole	7	15.6	56	31–67	Cured	1568	365–4745
Trimethoprim	4	8.9	48	25–62	Cured	1976	365–2373
Kanamycin	13	28.9	54	28–73	Cured	1219	350–2221
Ciprofloxacin[a]	11	24.4	51	30–72	Cured	740	205–1978
Norfloxacin	2	4.4	51	47–55	Cured	1089	1085–1093
Cephalexin	1	2.2	59		Cured	750	
Prostatectomy	3	6.7	60	58–70	Cured	2249	442–2525
Observation	4	8.9	46	38–55	Improved		

As of March 1992, 41/45 (91%) cured.
[a] Two of the ciprofloxacin patients have not yet reached a 12-month follow-up; however, they are symptomless and the urine and EPS cultures remain sterile following completion of treatment.

Table 7. Treatment of chronic bacterial prostatitis

Drug	Dosage	Duration of treatment
Kanamycin (intramuscular)	1000 mg, b.i.d.	3 days
	500 mg, b.i.d.	11 days
Cotrimoxazole	160 mg TMP + 800 mg SMX b.i.d.	5 months
Trimethoprim	100 mg t.i.d.	5 months
Ciprofloxacin	500 mg b.i.d.	5 months
Norfloxacin	400 mg b.i.d.	5 months

TMP, trimethoprim; SMX, sulfamethoxazole.

quinolones ciprofloxacin and norfloxacin (Table 7). Surgery by a modified retropubic prostatectomy will probably be necessary in very few cases and in only those patients with an associated pathology such as benign hyperplasia of the prostate who do not respond to any of the above antibacterial regimens. The younger patient who does not respond to antibacterial treatment can be maintained symptomless by daily administration of low-dose antibacterials such as 50 mg nitrofurantoin macrocrystals or trimethroprim according to the sensitivity of the pathogen.

It should be emphasized that cure of CBP can be assured only if repeated urine and prostatic secretion cultures remain sterile for at least 12 months following completion of treatment.

Finally, we would advise every urologist treating CBP to demonstrate enough patience and dedication to follow up the patient until bacteriologic cure is obtained, often a quite protracted process in the successful treatment of CBP.

References

Anderson RU, Fair WR (1976) Physical and chemical determinations of prostatic secretion in benign hyperplasia, prostatitis and adenocarcinoma. Invest Urol 14:137–140

Anderson RU, Weller C (1979) Prostatic secretion leukocyte studies in nonbacterial prostatitis (prostatosis). J Urol 121:292–294

Bergeron MG, Thabet M, Roy R, Lessard C, Foucault P (1985) Norfloxacin penetration into human renal and prostatic tissue. Antimicrob Agents Chemother 28:349–350

Bologna M, Vaggi L, Forchetti CM, Martini E (1983) Bactericidal intraprostatic concentrations of norfloxacin (Letter to the Editor). Lancet 2:280

Carroll PT, Robb CA, Tippett LO, Langsten JB (1971) Antibacterial activity of diaveridine, trimethoprim, and selected sulfonamides in prostatic fluid. Invest Urol 8:686–694

Cox CE (1989) Ofloxacin in the management of complicated urinary tract infections, including prostatitis. Am J Med 87 Suppl 6C:61S–68S

Dalhoff A, Weidner W (1984) Diffusion of ciprofloxacin into prostatic fluid. Eur J Clin Microbiol 5:360–362

Dan M, Golomb J, Gorea A, Braf Z, Berger SA (1986) Concentration of ciprofloxacin in human prostatic tissue after oral administration. Antimicrob Agents Chemother 30:88–89

Fair WR, Crane DB, Schiller N, Heston WDW (1979) A re-appraisal of treatment in chronic bacterial prostatitis. J Urol 121:437–441

Frimodt-Møller PC, Dørflinger T, Madsen PO (1984) Distribution of ciprofloxacin in the dog prostate and various tissues. Urol Res 12:283–286

Gombert ME, du Bouchet L, Audicino TM, Berkowitz LB, Macchia RJ (1987) Brief report: prostatic tissue concentrations of ciprofloxacin after oral administration. Am J Med 82 Suppl 4A:130–132

Granato JJ Jr, Gross DM, Stamey TA (1973) Trimethoprim diffusion into prostatic and salivary secretion of the dog. Invest Urol 11:205–210

Larsen EH, Gasser TC, Dørflinger T, Madsen PO (1986) The concentrations of various quinolone derivatives in the human prostate. In: Weidner W, Brunner H, Krause W, Rothauge CF (eds) Therapy of prostatitis: experimental and clinical data. Zuckschwerdt Munich, pp 40–44

Madsen PO, Kjaer TB, Baumueller A (1976) Prostatic tissue and fluid concentrations of trimethoprim and sulfamethoxazole: experimental and clinical studies. Urology 8:129–132

McGuire EJ, Lytton B (1976) Bacterial prostatitis: treatment with trimethoprim-sulfamethoxazole. Urology 7:499–500

McNeal JE (1968) Regional morphology and pathology of the prostate. Am J Clin Pathol 49:347–357

Meares EM Jr (1975) Long-term therapy of chronic bacterial prostatitis with trimethoprim-sulfamethoxazole. Can Med Assoc J 112 Suppl :22S–25S

Meares EM Jr (1982) Prostatitis: review of pharmacokinetics and therapy. Rev Infect Dis 4:475–483

Meares EM Jr (1986) Chronic bacterial prostatitis: role of transurethral prostatectomy (TURP) in therapy. In: Weidner W, Brunner H, Krause W, Rothauge CF (eds) Therapy of prostatitis: experimental and clinical data. Zuckschwerdt, Munich, pp 193–197

Meares EM, Stamey TA (1968) Bacteriologic localization patterns in bacterial prostatitis and urethritis. Invest Urol 5:492–518

Naber KG (1989) The role of quinolones in the treatment of chronic bacterial prostatitis. Infection 19 Suppl 3:S170–S177

Naber KG, Sörgel F, Kees F, Jaehde U, Schumacher H (1989) Pharmacokinetics of ciprofloxacin in young (healthy volunteers) and elderly patients, and concentrations in prostatic fluid, seminal fluid and prostatic adenoma tissue following intravenous administration. Am J Med 87 Suppl 5A:57S–59S

Oosterlinck W, Defoort R, Renders G (1975) The concentration of sulfamethoxazole and trimethoprim in human prostate gland. Br J Urol 47:301–304

Pfau A (1986) Prostatitis: a continuing enigma. Urol Clin North Am 13:695–715
Pfau A (1991) The treatment of chronic bacterial prostatitis. Infection 19 Suppl 3:S160–S164
Pfau A, Sacks T (1976) Chronic bacterial prostatitis: new therapeutic aspects. Br J Urol 48:245–253
Pfau A, Perlberg S, Shapiro A (1978) The pH of prostatic fluid in health and disease: implications of
    treatment in chronic bacterial prostatitis. J Urol 119:384–387
Reeves DS, Ghilchik M (1970) Secretion of the antibacterial substance trimethoprim in the prostatic
    fluid of dogs. Br J Urol 42:66–72
Robb CA, Carroll PT, Tippett LO, Langston JB (1971) The diffusion of selected sulfonamides,
    trimethoprim, and diaveridine into prostatic fluid of dogs. Invest Urol 8:679–685
Sabbay J, Hoagland VL, Cook T (1986) Norfloxacin versus cotrimoxazole in the treatment of
    recurring urinary tract infections in men. Scand J Infect Dis Suppl 48:48–53
Schaeffer AJ, Darras FS (1990) The efficacy of norfloxacin in the treatment of chronic bacterial
    prostatitis refractory to trimethoprim-sulfamethoxazole and/or carbenicillin. J Urol
    144:690–693
Stamey TA (1980) Urinary infections in males. In: Stamey TA (ed) Pathogenesis and treatment of
    urinary tract infections. Williams and Wilkins, Baltimore, pp 342–429
Stamey TA, Pfau A (1963) Some functional, pathologic, bacteriologic, and chemotherapeutic
    characteristics of unilateral pyelonephritis in man. II. Bacteriologic and chemotherapeutic
    characteristics. Invest Urol 1:162–172
Stamey TA, Meares EM Jr, Winningham DG (1970) Chronic bacterial prostatitis and the diffusion
    of drugs into prostatic fluid. J Urol 103:187–194
Stamey TA, Bushby SRM, Bragonje J (1973) The concentration of trimethoprim in prostatic fluid:
    Nonionic diffusion or active transport? J Infect Dis 128 Suppl: S686–S690
Weidner W, Schiefer HG, Brähler E (1991) Refractory chronic bacterial prostatitis: a re-evaluation
    of ciprofloxacin treatment after a median follow-up of 30 months. J Urol 146:350–352
Winningham DG, Nemoy NJ, Stamey TA (1968) Diffusion of antibiotics from plasma into prostatic
    fluid. Nature 219:139–143
Wright WL, Larking P, Lovell-Smith CJ (1982) Concentration of trimethoprim and sulphamethoxa-
    zole in the human prostate gland after intramuscular injection. Br J Urol 54:550–551

The Role of Quinolones in the Treatment of Chronic Bacterial Prostatitis*

K.G. Naber

Introduction

Bacterial prostatitis is a rare infection but one difficult to treat (Meares 1980); only a few antibiotics are suitable for sufficiently penetrating prostatic fluid (Stamey et al. 1970). Usually cotrimoxazole and to a lesser extent trimethoprim alone have been used, but with poor results (Table 1). Other antibiotics have also not improved the clinical outcome in patients followed-up for a sufficient period of time (Table 2). One exception seems to be the study by Mobley (1974) in which patients were treated initially with a 2-week course of 500 mg erythromycin orally four times daily combined with 10 g sodium bicarbonate with each dose of erythromycin, a lipid soluble basic macrolide with a pK_a higher than 8.6. Since erythromycin is not active at acid pH because virtually all of the molecules are charged, the author added sodium bicarbonate for urine alkalinization to increase its activity and antibacterial spectrum (Sabath et al. 1968; Zinner et al. 1971). Whether the addition of sodium bicarbonate influenced the pH of the prostatic fluid was not measured in the study. According to studies by Pfau et al. (1978), Anderson and Fair (1976) and Blacklock and Beavis (1974), the pH of prostatic fluid in patients with chronic bacterial prostatitis is alkaline rather than acidic, and therefore significantly different from the lower pH secretion observed in dogs (Meares 1975b) and in healthy males.

The newer quinolones such as zwitterions with pK_a's in acid as well as in alkaline mileu (Table 3) should theoretically be concentrated in acid and alkaline prostatic fluid. Because of their unique and favorable pharmacokinetic properties and their broad antibacterial spectrum, these antibacterial drugs may be a good alternative in the treatment of chronic bacterial prostatitis.

Concentrations of Quinolones in Prostatic Tissue and Secretions and in Seminal Secretions

In contrast to β-lactam antibiotics, concentrations of the newer quinolones in prostatic fluid, prostatic tissue, and seminal fluid are relatively high in

---

* A modified version of this chapter was first published in Hooper DC, Wolfson JS (eds) Quinolone antimicrobial Agents, 2nd edition, 1993. ASM Press, Washington, D.C., pp 285–297.

176   K.G. Naber

comparison to the corresponding plasma concentrations. Under steady-state
conditions in a dog model Madsen et al. (1978), Dørflinger et al. (1986), and
Gasser et al. (1987) demonstrated that the mean prostatic fluid to plasma
concentrations ratio was 0.34 for norfloxacin, 0.67 for ciprofloxacin, 1.12 for
fleroxacin, and 1.35 for enoxacin. Investigations in humans are somewhat

Table 1. Eradication of pathogens in patients with chronic bacterial prostatitis treated with
cotrimoxazole (trimethoprim 160 mg and sulfamethoxazole 800 mg twice daily) or trimethoprim
100 mg three times daily (from Hanus and Danzinger 1984)

Duration (days)	n	Bacteriological cure (%)	Follow-up (months)	Reference
10	10	0	3	Smith et al. (1979)
14	9	14	6	Meares (1978)
14	13	15	6	Meares (1973)
28	18	33	3	Drach (1974)
90	19	31	3	Meares (1975a)
90	13	38	6	Meares (1978)
90	15	40	12	McGurie and Lytton (1976)
90	8	50	3	Smith et al. (1979)
90	15	67	12	Paulson and White (1978)
120–140	15	40	12	Pfau (1986)
120–180	8[a]	50	12	Pfau (1986)

In all patients the infection was localized to the prostate according to the technique of Meares and
Stamey (1968).
[a] Trimethoprim.

Table 2. Eradication of pathogens in patients with chronic bacterial prostatitis treated with various
antibiotics (from Hanus et al. 1984)

Drug	Dosage (mg)	Duration	n	Bacteriol. cure (%)	Follow-up	Reference
Minocycline	100 b.i.d.	14[a]	14	70	12	Paulson and White (1978)
Erythromycin	500 q.i.d.	14	26	88	6–18	Mobley (1974)
Cephalexin	500 q.i.d.	28	9	22	1	Oliveri et al. (1979)
Carbenicillin	764 q.i.d.	28	22	68	1	Oliveri et al. (1979)
Cephalexin	500 q.i.d.	28	5	40	1	Mobley (1981)
Carbenicillin	764 q.i.d.	28	12	67	1	Mobley (1981)

In all patients the infection was localized to the prostate according to the technique of Meares and
Stamey (1968).
[a] Four patients withdrawn because of side effects.

Table 3. pK_a and pK_b values of newer quinolones

Drug	pK_a	pK_b
Ciprofloxacin	6.0	8.8
Enoxacin	6.0	8.5
Fleroxacin	5.7	8.0
Lomefloxacin	6.0	9.0
Norfloxacin	6.3	8.8
Ofloxacin	5.7	7.9
Pefloxacin	6.2	7.4–7.7
Temafloxacin	5.7	8.7
Sparfloxacin	6.3	9.3

hindered by the fact that prostatic fluid can usually be obtained in small amounts only by prostatic massage. Low-level contamination with urine containing high concentrations of these quinolones can therefore alter the results tremendously.

In our studies of drug levels in prostatic fluid (Naber et al. 1987a, 1988, 1989a–c, 1990a, b) we made sure that volunteers did not void urine before the prostatic sample was taken. In addition, a renal contrast medium, for example, ioxitalamic acid or iohexol, excreted almost exclusively by glomerular filtration was administered intravenously at the same time as the drug and served as an internal standard. In many experiments the prostatic fluid to plasma concentration ratios of the contrast medium were markedly below unity. Significant urinary contamination is considered to have occurred if this ratio becomes unexpectedly high (above unity). However, only experiments up to 4 h after a single dose can be analyzed in this manner because the subject must then void, resulting in urinary contamination of the urethra.

After administration of a single dose, the following median prostatic fluid to plasma concentration ratios were found (Table 4): for 800 mg oral norfloxacin, 0.12 (1–4 h); for 200 mg intravenous ciprofloxacin, 0.26 and 0.18 (0.5–2 h and 4 h), respectively; for 400 mg oral fleroxacin, 0.28 (2–4 h); for 400 mg oral temafloxacin[1], 0.36 (4 h); for 400 mg oral and 428 mg intravenous enoxacin 0.39 and 0.47 (2–4 h), respectively; and for 400 mg oral lomefloxacin 0.48 (4 h).

Data on the penetration of ciprofloxacin (Dalhoff and Weidner 1984; Boerema et al. 1985) and ofloxacin (Kumon et al. 1985; Suzuki et al. 1984) into prostatic fluid of healthy volunteers and patients have been reported, but no effort was made in these studies to assess possible urinary contamination. The high prostatic fluid to plasma ratios reported for some individuals may not reflect true concentrations in prostatic fluid.

Concentrations of ciprofloxacin in seminal fluid were measured by Dalhoff and Weidner (1984) and concentrations of ofloxacin by Mizoguchi et al. (1985), and Schramm (1986), with levels usually exceeding corresponding plasma concentrations several-fold. We measured the penetration of five newer quino-

---

[1] Because of severe and unexpected side effects, this drug was withdrawn worldwide in 1992.

178 K.G. Naber

Table 4. Concentrations of newer quinolones in prostatic fluid of volunteers (median concentration ratio, range; from Naber et al. 1987a, 1988, 1990b)

Drug	Dose (mg)	Time (h)	n	Plasma (mg/l)	Prostatic fluid (mg/l)	Prostatic fluid/ plasma ratio
Norfloxacin	800 p.o.	1–4	8 (2)	1.40 (0.69–2.71)	0.14 (0.08–0.43)	0.12 (0.08–0.19)
Ciprofloxacin	200 i.v.	0.5–2	10 (1)[a]	0.67 (0.45–1.12)	0.16 (0.10–0.50)	0.26 (0.15–0.53)
	200 i.v.[b]	4	8	0.44 (0.35–0.59)	0.08 (0.03–0.19)	0.18 (0.05–0.33)
Fleroxacin	400 p.o.	2–4	8	3.71 (3.30–4.70)	1.00 (0.84–1.69)	0.28 (0.22–0.37)
Temafloxacin	400 p.o.	4	4	2.23 (1.70–2.65)	0.78 (0.56–0.92)	0.36 (0.29–0.40)
Enoxacin	400 p.o.	2–4	10	1.09 (0.51–1.91)	0.39 (0.18–1.33)	0.39 (0.27–1.22)
	428 i.v.	2–4	9 (1)[a]	0.26 (1.10–1.71)	0.57 (0.29–0.96)	0.47 (0.20–0.56)
Lomefloxacin	400 p.o.	4	5	1.81 (1.39–3.00)	1.38 (0.60–3.06)	0.48 (0.40–1.53)

[a] A prostatic fluid/plasma value above unity for ioxitalamic acid was taken as the index for urinary contamination; results for patients with these values are not included in the table.
[b] Short and steady-state infusion.

lones into seminal fluid of volunteers (Table 5; Naber et al. 1988, 1989a–c, 1990a,b). Ciprofloxacin (200 mg intravenously) showed the highest seminal fluid to plasma ratio and fleroxacin (400 mg orally) the highest absolute concentrations. Drug concentrations in fraction 2 of the split ejaculate were usually somewhat higher than those in fraction 1, but were significantly higher ($p < 0.05$) only after intravenous administration (over 60 min) of 428 mg enoxacin.

Drug concentrations in prostatic tissue are usually measured in patients undergoing transurethral resection of the prostate and thus actually represent concentrations in prostatic adenoma tissue. Levels in prostatic tissue have been studied for most of the newer quinolones.

In general, tissue concentrations exceeded the corresponding plasma concentrations, with some differences between the quinolones. The results are not directly comparable, however, because different techniques of tissue preparation and analysis were used. Our results (Naber et al. 1987a, b, 1988, 1989a–c) with five quinolones are presented in Table 6.

In the three studies in which the stomacher and Ultra Turrax (Typ-Lab-Blender 80, Kleinfeld, Hannover; and Typ TP 18-10, IKA, Staufen, Germany) preparation techniques were used at the same time; concentrations found after using the Stomacher technique were generally lower. This difference could be explained by the fact that cells in which high concentrations of quinolones are expected were more thoroughly broken down by the Ultra Turrax technique.

For ciprofloxacin and enoxacin the prostatic tissue concentrations are about twice as high as the plasma concentrations; for norfloxacin they are about 1.5 times as high, and for ofloxacin and fleroxacin they are about 10% higher. Because of higher plasma concentrations ofloxacin and fleroxacin show the highest absolute tissue levels.

Table 5. Concentrations of newer quinolones in plasma (P) and seminal fluid (SF)[a] of volunteers (median concentration ratio, range; from Naber et al. 1988, 1990b)

Drug	Dose (mg)	Time (h)	n	P (mg/l)	Seminal fluid fraction 1			Seminal fluid fraction 2		
					SF1 (mg/l)	SF1/P		SF2 (mg/l)	SF2/P	
Lomefloxacin	400 p.o.	4	6	1.75 (1.39–3.00)	1.80 (1.48–2.65)	1.0 (0.7–1.3)		2.04 (1.87–2.65)	1.3 (1.0–1.4)	
	400 p.o.	24	6	0.19 (0.16–0.24)	0.17 (0.08–0.51)	1.1 (0.4–2.2)		0.20 (0.16–0.32)	1.1 (0.9–1.3)	
Temafloxacin	400 p.o.	4	12	2.16 (1.32–3.49)	2.30 (1.38–4.06)	1.1 (0.8–1.5)		2.52 (1.66–5.62)	1.3 (1.0–2.1)	
	400 p.o.	12	6	0.93 (0.69–1.17)	1.39 (0.68–4.96)	1.4 (0.8–5.3)		1.31 (0.82–1.77)	1.3 (1.0–2.0)	
Fleroxacin	400 p.o.	2–4	8	3.71 (2.98–4.70)	5.52 (3.05–8.13)	1.3 (0.8–2.2)		5.80 (3.95–8.61)	1.7 (1.9–2.3)	
	400 p.o.	12	4	1.69 (1.23–1.87)	2.76 (1.78–2.89)	1.5 (1.4–1.8)		2.89 (1.96–3.11)	1.7 (1.6–1.8)	
Enoxacin	400 p.o.	2–4	11	1.00 (0.51–1.91)	2.07 (1.21–4.60)	2.2 (1.4–3.3)		2.19 (1.13–3.17)	2.2 (1.5–3.3)	
	428 i.v.	2–4	11	1.24 (0.86–1.71)	2.53 (1.63–3.89)	2.1 (1.6–2.4)		3.50 (1.69–5.78)	2.8 (1.6–3.7)	
Ciprofloxacin	200 i.v.	4	8	0.44 (0.35–0.58)	2.53 (1.75–4.11)	5.8 (4.0–8.6)		2.53 (1.75–4.14)	7.1 (3.0–10.6)	
	200 i.v.	12	4	0.09 (0.06–0.10)	0.61 (0.54–1.38)	7.9 (6.7–13.8)		0.70 (0.44–1.37)	9.4 (4.9–13.7)	

[a] Seminal fluid was collected as a split ejaculate in fractions 1 and 2.
[b] Short and steady-state infusion.

Table 6. Concentrations of newer quinolones in plasma and prostatic tissue of elderly patients undergoing transurethral (median concentration ratio, range; from Naber et al. 1987a, 1989c)

Drug	Dose (mg)	Time (h)	n	Plasma (mg/l)	Prostatic tissue (mg/kg)	Tissue/plasma ratio
Ofloxacin	400 p.o.	2.0–4.5	7	3.99 (2.80–4.86)	4.08 (2.40–5.58)[a]	1.12 (0.86–1.32)
	400 p.o.	14.5–19.5	10	1.87 (0.41–3.34)	1.20 (< 0.1–1.99)[b]	0.95 (0.57–1.81)[b]
Fleroxacin	400 p.o.	1.5–4.0	11	3.73 (0.44–5.54)	4.24 (2.98–6.82)[a]	1.10 (1.00–1.92)[a]
Norfloxacin	800 i.v.	1.0–2.5	13	1.56 (0.40–5.07)	1.68 (0.68–4.30)[a]	1.52 (0.67–4.20)[a]
Ciprofloxacin	200 i.v.	1.0–2.5	14	0.81 (0.64–1.54)	1.71 (0.89–4.54)[a]	1.88 (1.30–4.24)[a]
	200 i.v.	1.0–2.5	14	0.81 (0.64–1.54)	1.87 (1.02–5.81)[b]	2.57 (1.41–5.43)[b]
Enoxacin	400 p.o.	1.0–4.0	7	0.95 (0.14–2.07)	1.65 (0.29–4.29)[a]	1.91 (1.26–2.25)[a]
			12	0.96 (0.14–2.07)	2.25 (0.37–5.02)[b]	2.56 (0.37–5.02)[b]

[a] Values obtained by the Stomacher method.
[b] Values obtained by the Ultra-Turrax method.

Results of Clinical Studies

Numerous studies have been conducted, with newer quinolones; Tables 7–10 report those in which the diagnostic procedure for determining prostatitis was mentioned. Patients with prostatitis treated as a subgroup had to be evaluated separately. To present the results of the studies in a comparative way, the bacteriological cure rate per patient, i.e., number of percentage of patients without pathogens at the site of infection, was calculated for the total time of follow-up. Patients dropping out earlier without pathogens at the site of infection were rated as unevaluable and were not included; patients dropping out any time during the follow-up period and presenting pathogens at the site of infection were rated as failure in terms of the least favorable outcome. Therefore the number of patients and the bacteriological cure rates may differ from the figures presented in the reports by the authors.

The presentation of clinical results also differed among the studies. In some studies clinical cure and improvement were considered as success, making a comparable evaluation difficult. In a considerable number of patients clinical results did not correlate well with bacteriological results, especially in the case of a short follow-up period. For all these reasons in the following analysis only the "objective" bacteriological results were considered. However, even these results are difficult to compare since in some studies not only chronic but also acute prostatitis episodes were treated, and the results were not reported separately. In addition, the investigators did not use the same criteria for the diagnosis of chronic bacterial prostatitis. The standard four-specimen technique according to Meares and Stamey (1968) for localizing the infection to the prostate was not used by all the investigators. French investigators usually diagnosed a prostatitis only according to clinical symptoms and digital rectal examination of the prostate in combination with an exacerbation of a UTI. The causative pathogens were cultured from a clean-catch midstream specimen of urine (> 10^4 cfu/ml; Guibert and Acar 1986; Guibert et al. 1986, 1987). In two studies (Bischoff 1985; Bischoff et al. 1989) the pathogens were cultured only from an ejaculate specimen. There was also a wide range of treatment duration, from 7 to 259 days, and the follow-up periods ranged from evaluation during treatment or immediately at the end of treatment (Japanese studies) to as long as 1 year or longer after completion of therapy (Weidner et al. 1987, 1991; Pfau 1991; Purt et al. 1989). In two studies no information concerning the follow-up period was available (Asbach and Melekos 1986; Okada 1985). Therefore the results must be interpreted with great caution.

If only studies are considered in which patients were included according to the standard localization of the infection (Meares and Stamey 1968) and with a follow-up of at least 1 month, only few studies remain for detailed discussion.

Norfloxacin

There are only three studies with norfloxacin (Table 7; Bologna et al. 1985; Schaeffer and Darras 1990; Petrikkos et al. 1991) which meet the above criteria. Bologna et al. (1985) treated 20 patients aged 24–62 years. Twelve patients were infected by gram-negative rods (*Escherichia coli* 8, *Klebsiella pneumoniae* 2, *Pseudomonas aeruginosa* 2) and eight by gram-positive cocci (enterococci and *Staphylococcus aureus* in mono- and mixed infection). Norfloxacin 400 mg twice daily was administered for 10 days plus serratiopeptidase (20000 U twice daily for 10 days), a fibrinolytic enzyme, to prevent postinflammatory fibrinolytic damage. The patients were followed up for at least 5 weeks. Three patients (15%) suffered a relapse (*E. coli* 2, *Enterococcus* 1) and one patient (5%) a reinfection (*S. epidermidis*). Schaeffer and Darras (1990) treated 15 men who had chronic bacterial prostatitis (*E. coli* 13, *P. aeruginosa* 2) refractory to trimethoprim-sulfamethoxazole and/or carbenicillin with 400 mg norfloxacin twice daily for 28 days. One patient was lost to follow-up at 1 month. Of the 14 patients followed for at least 6 months, 9 (64%) were cured of the original infection (*E. coli* only), including 6 who remained uninfected for at least 2 years (1), 1 year (2), or 6 months (3). In three patients UTI recurred with new pathogens at 6, 560, and 820 days, respectively, after results of prostatic fluid cultures had initially been negative after therapy. Bacterial prostatitis with the original pathogen recurred in 5 patients within 2 months of completing therapy. The bacteria remained susceptible to norfloxacin but could not be eradicated with additional norfloxacin therapy over 30–90 days. Petrikkos et al. (1991) treated 42 patients with norfloxacin at a dose of 400 mg twice daily, reduced to 200 mg twice daily after 3 months, for a mean duration of 5.8 months. During the median follow-up of 8 months 60% of the patients remained uninfected.

K.G. Naber

Table 7. Eradication of pathogens (bacteriological cure) in patients with bacterial prostatitis treated with norfloxacin

Drug	Dose (mg)	Duration of therapy (days)	n	Bacteriological cure (%)	Follow-up months	Type	Reference
Norfloxacin	400 b.i.d.	28–42	25	92	1	Chronic	Sabbaj et al. (1986)
Trimethoprim-sulfamethoxazole	160/800 b.i.d.	15	15	67	1	Chronic	Sabbaj et al. (1986)
Norfloxacin	400 b.i.d.	10	20[a]	85	1	Chronic	Bologna et al. (1985)
Norfloxacin	400 b.i.d.	10	50	88	0.1	NS	Bischoff (1985)
Rosoxacin	150 b.i.d.	14	20[a]	20	NS	Bac/Chl	Asbach and Melekos (1986)
Norfloxacin	400 b.i.d.	14	15[a]	75	NS	Bac/Chl	Asbach and Melekos (1986)
Ofloxacin	200 b.i.d.	14	20[a]	75	NS	Bac/Chl	Asbach and Melekos (1986)
Norfloxacin	400 b.i.d.	28	14[a]	64	6	Chronic[b]	Schaeffer and Darras (1990)
Norfloxacin	400 b.i.d.	28	15[a]	93	0.2	E. coli	Rauch and Taylor (1990)
Carbenicillin	764 q.i.d.	28	10[a]	60	0.2	E. coli	Rauch and Taylor (1990)
Norfloxacin	200–400 b.i.d.	174	42[a]	60	8	Chronic	Petrikkos et al. (1991)

NS, Not specified; Bac/Chl, bacterial, chlamydial.
[a] Localization study performed.
[b] Refractory to trimethoprim-sulfamethoxazole ± carbenicillin.

Ciprofloxacin

There are six studies with ciprofloxacin (Table 8; Weidner et al. 1987, 1991; Childs 1987; Pfau 1987, 1991; Langenmeyer 1987, Heidler 1990) meeting the above criteria. Childs (1987) collected data on 42 adult men aged from 19 to 85 years with documented chronic bacterial prostatitis. The most frequently isolated organisms were *E. coli* (17), *P. aeruginosa* (13), *Serratia marcescens* (2), *K. pneumoniae* (2), *Proteus vulgaris* (2), and *P. mirabilis* (2). The patients were treated with oral ciprofloxacin at a dosage of 500 mg twice daily for periods ranging from 10 to 259 days. Most patients were treated for a period of either 20–29 days (United States) or for 85 days (Europe); six had 10–14 days of therapy, and one had a 259-day course. In 29 of 37 evaluable patients (78%) the pathogens remained eradicated during the follow-up period of at least 10 weeks after completion of therapy. One patient required surgery for persisting symptoms.

Weidner et al. (1987) evaluated 15 men with chronic bacterial prostatitis (duration of symptoms more than 1 year) who had previously been treated with trimethoprim or trimethoprim-sulfamethoxazole for at least 6 weeks without showing any improvement. The patients were treated with oral ciprofloxacin 500 mg twice daily for 2 weeks. Eradication for up to 1 year after completion of therapy could be achieved in 9 of 15 (60%). For six patients (*E. coli* prostatitis) who had acquired infections with *Chlamydia* or *Ureaplasma* during follow-up, an additional therapy with tetracycline hydrochloride (1000 mg daily for 1 week) was prescribed. In a second study Weidner et al. (1991) evaluated 16 men with confirmed chronic bacterial prostatitis treated with oral ciprofloxacin 500 mg twice daily for 4 weeks. All the men had been pretreated either with cotrimoxazole, trimethoprim, or norfloxacin (two cases). Two patients stopped treatment earlier because of central nervous system side effects. After a median follow-up of 30 (21–36) months, 10 of 16 patients were considered cured. Langenmeyer et al. (1987) treated 32 men for 28 days with ciprofloxacin 500 mg twice daily, with a cure rate of 75% after 2-month follow-up. Heidler (1990) treated 34 patients between 21 days and 42 days (if not free of symptoms after 21 days), with a dose of 250 mg twice daily and obtained a bacteriological cure of 62% after 6 months. Pfau (1987, 1991) cured six of seven patients (84%) with ciprofloxacin 500 mg twice daily, with a follow-up period of at least 12 months.

Ofloxacin

With ofloxacin (Table 9), localization studies were performed in four investigations (Asbach and Melekos 1986; Pust et al. 1989; Corrado 1991; Suzuki et al. 1984). However, in three studies it was not reported how long the patients were followed up, or the evaluation was performed at completion of therapy. Therefore, the success rates obtained cannot be compared with those of other

Table 8. Eradication of pathogens (bacteriological cure) in patients with bacterial prostatitis treated with ciprofloxacin

Drug	Dose (mg)	Duration of therapy (days)	n	Bacteriological cure (%)	Follow-up months	Type	Reference
Ciprofloxacin	100 t.i.d.	12,17	2	100	NS	Chronic	Okada (1985)
Ciprofloxacin	250 b.i.d.	7	10	60	1	Acute/chronic	Zamfirescu and Chysky (1985)
Ciprofloxacin	500 b.i.d.	84	15	67	3	P. aeruginosa	Guibert et al. (1986)
Ciprofloxacin	500 b.i.d.	28 or 84	26	77	1	NS	Guibert et al. (1986)
Ciprofloxacin	500 b.i.d.	14	15[a]	60	12	Chronic[b]	Weidner et al. (1987)
Ciprofloxacin	500 b.i.d.	28	16[a]	63	21–36	Chronic[b]	Weidner et al. (1991)
Ciprofloxacin	500 b.i.d.	10–259	37[a]	78	2.5	Chronic	Childs (1987)
Ciprofloxacin	500 b.i.d.	28	32[a]	75	2	Chronic	Langenmeyer et al. (1987)
Ciprofloxacin	400–600/day	7–21	21[a]	83	0	Acute/chronic	Matsumoto et al. (1987)
Ciprofloxacin	250 b.i.d.	14	40	78	6	NS	Bischoff and Bischoff (1989)
Trimethoprim-sulfamethoxazole	160/800 b.i.d.	14	40	61	6	NS	Bischoff and Bischoff (1989)
Ciprofloxacin	500 b.i.d.	60–150	7[a]	86	12	Chronic	Pfau (1987, 1991)
Ciprofloxacin	250 b.i.d.	21–42	34[a]	62	6	Chronic	Heidler (1990)
Ciprofloxacin	300 b.i.d.	14	20[a]	100	0	Chronic	Yoshida et al. (1991)
Ciprofloxacin	200 b.i.d.	14	20[a]	75	0	Chronic	Suzuki et al. (1991)

NS, Not specified.
[a] Localization study performed.
[b] Refractory to trimethoprim ± sulfamethoxazole.
[c] Combined with UTI.

Table 9. Eradication of pathogens (bacteriological cure) in patients with bacterial prostatitis treated with ofloxacin

Drug	Dose (mg)	Duration of therapy (days)	n	Bacteriological cure (%)	Follow-up (months)	Type	Reference
Ofloxacin	100–200 t.i.d.	5–21	22[a]	82	0	Acute/chronic	Suzuki et al. (1984)
Ofloxacin	200 b.i.d.	40	14	79	3–12	NS	Guibert and Acar (1986)
Ofloxacin	200 b.i.d.	60	23	91	7–13	Acute/chronic	Remy et al. (1988)
Rosoxacin	150 b.i.d.	14	20[a]	20	NS	Bac/Chl	Asbach and Melekos (1986)
Norfloxacin	400 b.i.d.	14	15[a]	75	NS	Bac/Chl	Asbach and Melekos (1986)
Ofloxacin	200 b.i.d.	14	20[a]	75	NS	Bac/Chl	Asbach and Melekos (1986)
Ofloxacin	300 b.i.d.	42	43[a]	85	NS	NS	Corrado (1991)
Carbenicillin	764 t.i.d.	42	42[a]	53	NS	NS	Corrado (1991)
Ofloxacin	200 b.i.d.	14	21[a]	67	12	Chronic	Pust et al. (1989)

NS, Not specified; Bac/Chl, bacterial/chlamydial.
[a] Localization study performed.

Table 10. Eradication of pathogens (bacteriological cure) in patients with bacterial prostatitis treated with quinolones

Drug	Dose (mg)	Duration of therapy (days)	n	Bacteriological cure (%)	Follow-up months	Type	Reference
Perfloxacin	400 b.i.d.	NS	31	65	3	NS	Desplaces et al. (1986)
Perfloxacin	400 b.i.d.	28	31	74	1	Acute/chronic	Guibert et al. (1990)
Enoxacin	200 t.i.d.	14	97[a]	55	0	Chronic	Kumamoto et al. (1986)
Enoxacin	400 b.i.d.	28	38[a]	55	1	Chronic	Christensen et al. (1989)
Carbenicillin	764 b.i.d.	28	46[a]	53	1	Chronic	Christensen et al. (1989)
Temafloxacin	400 b.i.d.	28	76[a]	72	1	Chronic	Cox and Childs (1991)
Temafloxacin	400 b.i.d.	28	42[a]	68	1	Chronic	Naber et al. (1991)
Rufloxacin	200 q.i.d.	28	24[a]	79	1	Chronic	Boerema et al. (1990)
Fleroxacin	200–300 q.i.d.	7–26	11[a]	100	0	Chronic	Nishitani et al. (1991)

[a] Localization study performed.

studies. In one study (Pust et al. 1989) the patients were followed up to 1 year with a final cure rate of 67%.

Other Quinolones

Of the studies with other quinolones (Table 10), the comparative study with enoxacin versus carbenicillin (Christensen et al. 1990), the two studies with temafloxacin (Cox and Childs 1991; Naber et al. 1991), and the study with rufloxacin (Boerema et al. 1991) fulfilled the above criteria. In the other studies either the infection was not localized or the evaluation was performed at completion of therapy.

Christensen et al. (1990) analyzed data on patients treated with oral enoxacin 400 mg twice daily versus oral carbenicillin 764 mg four times daily for 28 days. Four to six weeks after therapy 8 of 9 (89%) gram-negative rods were eradicated by enoxacin as compared with 7 of 17 (41%) by carbenicillin. Of the gram-positive cocci 13 of 29 (45%) were eradicated by enoxacin and 17 of 28 (61%) by carbenicillin. The overall eradication rates of 55% and 53%, respectively, were almost identical.

In the two studies with temafloxacin (Cox and Childs 1991; Naber et al. 1991) 76 and 42 men were evaluated, resulting in bacteriological cure of 72% and 68%, respectively.

Boerema et al. (1991) analyzed an uncontrolled multicenter study with rufloxacin. Twenty-four men with chronic bacterial prostatitis treated orally with 400 mg once daily on the first day followed by 200 mg once daily over 4 weeks were evaluated. Up to 1 month after completion of therapy 79% of the patients showed bacteriological cure.

Conclusion

Although the newer quinolones appear to have been used to quite an extent for the treatment of chronic bacterial prostatitis, the analysis of the published studies has not yet established a definitive conclusion concerning the role of quinolones as compared with standard treatment. Results can be compared only for investigations in which the diagnosis was obtained by localization studies, and in which the patients were followed up for a sufficient length of time after completion of therapy, and only a few studies meet these criteria. Of these, only four – one with norfloxacin (Schaeffer and Darras 1990), four with ciprofloxacin (Weidner et al. 1987, 1991; Pfau 1987, 1991; Heidler 1990) and one with ofloxacin (Pust et al. 1989) – presented results obtained during a follow-up period of at least 6 months. The results of these studies seem to be comparable.

In general, the therapeutic results are good in chronic prostatitis due to *E. coli* or other Enterobacteriaceae but not in prostatitis due to *P. aeruginosa* or enterococci. For the chronic prostatitis caused by *E. coli* a treatment duration of 1 month seems to be superior than the usual 3-month treatment period with cotrimoxazole. There is a need for further, especially controlled studies with valid protocols to elucidate the role of the newer quinolones in the treatment of chronic bacterial prostatitis.

References

Anderson RU, Fair WR (1976) Physical and chemical determinations of prostatic secretion in benign hyperplasia, prostatitis and adenocarcinoma. Invest Urol 14:137–140

Asbach HW, Melekos M (1986) Zur Behandlung der Urethro-Adnexitis des Mannes mit Gyrasehemmern. In: Adam D, Knothe H, Lode H, Stille W (eds) Ofloxacin, Fortschr Antimicrob Antineopl Chemother FAC 5-5. Futuramed, Munich, pp 857–859

Bischoff W (1985) Norfloxacin-Behandlung der akuten Zystitis der Frau und der bakteriellen Prostatitis. Fortschr Med 103:225–228

Bischoff W, Bischoff H (1989) Bacterial prostatitis: efficacy of ciprofloxacin versus sulfonamide-trimethoprim therapy (poster). International Congress on Chemotherapy, Jerusalem, p 213

Blacklock NJ, Beavis JP (1974) The response of fluid pH in inflammation. Br J Urol 46:537–542

Bologna M, Vaggi L, Flammini D, Carlucci G, Forchetti CM (1985) Norfloxacin in prostatitis: correlation between HPLC tissue concentrations and clinical results. Drugs Exp Clin Res 11:95–100

Boerema JB, Dalhoff A, Debruyne FMY (1985) Ciprofloxacin distribution in prostatic tissue and fluid following oral administration. Chemotherapy 31:13–18

Boerema JB, Bischoff W, Focht J, Naber KG (1991) An open multicentre study on the efficacy and safety of rufloxacin in patients with chronic bacterial prostatitis. J Antimicrob Chemother 28:587–597

Childs SJ (1987) Treatment of chronic bacterial prostatitis with ciprofloxacin. Infect Surg 6:649–651

Christensen MM, Knes JM, Madsen PO (1990) Chronic prostatitis: pharmacokinetics of enoxacin and clinical trial results. In: Rubinstein E, Adam D (eds) Recent advances in chemotherapy. Proceedings of the 16th International Congress on Chemotherapy, Jerusalem 1989. Antimicrobial section 1. Lewin-Epstein, Jerusalem, pp 267.1–267.2

Corrado ML (1991) Worldwide clinical experience with ofloxacin in urological cases. Urology Suppl 27:28–32

Cox CE, Childs SJ (1991) Treatment of chronic bacterial prostatitis. Am J Med 91 Suppl 6A:134S–139S

Dalhoff A, Weidner W (1984) Diffusion of ciprofloxacin into prostatic fluid. Eur J Clin Microbiol 3:360–366

Desplaces N, Gutmann L, Carlet J, Guibert J, Acar JF (1986) The new quinolones and their combinations with other agents for therapy of severe infections. J Antimicrob Chemother 17 Suppl A:25–39

Dørflinger T, Larsen EH, Gasser TC, Madsen PO (1986) The concentration of various quinolone derivatives in the dog prostate. In: Weidner W, Brunner H, Krause W, Rothauge CF (eds) Therapy of prostatitis. Zuckschwerdt, Munich, pp 35–39

Drach GW (1974) Trimethoprim-sulfamethoxazole therapy of chronic bacterial prostatitis. J Urol 111:637–639

Gasser TC, Graversen PH, Madsen PO (1987) Fleroxacin (Ro 23-6240) distribution in canine prostatic tissue and fluids. Antimicrob Agents Chemother 31:1010–1013

Guibert J, Acar JF (1986) Ofloxacin (RU 43280): evaluation clinique dans les infections urinaires et prostatiques. Pathol Biol (Paris) 34:494–497

Guibert J, Destrée D, Konopka C, Acar J (1986) Ciprofloxacin in the treatment of urinary tract infection due to enterobacteria. Eur J Clin Microbiol 5:247–248

Guibert JM, Destrée DM, Acar JF (1987) Ciprofloxacin (BAY 09867): clinical evaluation in urinary tract infections due to Pseudomonas aeruginosa. Chemioterapia 6 Suppl:524–525

Guibert J, Boutelier R, Guyot A (1990) A clinical trial of pefloxacin in prostatitis. J Antimicrob Chemother 26 Suppl B:161–166

Hanus PM, Danzinger LH (1984) Treatment of chronic bacterial prostatitis. Clin Pharm 3: 49–55

Heidler H (1990) Clinical effects of ciprofloxacin: clinical results in chronic bacterial prostatitis. In: Lode H (ed) Ciprofloxacin in clinical practice: new light on established and emerging uses. Schwer, Stuttgart, pp 53–56

Kumamoto Y, Sakai S, Tamate H, Gohro T, Inoke T, Tabata S, Tanda H, Kato S, Saka T, Hemmi I (1986) Therapeutic studies on chronic prostatitis – use of AT-2266. Hinyokika Kiyo 32:1213–1223

Kumon H, Mizuno A, Kishi M, Miyata K, Ohmori H (1985) The concentration of ofloxacin in human prostatic tissue and fluid. In: Ishigami J (ed) Recent advances in chemotherapy. Proceedings of the 14th International Congress of Chemotherapy, sect 2. University of Tokyo Press, Tokyo, pp 1767–1768

Langenmeyer TN, Ferwerda WH, Hoogkamp-Korstanje JA, de Leur EJ, van Oort H (1987) Treatment of chronic bacterial prostatitis with ciprofloxacin. Pharm Weekbl [Sci] 9 Suppl:78–81

Madsen PO, Baumüller A, Hoyme U (1978) Experimental models for determination of antimicrobials in prostatic tissue, interstitial fluid and secretion. Scand J Infect Dis 1 Suppl 4:145–150

Matsumoto T, Tanaka M, Kumazawa J, Hara S, Iwakawa A, Ito K, Nagayoshi H, Hirano H, Sato S, Omoto T, Amano T, Soejima T, Jinnouchi K, Mikuriya M, Nakao T, Nanri K, Hirata H, Miyazaki N, Nagayama A (1987) Clinical studies of ciprofloxacin (BAY 09867) in the treatment of prostatitis and acute epididymitis. Nishinikou J Urol 49:673–690

McGurie EJ, Lytton B (1976) Bacterial prostatitis. Treatment with trimethoprim-sulfamethoxazole. Urology 7:499–500

Meares EM Jr (1973) Observations on activity of trimethoprim-sulfamethoxazole in the prostate. J Infect Dis 129 Suppl:679–685

Meares EM Jr (1975a) Long-term therapy of chronic bacterial prostatitis with trimethoprim-sulfamethoxazole. Can Med Assoc J 112 Suppl:22–25

Meares EM Jr (1975b) Prostatitis. A review. Urol Clin North Am 2:3–27

Meares EM Jr (1978) Serum antibody titers in treatment with trimethoprim-sulfamethoxazole for chronic prostatitis. Urology 11:141–146

Meares EM Jr (1980) Prostatitis syndromes. New perspectives about old woes. J Urol 123:141–147

Meares EM, Stamey TA (1968) Bacteriologic localization patterns in bacterial prostatitis and urethritis. Invest Urol 5:492–518

Mizoguchi H, Maeda A, Thimizu T, Ishigami J (1985) An appraisal of ofloxacin level in semen. In: Ishigami J (ed) Recent advances in chemotherapy. Proceedings of the 14th International Congress of Chemotherapy, sect 2. University of Tokyo Press, Tokyo, pp 1793–1794

Mobley DF (1974) Erythromycin plus sodium bicarbonate in chronic bacterial prostatitis. Urology 3:60–62

Mobley DF (1981) Bacterial prostatitis: treatment with carbenicillin indanyl sodium. Invest Urol 19:31–33

Naber KG, Sörgel F, Kees F, Schumacher H, Metz R, Grobecker H (1987a) Norfloxacin concentration in prostatic adenoma tissue (patients) and in prostatic fluid in patients and volunteers. 15th International Congress of Chemotherapy, Landsberg

Naber KG, Adam D, Kees F (1987b) In vitro activity and concentrations in serum, urine, prostatic secretion and adenoma tissue of ofloxacin in urological patients. Drugs 34 Suppl 1:44–50

Naber KG, Sörgel F, Kees F, Jaehde U, Schumacher H, Metz R, Grobecker H (1988) In vitro activity of fleroxacin against isolates causing complicate urinary tract infections and concentrations in seminal and prostatic fluid and in prostatic adenoma tissue. J Antimicrob Chemother 21 Suppl D:199–207

Naber KG, Sörgel F, Kees F, Schumacher H, Sigl G, Zürcher J, Berger S (1989a) Enoxacin-Konzentrationen in der Samenflüssigkeit, im Prostatasekret und im Prostatadenomgewebe nach oraler Gabe oder intravenöser Infusion. Infection 17 Suppl 1:30–36

Naber KG, Sörgel F, Kees F, Jaehde U, Schumacher H (1989b) Pharmakokinetik von Ciprofloxacin bei Probanden und älteren Patienten und Konzentrationen im Prostatasekret, Ejakulat und im Prostataadenomgewebe nach intravenöser Gabe. In: Adam D, Dalhoff A, Wiedemann B (eds) Ofloxacin. Fortschr Antimicrob Antineopl Chemother FAC 8-1. Futuramed, Munich, pp 75–87

Naber KG, Sörgel F, Kees F, Jaehde U, Schumacher H (1989c) Brief report: pharmacokinetics of ciprofloxacin in young (healthy) volunteers and elderly patients, and concentrations in prostatic fluid, seminal fluid, and prostatic adenoma tissue following intravenous administration. Am J Med 87 Suppl 5A:57–59

Naber KG, Sörgel F. Sigl G, Schumacher H, Metz R (1990a) Lomefloxacin: Penetration into prostatic and seminal fluid in volunteers (Poster). 3rd Int Symp on New Quinolones, Vancouver, Abstract no 248

Naber KG, Sörgel F, Sigl G, Schumacher H, Jürcher J (1990b) Penetration of temafloxacin into prostatic and seminal fluid in volunteers. Eur J Clin Microb Infect Dis 29–30

Naber KG, Boerema JBJ, Bischoff W, Blenk H, Focht J, Carpentier P, Sylvester J (1991) An assessment of temafloxacin in the treatment of chronic bacterial prostatitis. J Antimicrob Chemother 28 Suppl C:87–96

Nishitani Y, Uno S, Tsugawa M, Kondo K, Kumon H, Ohmori H (1991) Fleroxacin in the treatment of bacterial prostatitis. (extended abstract). 17th International Congress of Chemotherapy, June 23–28, Berlin

Okada K (1985) Clinical studies on BAY 09867 in the field of urology. Chemotherapy (Tokyo) 33 Suppl 7:601–611

Oliveri RA, Sachs RM, Castl PG (1979) Clinical experiences with geocillin in the treatment of bacterial prostatitis. Curr Ther Res 25:415–421

Paulson DF, White RD (1978) Trimethoprim-sulfamethoxazole and minocyclinehydrochloride in the treatment of culture-proved bacterial prostatitis. J Urol 120:184–185

Petrikkos G, Peppas T, Giamarellou H, Poulios K, Zouboulis P, Sfikakis P (1991) Four year experience with norfloxacin in the treatment of chronic bacterial prostatitis (Abstr 1302). 17th International Congress of Chemotherapy, June 23–28, Berlin

Pfau A (1986) Prostatitis. A continuing enigma. Urol Clin North Am 13:695–715

Pfau A (1987) Therapie der unteren Harnwegsinfektionen beim Mann unter besonderer Berücksichtigung der chronischen bakteriellen Prostatitis. Aktuel Urol 18:31–33.

Pfau A (1991) The treatment of chronic bacterial prostatitis. Infection 19 Suppl 3:160–164

Pfau A, Perlberg S, Shapiro A (1978) The pH of the prostatic fluid in health and disease: implications of treatment in chronic bacterial prostatitis. J Urol 119:384–387

Pust RA, Ackenhiel-Koppe HR, Gilbert T, Weidner W (1989) Clinical efficacy of ofloxacin (Tanviol) in patients with chronic bacterial prostatitis: preliminary results. J Chemotherm 1 Suppl 4:869–871

Rauch AM, Taylor VI (1990) Effective treatment of E. coli prostatitis with norfloxacin (Poster No. 254) 3rd Int Symp New Quinolones, Vancouver

Remy G, Rouger C, Chavanet P, Bernard E, Dellamonica P, Portier H (1988) Use of ofloxacin for prostatitis. Rev Infect Dis 10 Suppl 1:173–174

Sabath LD, Gerstein D'A, Loder FB, Finland M (1968) Excretion of erythromycin and its enhanced activity in urine against gram-negative bacilli with alkalinization. J Lab Clin Med 72:916–923

Sabbaj J, Hoagland VL, Cood T (1986) Norfloxacin versus co-trimoxazole in the treatment of recurring urinary tract infections in men. Scand J Infect Dis Suppl 48:48–53

Schaeffer AJ, Darras FS (1990) The efficacy of norfloxacin in the treatment of chronic bacterial prostatitis refractory to trimethoprim-sulfamethoxazole and/or carbenicillin. J Urol 144: 690–693

Schramm P (1986) Ofloxacin concentration in human ejaculate and influence on sperm motility. Infection 14 Suppl 4:274–275

Smith JW, Jones SR, Reed WP, Tice AD, Deuprée RH, Kaijser B (1979) Recurrent urinary tract infections in men. Ann Intern Med 91:544–548

Stamey TA, Meares EM Jr, Winningham DG (1970) Chronic bacterial prostatitis and the diffusion of drugs into prostatic fluid. J Urol 103:187–194

Suzuki K, Tamai H, Naide Y, Ando K, Moriguchi R (1984) Laboratory and clinical study of ofloxacin in the treatment of bacterial prostatitis. Hinyokika Kiyo 30:1505–1518

Suzuki K et al. (1991) Ciprofloxacin in treatment of chronic prostatitis (Abstr 1304). 17th International Congress of Chemotherapy, June 23–28, Berlin

Weidner W, Schiefer HG, Dalhoff A (1987) Treatment of chronic bacterial prostatitis with ciprofloxacin. Results of a one-year follow-up study. Am J Med 82 (Suppl 4A):280–283

Weidner W, Schiefer HG, Brähler E (1991) Refractory chronic bacterial prostatitis: a re-evaluation of ciprofloxacin treatment after a median follow up of 30 months. J Urol 146:350–352

Yoshida K, Uchijima Y, Saitoh H, Negishi T, Yamada T, Watanabe T, Kawakami K (1991) Abstract No. 1303. 17th International Congress of Chemotherapy, June 23–28, Berlin

Zamfirescu C, Chysky V (1985) Behandlung von refraktären Harnwegsinfektionen und Prostatitis bei nicht hospitalisierten Patienten mit Ciprofloxacin. Urologe [B] 25:330–333

Zinner SH, Sabath LD, Casey JL, Finland M (1971) Erythromycin and alkalinization of the urine in the treatment of urinary tract infections due to gram-negative bacilli. Lancet 1:1267–1268

In Loco Antibiotics in Chronic Bacterial Prostatitis

L. Baert and D. De Ridder

Introduction

Chronic bacterial prostatitis (CBP) is a rare pathological entity. Bacterial prostatitis is the most difficult form to treat. Many efforts have been made to find a way of curing this disease: long-term antibiotics, suppressive regimes of antibiotics, and surgical treatment with transurethral resection. In loco injection of antibiotics via perineal route offers a good therapeutic alternative for these classic treatments. However, since new quinolones have appeared and are easily available, the indications for in loco injections have diminished. This review analyzes the theoretical background, the principles involved, and the literature of the past decade.

Theoretical Considerations

Chronic Bacterial Prostatitis

The diagnosis of CBP must be based on accurate lower urinary tract localization studies and examination of the prostatic fluid (Baert et al. 1983a, b, 1991; Meares 1991). Some authors also accept ejaculate cultures as diagnostic (Blacklock 1991). The localization studies as described by Meares and Stamey can easily be modified and so reach higher accuracy by replacing the VB2 specimen by a suprapubic puncture sample (Baert et al. 1983). The diagnosis of CBP can be made only when at least 10 000 colonies/ml are counted in the VB3 specimen or at least 100 colonies in the expressed prostatic secretion. The VB3 to VB1 ratio must be 10 or higher, and the VB2 or suprapubic puncture specimen must remain sterile. Only when suprapubic puncture, expressed prostatic secretion (EPS), and VB3 culture show no growth, can cultures be regarded as negative. In most cases *Escherichia coli* is the pathogenic organism. Other gram-negative organisms may also be found. Whether gram-positive organisms may be pathogens or urethral contamination remains controversial.

Microscopic examination of the expressed prostatic secretions is also indispensable for the accurate diagnosis of CBP. However, this examination can be misleading when the condition of the urethra is not evaluated at the same time. In cases of urethritis, urethral stricture, urethral diverticulum, ejaculation, and sexual intercourse, the urethral surface sheds inflammatory cells. These cells can contaminate the expressed fraction and give the impression that the prostate is inflamed (Meares 1991).

To localize the site of infection the physician should always compare the microscopic appearance of the prostatic secretion with smears of the VB1 and VB2 sediments.

Despite some controversy more than 15–20 white blood cells per high-power field in the EPS are considered as diagnostic of prostatic infection. The most convincing sign of prostatitis is the finding of both excessive numbers of white blood cells and macrophages containing fat droplets (oval fat bodies) in the EPS, as well as a variable decrease of the so-called lecithin bodies (Baert et al. 1983a, b).

CBP is often associated with prostatic calculi. These are composed mainly of cellular debris from the prostate and constituents found only in urine (Klimas et al. 1985). Intraprostatic reflux is seen as an important pathogenic factor (Kirby et al. 1982; Klimas et al. 1985; Meares 1991). Once infected, these calculi may be responsible for relapsing prostatitis or urinary tract infections. As with infected kidney stones, antibiotics can mend but not cure the infection.

The Plasma-Prostate Barrier

The treatment of choice for CBP during the past decade has been trimethoprim-sulfamethoxazole for a prolonged course of 6–12 weeks (McGuire 1984; Schaeffer 1984). With this therapeutic regime there is still a failure rate of 40%–60% (Meares 1991; Schaeffer 1984). The failure rate does not seem to be related to bacterial resistance (Schaeffer 1984). This form of therapy is based on dog model studies. The diffusion of antimicrobial agents from the plasma to the prostatic fluid was studied in dogs with surgically created prostatic fistulas (Goldfarb 1984; McGuire 1984; Schaeffer 1984). Most agents known at that time which were useful against gram-negative uropathogens showed poor diffusion. Trimethoprim, however, reached levels in the prostatic fluid that exceeded plasma levels by three- to tenfold. Unfortunately, the pharmacokinetics observed in these dog experiments do not accurately reflect the situation of the infected human prostate. In dogs the prostatic fluid is more acid than the plasma (pH 6.4). The expressed prostatic secretion in normal man is slightly alkaline (mean pH 7.31). With prostatic infection the pH of the prostatic fluid increases markedly (mean pH 8.34; Baert et al. 1991; Fair and Cordonnier 1977; Fair et al. 1978). Thus the hydrogen ion concentration of canine and human prostatic fluid may be dissimilar by a factor of 100-fold.

The major determinants for a drug to diffuse across a lipid membrane are the lipid solubility and the degree of ionization. Only non-ionized lipid soluble particles diffuse across a lipid membrane and equilibrate on both sides of a stable system. The diffusion of a charged drug depends on the pH, the higher concentration being on the side of the higher degree of ionization. This phenomenon is called ion trapping. When the prostatic fluid is more acid than the plasma, as in the dog, antimicrobial bases (trimethoprim-sulfamethoxazole) ionize to a greater extent in prostatic fluid than in plasma. Accordingly, ion trapping occurs at the prostatic side of the membrane. Therefore their concentration in prostatic fluid is higher than in plasma (McGuire 1984; Pfau 1991; Schaeffer 1984; Fair et al. 1978; Baert et al. 1983a, b; Meares 1991). In the human prostate, however, the situation is different. The prostatic fluid is alkaline, and bases do not accumulate in the prostatic fluid. The newer antimicrobial agents such as the quinolones and fluoroquinolones are mostly acid; for example, ciprofloxacin has a pK_a of 7.3. Theoretically these drugs should accumulate on the prostatic side of the lipid membrane, which has been confirmed (Weidner and Schiefer 1987; Naber 1991; Pfau 1991). Although many drugs reach significant therapeutic levels in the interstitium and stroma, the drug level in the prostatic fluid correlates best with therapeutic success or failure (Meares 1982, 1991).

In Loco Injections

In loco injection of an antiseptic fluid into the infected prostate was first performed by Ritter and Lippow in 1938, who used electrogel, a colloidal solution containing 0.04% silver, via transurethral route (Jiménez-Cruz et al. 1988; Ritter and Lippow 1938). This method was forgotten until the work of Baert and colleagues, who published the first well-documented study on this subject (Plomp et al. 1980). The method was never accepted on a wide scale. Mostly it has been European centers which have followed the example (Chantrie 1983; Jiménez-Cruz et al. 1988; Wyndaele 1985).

The method is quite simple. With a spinal needle the prostate lobes are punctured under rectal digital control via the perineum after local anesthesia (Baert et al. 1983; Chantrie 1983). Some authors as Jiménez-Cruz use echographic control and inject the antibiotic only in hypoechogenic lesions (Jiménez-Cruz et al. 1988). All authors use aminoglycosides as antibiotic drug, except one who used amoxicilline (Chantrie 1983). Patients experience only minor discomfort or pain during an acute exacerbation of CBP. There is a risk of dissemination of the infection and septicemia. Local necrosis was never noted. Hematuria and hemospermia are always present after the treatment and can last some weeks.

Occasionally urinary retention was observed (Plomp et al. 1980). In an attempt to bypass the plasma-prostate barrier, in loco injections of antimicrobial agents formed a logical step at a time when quinolones were not yet available. The drug was delivered at the site. Most authors believe that intraprostatic injections of antibiotics create an antimicrobial medium dispersed within and around the substance of the prostate gland, part of which is absorbed

Table 1. Results of in loco injections for CBP

Reference	n	Medication	Cure	
			3 months	6 months
Baert and Leonard (1988)	24	Gentamicin, cefazolin	–	70%
Baert et al. (1983b)	3	Thiamphenicol	–	0%
Chantrie (1983)	20	Amoxicillin	85%	?
Jiménez-Cruz et al. (1988)	51	Amikacin, tobramycin	71.4%	58.8%
Wyndaele (1985)	5	Gentamicin	0%	0%
Plomp et al. (1980)	29	Thiamphenicol	–	66%

by the cells while another part remains in the interstitial spaces, and the remainder eventually reaches the systemic circulation (Baert and Leonard 1988). As mentioned above, the concentration of antibiotic in the prostatic fluid correlates best with the therapeutic success or failure.

Plomp and Baert noted after thiamphenicol injection a concentration in the prostatic fluid of 1000–4000 $\mu g/ml$. The minimal inhibitory concentration for *E. coli* yields from 12.5 to 100 $\mu g/ml$. They also measured the serum levels of thiamphenicol, which decreased in 24 h from 25 to 0.3 $\mu g/ml$ (thiamphenicol half-life is 3.6 h). There was no correlation between the antibiotic concentration in the prostatic fluid and the time after injection (Baert et al. 1983; Plomp et al. 1980). They concluded that for the most strains of *E. coli* the minimal inhibitory concentration was reached. The same authors demonstrated that aminoglycosides are absorbed by the prostatic cell by confirming the presence of lamellar structures within the lysosomes of the prostatic cells which proved to be of amino sugar composition (Baert and Leonard 1988; Plomp et al. 1980).

Recently Shafik (1991) published data on anal submucosal injection of antibiotics for CBP. The drug reaches the prostate in high concentration via unidirectional hemorrhoidogenital veins and achieves therapeutic concentrations in and around the prostate. In a report on 11 patients he reported a 100% cure rate. However, further investigations are necessary to evaluate this route of drug delivery and its efficacy in treating CBP.

The overall cure rate reported in most well-documented studies is 66%–71.5%. The different authors and studies are listed in Table 1. Comparing one study with another is almost impossible since "cure" is not well defined in most studies. We should rather talk about long-term remissions (Baert and Leonard 1988; Jiménez-Cruz 1988; Meares 1991).

Conclusion

In loco injection of antibiotics for CBP was a logical step in trying to bypass the plasma-prostate barrier at a time before quinolones became available.

Only recently the scientific background for this so-called barrier was understood: the role of pH in the infected prostate and the limitations of the dog model. Since new drugs such as the quinolones and especially the fluoroquinolones are available which show good penetration in the infected prostate and are highly effective against the micro-organisms involved, there remains only limited place for in loco injections. Moreover, in the presence of infected prostatic calculi no antibiotic can really cure the patient but can only offer long-term remissions. Only radical treatment can cure the patient by means of a transurethral resection of the prostate or a radical prostatectomy. Indications for in loco injection of antibiotics into prostate are thus limited to patients who cannot be treated with quinolones, for example, in the case of allergy, or who are too young or have too high a surgical risk to be treated surgically.

References

Baert L, Leonard A (1988) Chronic bacterial prostatitis: 10 years of experience with local antibiotics. J Urol 140:755–757

Baert L, Mattelaer J, de Nollin P (1983a) Prostatitis update. Acta Urol Belg 51(3):345–357

Baert L, Mattelaer J, de Nollin P (1983b) Treatment of chronic bacterial prostatitis by local injection of antibiotics into prostate. Urology 21(4):370–375

Baert L, Van Poppel H, Vandeursen H (1991) Review of modern trends in the treatment of chronic bacterial prostatitis. Infection 19 Suppl 3:S157–S159

Blacklock NJ (1991) The anatomy of the prostate: relationship with prostatic infection. Infection 19 Suppl 3:S111–S114

Chantrie (1983) L'amoxicilline en injection locale dans le traitement de prostatite chronique. Acta Urol Belg 51(4):538–542

Fair W, Cordonnier JJ (1977) The pH of prostatic fluid: a reappraisal and therapeutic implications. J Urol 120:695–698

Fair W, Crane DB, Schiller N, Heston WDW (1978) A reappraisal of treatment in chronic bacterial prostatitis. J Urol 121:437–441

Goldfarb M (1984) Clinical efficacy of antibiotics in treatment of prostatitis. Urology 24(6):12–13

Jiménez-Cruz JF, Boronat Tormo F, Callego Gomèz J (1988) Treatment of chronic prostatitis: intraprostatic antibiotic injection under echography control. J Urol 139:967–970

Kirby RS, Lowe D, Bultitude MI, Shuttleworth KED (1982) Intraprostatic urinary reflux: an etiological factor in abacterial prostatitis. Br J Urol 54:729–731

Klimas R, Bennett B, Gardner WA (1985) Prostatic calculi: a review. Prostate 7:91–96

McGuire E (1984) Theoretical basis for treatment of prostatitis. Urology 24(6):10–11

Meares EM Jr (1982) Prostatitis: review of pharmacokinetics and therapy. Rev Infect Dis 4:475

Meares EM Jr (1991) Prostatitis. Med Clin North Am 75(2).405–424

Naber KG (1991) The role of quinolones in the treatment of chronic bacterial prostatitis. Infection 19 Suppl 3:S170–S177

Pfau A (1991) The treatment of chronic bacterial prostatitis. Infection 19 Suppl 3:S160–S164

Plomp TA, Baert L, Maes RA (1980) Treatment of recurrent chronic bacterial prostatitis by local injection of thiamphenicol into prostate. Urology 15(6):542–547

Ritter SJ, Lippow C (1938) Pathological and bacteriological processes present in prostatitis and tissue reaction to therapy. J Urol 39:111

Schaeffer AJ (1984) Pharmacokinetics of antibiotics used in the treatment of prostatitis. Urology 24(6):S8–S9

Shafik A (1991) Anal submucosal injection: a new route for drug administration. VI. Chronic prostatitis: a new modality of treatment with report of eleven cases. Urology 37(1):64–67
Weidner W, Schiefer HG, Dalhoff A (1987) Treatment of chronic bacterial prostatitis with ciprofloxacin. Results of a one year follow-up study. Am J Med 82 (Suppl 4A):280–283
Wyndaele JJ (1985) Chronic prostatitis in spinal cord injury patients. Paraplegia 23:164–169

Radical Transurethral Prostatectomy for Chronic Bacterial Prostatitis

L. Baert and D. Herremans

Introduction

Chronic bacterial prostatitis (CBP) is defined as persistence of the same pathogen in the prostatic secretions despite courses of antimicrobial therapy. The most characteristic finding is relapsing recurrent urinary tract infections (UTI), and the diagnosis is best confirmed using bacteriological localization cultures and examination of the expressed prostatic secretion (EPS) after prostatic massage, as described by Meares and Stamey (1968). In older patients CBP is frequently associated with other prostatic diseases, such as benign prostatic hyperplasia (BPH) and carcinoma. Lower urinary tract obstructions such as sphincter dyssynergia and strictures are more common in younger patients.

In CBP both the nature of the pathology and the pathological anatomy (focal character, infected calculi, duct obstructions) present difficulties in the cure in some cases and support treatment by surgery, including transurethral resection of the prostate (TURP) or radical prostatectomy. The basis of effective treatment is the removal of all infectious foci and the promotion of drainage of inflammatory products, together with prevention of a high-pressure zone of urine in the prostatic urethra. Although radical prostatectomy offers the greatest certainty of complete eradication, the risk of complications limits its acceptability in a benign disease such as CBP.

Rationale for Transurethral Resection in CBP

A major explanation for the chronicity of prostatitis is the presence of prostatic calculi and duct obstructions. Calculi are commonly found in the prostate and may become infected during an episode of bacterial prostatitis (Fox 1963; Eyken et al. 1974; Meares 1974). Fox found by careful examination of surgical and postmortem specimens that small prostatic calculi, often invisible on X-ray films, occur in almost every adult prostate. These stones are usually not associated with prostatic infection and cause no symptoms so long as they remain uninfected and confined to the prostate.

Sutor and Wooley (1974) and Ramirez et al. (1980) studied prostatic calculi using crystallography and found that many constituents precipitate from urine and not from the prostatic fluid. This implicates intraprostatic urinary reflux in the formation of prostatic calculi. More recently, Kirby et al. (1982) provided more direct proof of intraprostatic reflux; they instilled a carbon particle solution into the bladder of men just before TURP for BPH and into the bladder of men having nonbacterial prostatitis. They demonstrated that reflux occurs commonly (70% of men who underwent surgery and 100% of men with nonbacterial prostatitis) and is probably important in the pathogenesis of prostatic calculi. Similarly, urethroprostatic reflux may transport bacteria from infected urine into the prostate with resultant bacterial prostatitis and infection of the prostatic calculi.

We may speculate that besides a poor tissue penetration of the antibiotic agent (a problem solved with the use of the new generation of quinolones (Naber 1991; Madsen and Aagaard 1991)) unrecognized infected prostatic stones play an important role in our inability to cure many patients with CBP by antibacterial therapy (Meares 1981; Fitzpatrick and Krane 1989). Generally the development of resistance can be excluded as the cause of treatment failure. In most prospective studies that have employed various antimicrobial agents, the cure rates have been less than 50%, despite favorable results of in vitro susceptibility testing of prostatic pathogens (Meares 1986). The infecting bacteria reside within the stones and are therefore protected from the action of antimicrobial agents. The infected calculi may serve as persistent foci for bacteria in the male lower urogenital tract. Antibiotic treatment in these patients can at best be only suppressive, relapses sometimes occurring whenever drugs are discontinued and sometimes despite drugs (Eyken et al. 1974; Smart and Jenkins 1973). Similarly to infected renal calculi, the infection associated with infected prostatic calculi cannot be cured unless the stones are removed successfully by surgical means (Meares 1987). These principles form the basis and rationale for the surgical management of CBP.

Anatomical Aspects of Prostatitis

A full understanding of the anatomical features of CBP and related predisposing factors is absolutely essential in the choice of an effective and justified therapeutic modality. McNeal (1972) subdivided the prostate into central and peripheral zones on the basis of histological differences in the ducts, stroma, and epithelium. He also drew attention to the markedly greater frequency with which the peripheral zone is involved in inflammation and infection. This can be accounted for on the grounds of an ascending route of infection and various anatomical factors, described by Blacklock (1974, 1991). Micro-organisms present within the prostatic urethra may be forced into the gland by any rise in pressure in the prostatic urethra during urination as a result of failure of relaxation of the external sphincter (dynamic obstructions, as neurogenic bladder, anxious bladder syndrome, anogenital stimuli, etc.) or some lower organic obstruction (stricture, phimosis, etc.). The ducts of the peripheral zone which drain into the posterolateral recess of the distal urethral segment at right angles to or oblique against the direction of the urinary flow are most vulnerable for reflux in these situations. By contrast, the ducts of the central zone, opening above the ejaculatory ducts on the verumontanum obliquely in the direction of flow, are forced shut in these circumstances, protecting them against reflux. The entry of these central ducts is valvular in nature, which also prevents such reflux. The course of the peripheral zone ducts is markedly curved laterally and ultimately anteriorly, which makes them vulnerable to occlusion by edema, scarring, or calculi.

In focal inflammation, which is the characteristic pathology in chronic prostatitis, ducts may be occluded isolating an infected segment at the periphery of the gland so that the prostatic secretions, with pus cells and micro-organisms, even do not evacuate in the EPS in spite of adequate prostatic massage (Blacklock 1973). This situation increases the likelihood of chronicity.

The aim in radical TURP for CBP is to resect as much infected glandular tissue, mainly apically localized, as possible, with preservation of continence. At the heart of success is proper patient selection and endoscopic skill in the precise resection in the apical region and near to the real prostatic capsule, as at radical operative prostatectomy a clear identification of the anatomic landmarks and an understanding of the variations in prostate size and shape is required. Myers (1991; Myers et al. 1987) described two basic configurations with or without anterior apical notch (the croissant and the more common doughnut shapes) and showed the anatomic relationship with the proximal and distal male continence mechanism. As McNeal (1972), they have shown the variations in the presentation of the apical peripheral zone distal to the verumontanum, which requires the most precise resection regarding continence, keeping in mind that this region is preferentially attained in prostatitis. Especially in men with CBP who also have BPH, considerable prostatic tissue at the apex of the gland extends distal to the level of the verumontanum, which normally serves as distal landmark for resection.

Surgical Aspects of TURP for CBP

To cure patients successfully of their CBP the resectionist must perform a radical procedure to remove all foci of infected tissue and prostatic calculi. Prostatitis involves especially the peripheral zone, so that the resection must be directed to this part of the gland. This may involve resection of prostatic tissue at the level of or just below the verumontanum, which is technically both difficult and dangerous for continence. The resection must also extend out as far as the so-called true capsule of the prostate, which at this level is a tenous fibromuscular layer (Kaye and Richter 1990; Blacklock 1974). Control of the resection by a finger in the rectum is essential and may additionally define indurated parts of the prostate which are foci of chronic inflammation. True capsular tissue should be exposed throughout the lateral area, along the floor and at the apices. Anteriorly and along the roof of the gland the radical character of the resection is less important than in the other areas (Meares 1986). Because of the multilocular focal character of the disease the apical predominance and the known variability of the apical prostate shape (Myers 1991) a number of resections may be necessary before all loculi of prostatitis are removed. Blacklock (1985) mentioned the possibility of operative control by the use of real-time ultrasound in the operating theater.

This surgical treatment is not recommended for use by surgeons without skill in TURP because resection of large portions of the true prostatic capsule results in large perforations and extensive periprostatic extravasation. The complications from small perforations are not a problem when isotonic irrigating fluid is used (Barnes et al. 1982).

If the internal sphincter is compromised by bladder neck resection the prostatic urethra remains in communication with the bladder cavity at all times and is therefore subject to any pressure changes within it. This situation makes the residual prostatic gland tissue continually at risk of infection or reinfection and is therefore contraindicated in patients with CBP (Blacklock 1991).

Appropriate antimicrobial therapy is essential to cover the operative and postoperative periods, and associated conditions which predispose, precipitate, or perpetuate the prostatitis must be managed before TURP can be considered.

Indications of Radical TURP for CBP

CBP as an important cause of relapsing recurrent UTI is difficult to cure by the use of conservative medical treatment alone. The cure rates mentioned in most studies have been less than 50% (Meares 1981, 1982; Sharer and Fair 1982; Stamey 1980). These poor clinical results are surely related to unfavorable pharmacokinetics and the presence of infected prostatic calculi, as explained above (Meares 1974, 1982, 1986; Sharer and Fair 1982; Stamey 1980; Eyken et al. 1974). Treatment by local injection of antibiotics into the prostate via the direct transperineal route attempted to cross the plasmaprostatic barrier (Baert et al. 1983; Meares 1986; Baert 1986), with higher percentages of complete cure or at least long-term remissions.

The new generation of quinolones possess an ideal antibacterial spectrum and a proven good penetration capacity in prostatic tissue (Naber 1991; Madsen and Aagaard 1991). Thus when multiple sessions of adequate treatment with these products, in combination with conservative measures such as regular ejaculation and prostatic massage, fail to cure, surgery must be considered a causally orientated therapy. Otherwise, patients not cured by medical therapy can be managed satisfactorily only by continuous suppressive treatment with long-term low-dose medication (Meares 1986). Suppressive therapy usually controls symptoms and prevents bacteriuria; however, the pathogen persists in the prostate, and discontinuation of treatment eventually leads to recurrent symptoms and bacteriuria.

Total prostatovesiculectomy can per definition cure all men suffering from CBP, with the risk of erectile impotence and urinary incontinence. Now that this radical procedure has become routine in the management of localized prostate cancer with minimization of the risk for incontinence, it can be justified in specific well-documented cases.

The rationale for radical TURP in CBP is based on the presence of duct obstructions and infected prostate calculi which act as permanent foci of infection. It must therefore be advised not to perform radical TURP in the management of patients who have nonbacterial chronic prostatitis or complaints of prostatodynia. In practice the diagnosis of bacterial prostatitis is not easy and is based mainly upon accurate lower tract localization studies, examination of the prostatic fluid, and the clinical history of recurrent, relapsing UTIs (Baert et al. 1983; Baert and Leonard 1988; Baert 1986). Only the hardcore group of patients with confirmed CBP, offering a stubborn resistance to long-term (at least 1-year) adequate medical therapy, can be considered for radical endoscopic resection.

Because radical TURP usually results in permanent retrograde ejaculation most ideal candidates are middle-aged or older patients who suffer from associated symptoms of prostatism due to BPH. Although prostatitis tends to occur in the sexually active phase of life, TURP is not indicated in younger men who wish to remain fertile. Patients must be informed that they will undergo an intervention possibly resulting in sterility but not impotence. The patient who wishes to remain fertile continues to be a problem, and suppression of symptoms with antibiotics should be continued until TURP can be undertaken.

Clinical Reports and Results

In the literature only few clinical reports have been published on the true role of radical TURP in the management of CBP. Cure rates range from 30% to 100%. Most reports are difficult to interpret because they lack proper bacteriological documentation to prove the bacterial character of the treated cases, and because many TURPs are standard and not radical.

Drach (1975) mentioned a significant improvement in approximately one-third of his patients. Stamey (1972) reported two patients with well-documented CBP associated with prostatic calculi, in whom the removal of calculi and prostatic tissue by TURP cured the prostatitis. On the other hand, this did not happen in three other well-documented cases, two not associated with prostatic calculi.

Smart and Jenkins (1973) published a series of 32 patients treated by TURP because of failure of conservative measures. Almost all patients presented symptoms of "prostatitis" and prostatic tenderness by rectal examination, but localization studies revealed urinary pathogens in only five. Twenty-three patients (72%) were rendered asymptomatic within 3 months following the operation while 19% improved. Five underwent more than one session of TURP. The most satisfactory results have been obtained in the patients with severe histological changes. The incidence of pathogenic bacteria in the prostatic secretion and the prostatic tissue was increased with the severity of the histological changes.

Barnes et al. (1982) reported the treatment by TURP of 49 patients with chronic prostatitis. The 33 patients who were followed up for 1 year or longer 67% were relieved of their symptoms and infection, 21% improved, and 12% received no benefit. However, patient selection was not well defined, with poor data about the bacterial aspect of the prostatitis. The authors admitted that too many TURPs for CBP have been performed, and that strict selection criteria must be used.

The best documented reports have been given by Meares (1986, 1987). He reported success in curing all ten patients with refractory CBP by "radical" transurethral prostatectomy combined with appropriate antimicrobial therapy. Localization cultures were positive for prostatic pathogens in nine patients. Two patients underwent a second TURP before symptomatic and bacteriological cure. Histological evidence of chronic prostatitis was present in all cases; BPH of variable degree was noted in seven resection specimens. The postoperative morbidity was deemed no different than that after routine TURP for BPH.

In our clinical department we treated five patients with confirmed CBP in the period from November 1986 to December 1990 (Tables 1, 2). All patients had positive localization culture results at admission for the surgical procedure and a history of infection lasting at least 1 year (mean 19.6 months). The mean age was 55.6 years. In two cases (patients 2 and 5) the CBP was a post-TURP complication after a TURP for BPH in another hospital. Patient 4 underwent three transurethral resections for CBP in another hospital and 2 in loco

Table 1. Data on five patients with CBP treated by TURP

Patient no.	Age (years)	Duration of symptoms (months)	Localization cultures	EPS	Urological antecedents
1	63	12	*Escherichia coli*	+	Orchitis BPH
2	71	48	*E. coli, Proteus mirabilis*	+	TURP (BPH), post-TURP prostatitis
3	58	12	*E. coli*	+	BPH vesicoureteral reflux
4	34	24	*E. coli*	+	TURP (3 ×), in loco antibiotics (2 ×)
5	52	12	*E. coli*	+	TURP (BPH), post-TURP UTI, TU drainage of prostatic abscess

Table 2. Results in five patients with CBP treated by radical TURP

Patient no.	Intervention	Complication	Calculi	Pathology	Follow-up
1	Radical TURP + vasectomy	None	+	BPH + inflammation	Symptoms: − Cultures: − 11 months
2	Radical TURP	None	+	BPH + inflammation	Frequency (±) Cultures: − 56 months
3	Radical TURP	None	+	BPH + inflammation	Symptoms: − Cultures: − 60 months
4	Radical TURP of apical rest	None	+	Inflammation	Symptoms: + + Cultures: multiresistant E. coli 6 months
5	Radical TURP + opening of seminal vesicles	None	+	BPH + inflammation	Second TURP after 10 months (UTI) Cultures: − Symptoms: + + 44 months

injections of antibiotics in our service because of persisting and relapsing UTI. Radical resection of the apical prostatic rest had only minimal influence on his subjective complaints and on the frequency of UTI. Another patient (patient 5) with antecedents of TURP for BPH and transurethral evacuation of a prostatic abscess (post-TURP prostatitis) needed a second TURP after 10 months and presented postoperatively with persisting irritable bladder symptoms, probably related to a sphincter dyssynergia, improving only minimally with medical therapy and bladder reeducation. Localization cultures, however, remained sterile. Three patients have remained free of symptoms as well as of infection after a mean follow-up period of 3.5 years. Prostatic calculi were present in all cases and pathological examination of the resection specimens also showed inflammation in all. We can thus report a bacteriological success rate of 80% (4/5 patients), and a symptomatic success rate of 60% (3/5 patients). The majority of our patients with CBP in this period were managed with in loco injections of antibiotics (Baert et al. 1976, 1983; Baert and Leonard 1988; Baert 1986).

Conclusion

The pathological entity of CBP remains clinically important as the major cause of relapsing UTI in men. Diagnostic confirmation can be made only by

simultaneous quantitative localization cultures and microscopic examination of the prostatic fluid. Efforts to cure CBP by medical therapy alone have been disappointing; cure rates seldom exceed 50%.

The typical pathological characteristics of CBP and the high frequency of infected prostatic calculi suggest a surgical solution such as TURP to cure the strictly selected hard-core group of patients who cannot be managed satisfactorily by long-term and adequate medical therapy. When all foci of infected tissue and calculi are successfully removed, radical TURP can cure patients of their CBP. However, since the peripheral zones typically contain the greatest foci, cure can be achieved only if the resection is very thorough, especially apically, with respect to the integrity of the striated sphincter to maintain urinary continence. Hence, a repeat resection may be required to achieve a cure in some patients.

It is necessary, however, for strict criteria to be used when deciding on whether a radial TURP for chronic bacterial prostatitis is indicated. (a) Sequential bacteriological localization cultures are of critical importance in reaching the correct diagnosis of CBP and cannot be replaced by any other method. Chronic abacterial prostatitis is absolutely no indication for prostatic resection. (b) CBP is not cured by long-term adequate medical treatment applied for at least 1 full year. (c) Psychosomatic problems must be eliminated to prevent a postoperative persistence of symptoms without bacteriological basis of residual infection. (d) A minimal endoscopic skill on the part of the surgeon is desirable to avoid major complications, such as incontinence or large perforations of the true prostatic capsule.

Long-term prospective follow-up studies are essential to draw any conclusions with respect to the ultimate role of radical TURP in the effective and scientifically based treatment of CBP.

References

Baert L (1986) Is the local administration of antibiotics into the prostatic gland in chronic bacterial prostatitis more than an attempt? In: Weidner W, Brunner H, Krause W, Rothauge CF (eds) Therapy of prostatitis. Zuckschwerdt, Munich, pp 59–66
Baert L, Leonard A (1988) Chronic bacterial prostatitis: 10 years of experience with local antibiotics. J Urol 140:755–757
Baert L, Soep H, Pijck J (1976) Chronic bacterial prostatitis. Annu Urol 10:39
Baert L, Mattelaer J, DeNollin P (1983) Treatment of chronic bacterial prostatitis by local injection of antibiotics into prostate. Urology 21(4):370–375
Baert L, Van Poppel H, Vandeursen H (1991) Review of modern trends in the treatment of chronic bacterial prostatitis (C.B.P.). Infection 19 Suppl 3:157–159
Barnes WR, Hadley HL, O'Donoghue EPN (1982) Transurethral resection of the prostate for chronic bacterial prostatitis. Prostate 3:215–219
Blacklock NJ (1974) Anatomical factors in prostatitis. Br J Urol 46:47–54
Blacklock NJ (1985) Surgical concepts in the treatment of chronic bacterial prostatitis. In: Brunner H, Krause W, Rothauge CF, Weidner W (eds) Chronic prostatitis. Schattauer, Stuttgart, pp 13–27

Blacklock NJ (1991) The anatomy of the prostate: relationship with prostatic infection. Infection 19 Suppl 3:111–114

Drach GH (1975) Prostatitis: man's hidden infection. Urol Clin North Am 2(3):499–520

Eyken S, Bultitude ME, Mayo ME, Lloyd-Davies RW (1974) Prostatic calculi as a source of recurrent bacteriuria in the male. Br J Urol 46:527–532

Fitzpatrick JM, Krane RJ (1989) Acute and chronic prostatitis and prostatodynia. In: The prostate. Churchill Livingstone, Edinburgh

Fox M (1963) The natural history and significance of stone formation in the prostate gland. J Urol 89:716–727

Gorelick JI, Senterfit LB, Vaughan ED Jr (1988) Quantitative bacterial tissue cultures from 209 prostatectomy specimens: findings and implications. J Urol 139:57–60

Kaye KW, Richter L (1990) Ultrasonographic anatomy of normal prostate gland: reconstruction by computer graphics. Urology 35(1):12–17

Kirby RS, Lowe D, Bultitude MI, Shuttleworth KED (1982) Intraprostatic urinary reflux: an aetiological factor in abacterial prostatitis. Br J Urol 54:729–731

Klimas R, Bennett B, Gardner WA (1985) Prostatic calculi: a review. Prostate 7:91–96

Madsen PO, Aagaard J (1991) Pharmacokinetics of quinolone derivatives in the prostate. Infection 19 Suppl 3:154–164

McNeal JE (1972) The prostate and prostatic urethra: a morphologic synthesis. J Urol 107:1008

Meares EM Jr (1974) Infection stones of the prostate gland: laboratory diagnosis and clinical management. Urology 4:560–566

Meares EM Jr (1981) Nephrology forum: prostatitis. Kidney Int 20:289

Meares EM Jr (1982) Review of pharmacokinetics and therapy. Rev Infect Dis 4:475

Meares EM Jr (1986) Chronic bacterial prostatitis: role of transurethral prostatectomy (TURP) in therapy. In: Weidner W, Brunner H, Krause W, Rothauge CF (eds) Therapy of prostatitis. Zuckschwerdt, Munich, pp 193–197

Meares EM Jr (1987) Acute and chronic prostatitis: diagnosis and treatment. Infect Dis Clin North Am 1(4):855–873

Meares EM Jr, Stamey TA (1968) Bacteriologic localization patterns in bacterial prostatitis and urethritis. Invest Urol 5:499

Myers RP (1991) Male urethral anatomy and radical prostatectomy. Urol Clin North Am 18(2):211–227

Myers RP, Goellner JR, Cahill DR (1987) Prostate shape, external striated urethral sphincter and radical prostatectomy: the apical dissection. J Urol 138:543

Naber KG (1991) The role of quinolones in the treatment of chronic bacterial prostatitis. Infection 19 Suppl 3:170–177

Pfau A, Sacks T (1976) Chronic bacterial prostatitis: new therapeutic aspects. Br J Urol 48:245–253

Ramirez TC, Ruiz JA, Gomez AZ, Orgaz R, Sampler SD (1980) A crystallographic study of prostatic calculi. J Urol 124:840–843

Sharer WC, Fair WR (1982) The pharmacokinetics of antibiotic diffusion in chronic bacterial prostatitis. Prostate 3:139

Smart CJ, Jenkins JD (1973) The role of transurethral prostatectomy in chronic prostatitis. Br J Urol 45:654–662

Stamey TA (1972) Urinary infections in males. In: Stamey TA (ed) Urinary infections. Williams and Wilkins, Baltimore, pp 164–165

Stamey TA (1980) Pathogenesis and treatment of urinary tract infections. Williams and Wilkins, Baltimore

Sutor DJ, Wooley SE (1974) The crystalline composition of prostatic calculi. Br J Urol 46:533–536

Thibault PH, Gattegno B, Jacob M, Leandri R, Scetbon V (1978) Traitement des prostatites récidivantes par la résection endoscopique. Société Française d'Urologie session of May 20

Thin RN, Simmons PD (1983) Chronic bacterial and non-bacterial prostatitis. Br J Urol 55:513–518

Radical Prostatectomy
for Chronic Bacterial Prostatitis

L. Baert and H. Van Poppel

Only few reports have dealt with indications for total prostatovesiculectomy in chronic prostatitis. Although prostatectomy for specific granulomatous prostatitis by syphilis or tuberculosis has been performed for years (Nesbit and Lynn 1949) and may still be indicated in some cases, the indication for surgery in nonspecific granulomatous prostatitis is much more controversial. Indeed, the clinical course of nonspecific granulomatous prostatitis is mostly benign; the disease is self-limited and can best be managed conservatively by corticosteroids (Bush et al. 1964). When obstructive symptoms occur, conventional surgery such as transurethral resection or adenomectomy – either retropubic or perineal – can be proposed (Kelalis et al. 1965; Schmidt 1965). Nongranulomatous bacterial prostatitis occurs in the vast majority of patients and can be extremely refractory to all kinds of treatment. Only in some carefully selected patients can a radical prostatovesiculectomy be proposed as the ultimate therapeutic measure.

Theoretically, surgical eradication of a prostate and seminal vesicles harboring a bacterial prostatitis should lead to complete remission. The disadvantages of an open surgical procedure and its possible complications have not made this curative treatment very popular. Although the risk of incontinence is low and can even be reduced to nonexistence in experienced hands, there is still the risk of erectile impotence. Dissection of the apex and posterior aspect of the prostate affected by recurrent infections is generally difficult, and no guarantee can be given that the neurovascular bundles can be kept intact.

Other authors and ourselves have performed radical prostatovesiculectomy in a few patients (Davis and Weigel 1990). Recurrent exacerbations of chronic bacterial prostatitis resulting in sepsis and necessity of repeated intravenous antibiotherapy that persist after other therapeutic measures such as radical transurethral resection or in local antibiotherapy constitute a definite indication for radical prostatovesiculectomy to be performed in an experienced center. The morbidity is comparable to that of radical prostatectomy for cancer although dissection of the seminal vesicles is generally tedious.

The occurrence of unsuspected adenocarcinoma of the prostate in patients undergoing cystoprostatectomy for other causes is well documented (Kabalin et al. 1989). Also the possible clinical and pathological confusion between granulomatous prostatitis and carcinoma has been extensively reported (Taylor et al. 1977; Presti and Weidner 1991; Bogomoletz 1985). On the other hand, unspecific nongranulomatous prostatitis has also been shown to be accompanied by carcinoma in about 15% of cases (Maksem et al. 1988).

It is noteworthy that in two patients reported in the paper by others (Davis and Weigel 1990) and in one of our patients (Figs. 1–3; whose recurrent infection caused relapsing hemolytic crises and paroxysmal nocturnal hemoglobinuria) who underwent radical prostatectomy for refractory bacterial prostatitis, an adenocarcinoma was found which was not diagnosed preoperatively. Although puncture biopsy could have missed the carcinoma by a sampling error, we believe that there is a place for either selective or random biopsy of the prostate when there is any suspicion of carcinoma on clinical examination, transrectal ultrasound, or prostate-specific antigen. The latter, indeed, has been proven to be significantly increased not only in severe acute but also in moderate and severe chronic prostatitis, in a range which could not be distinguished from that in patients with carcinoma (Block et al. 1991).

Even in very young patients (25 and 36 years old) adenocarcinoma was found to be associated with refractory prostatitis (Davis and Weigel 1990). Although there has been no evidence of a causal relationship between chronic prostatitis and malignant change, patients with chronic prostatitis should be followed up very carefully.

Radical prostatectomy has a place in the treatment of extremely refractory chronic bacterial prostatitis. A number of patients are not only asymptomatic

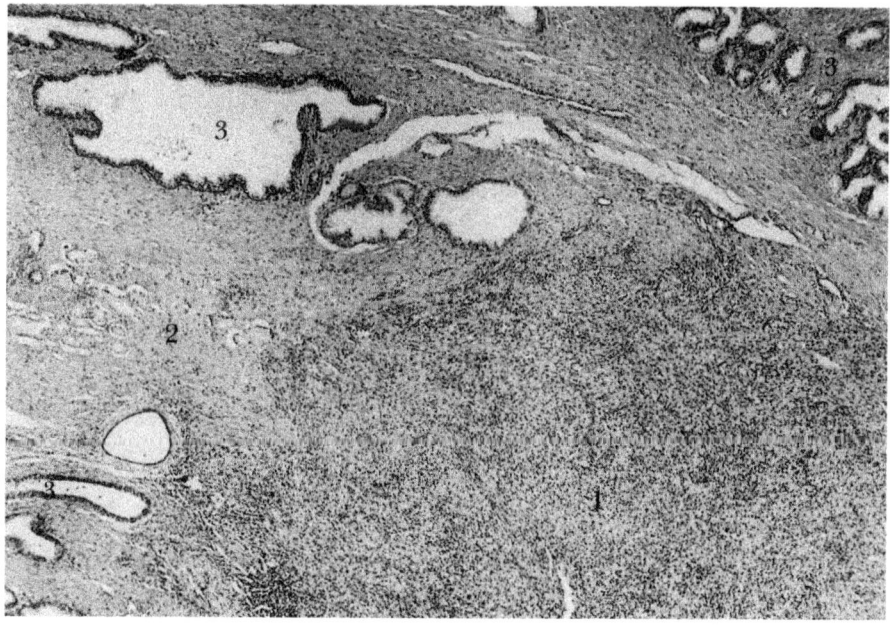

Fig. 1. *1*, Granulomatous prostatitis; *2*, adenocarcinoma; *3*, normal prostate parenchyma

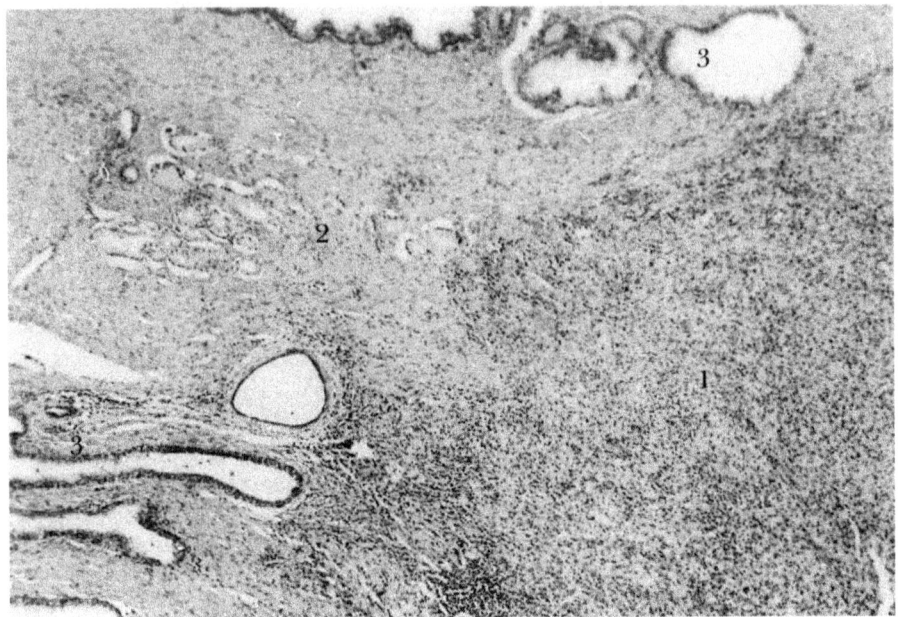

Fig. 2. *1*, Granulomatous prostatitis; *2*, adenocarcinoma; *3*, normal prostate parenchyma

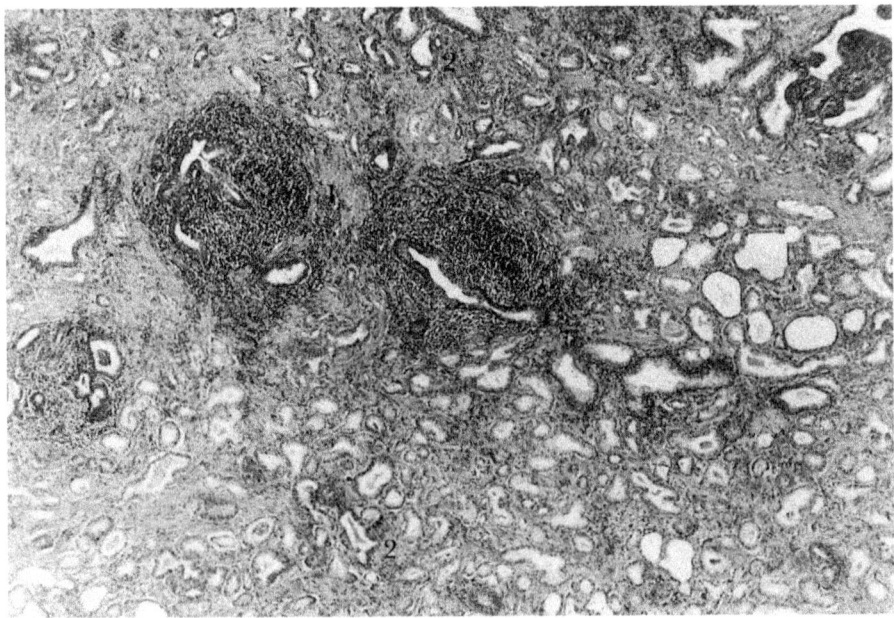

Fig. 3. *1*, Chronic (nongranulomatous prostatitis) nontumoral glands surrounded and infiltrated by a dene infiltration by lymphocytes; *2*, adenocarcinoma

after the operation but are also cured of an accompanying latent adenocarcinoma which in younger patients could have time to become clinically significant carcinoma. Patients with prostatitis should be thoroughly followed and undergo puncture biopsy when suspicion is raised of a possible malignancy.

References

Block T, Bruel J, Schmidt F, Rotter M, Busch R, Hartung R (1991) Influence of prostatic inflammation on prostate specific antigen (Abstr). 1st International Congress of the Dutch Urological Association, Rotterdam, p 33

Bogomoletz WV (1985) Pseudotumors and rare malignant tumors of the prostate. Bull Cancer (Paris) 72:423–428

Bush I, Orkin LA, Bauer S (1964) Steroid therapy in non specific granulomatous prostatitis. J Urol 92:303–305

Davis BE, Weigel JW (1990) Adenocarcinoma of the prostate discovered in 2 young patients following total prostatovesiculectomy for refractory prostatitis. J Urol 144:744–745

Kabalin JN, McNeal JE, Price HM, Freiha FS, Stamey TA (1989) Unsuspected adenocarcinoma of the prostate in patients undergoing cystoprostatectomy for other cancers: incidence, histology and morphometric observations. J Urol 141:1091–1093

Kelalis PP, Greene LF, Harrison EG Jr (1965) Granulomatous prostatitis. JAMA 191:287–289

Maksem JA, Johenning PW, Galang CF (1988) Prostatitis and aspiration biopsy. Cytology of prostate. Urology 23:263–268

Nesbit RM, Lynn JM (1949) Subtotal extirpation of the granulomatous prostate. J Urol 61:766–767

Presti B, Weidner N (1991) Granulomatous prostatitis and poorly differentiated prostate carcinoma. Their distinction with the use of immunohistochemical methods. Am J Clin Pathol 95:330–334

Schmidt JD (1965) Non specific granulomatous prostatitis; classification, review and report of cases. J Urol 94:607–609

Taylor EW, Wheelis RF, Correa RJ Jr, Gibbons RP, Mason JT, Cummings KB (1977) Granulomatous prostatitis: confusion clinically with carcinoma of the prostate. J Urol 117:316–318

Immunotherapy and Prostatitis

L. Baert and E. Van Thillo

Granulomatous prostatitis after intravesical immunotherapy with bacille Calmette-Guérin for superficial bladder cancer has been described many times (Stilmant et al. 1985; Torres et al. 1990; Oates et al. 1988; Pinsky et al. 1985); it is even a recognized complication of intravesical Calmette-Guérin immunotherapy. On the other hand, little has been described in the world literature on immunotherapy and infectious disease of the genitourinary tract.

The local immunological response to bacterial colonization of mucosal surfaces appears to constitute an important mechanism for the prevention of infection. The prostate gland secretes fluid that contains immunoglobulins, i.e., IgA, and the prevention of prostatic infection may be mediated in part by the antibacterial effects of these immunoglobulins (Fowler und Mariano 1984). The prostate gland is usually colonized during episodes of urinary tract infection, but it seems that symptomatic or chronic infections are prevented by the secretion of antigen-specific IgA (Fowler und Mariano 1984). On the other hand, the finding of IgM and IgA antibodies, complement, and fibrinogen deposition within the prostate of chronic abacterial prostatitis patients, but not controls, suggests that these antibodies are formed in response to an extrinsic antigen. Possible candidates include remnants or products, urinary constituents, and auto-antibodies (Doble et al. 1990). The immune response of the prostate to bacterial infection has the characteristics of secretory immunity (Fowler 1991).

In recurrent urogenital infections in which no curable cause can be found, long-term antibiotic therapy is often the only possible form of treatment. Little is known of immunotherapy in cases of (chronic) prostatitis.

Patients with Chronic Urogenital Infections Can Be Treated with a Vaccine

A vaccine active against *Escherichia coli*, *Proteus*, *Klebsiella*, and *Streptococcus faecalis* has been used in 25 patients with chronic urogenital infection. This Sulco Urovak vaccine was very well tolerated and a bacteriological control in the 6th week after vaccination showed sterile urine in 68% of the patients (Donovski 1989).

Vaccination with formalin-treated cells of *E. coli* serotype 06 would give protection to chronic bacterial pyelonephritis due to *E. coli* 06, as high levels of antibody to *E. coli* lipopolysaccharide were found in vaccinated animals (Brooks et al. 1977). This raises the question of whether vaccination ought to be considered for patients predisposed to chronic bacterial urogenital infection.

Immunotherapy with Immunomodulators Has Seldom Been Described

Jecht (1978) described eight patients suffering from chronic epididymitis, prostatitis, and urethritis who were treated with levamisole. A definite and lasting improvement was seen in six of the eight patients.

The addition of miramistin to the traditional anti-inflammatory treatment would result in stimulation of the absorptive capacity of phagocytes and improve the results of treatment of patients with chronic urethroprostatitis, as published by Russian investigators (Vozianov et al. 1990).

Some Chinese investigators have adopted the method of seminal consolidation and turbidity excretion in a specific prescription for the treatment of 133 cases of chronic prostatitis. Besides direct bacteriostatic and bacteriocidal effects, the prescription would also strengthen or regulate local immunological functions (Zhu 1989).

The Combination of a Vaccine with an Immunostimulant Could Be More Effective

Henocq et al. (1985) evaluated the effectiveness of vaccination consisting of antigen therapy and an immunostimulant (P 40) in 20 patients. The recurrent urogenital infections were controlled in the cases in which this combination was used; in half of the cases maintenance vaccination was required for a period of 2–3 years. The preventive effect of P 40 on infections of the lower urinary tract seemed to be mostly mediated by the stimulation of phagocytosis, although both humoral and cellular immunity may also be involved. P 40 is a fraction of delipidated whole cells of *Corynebacterium granulosum* and exhibits immunostimulating and adjuvant activities. P 40 fraction indeed was shown to increase the granulopexic capacity of the reticuloendothelial system and to augment the resistance to bacterial infections (Henocq et al. 1985).

Little has been published about immunotherapy and prostatitis. Its value is still a point of discussion. More prospective randomized studies are necessary to define the value of this infrequent therapy for (chronic) urogenital infections.

References

Brooks SJ, Lyons JM, Braude Al (1977) Immunization against retrograde pyelonephritis: vaccination against chronic pyelonephritis due to Escherichia coli. J Infect Dis 136:633–639

Doble A, Walker MM, Harris JRW et al. (1990) Intraprostatic antibody deposition in chronic abacterial prostatitis. Br J Urol 65:598–605

Donovski L (1989) Immunotherapy with Solco Urovac vaccine in chronic genitourinary infection. Khirurgiia (Sofiia) 42:28–30

Fowler JE Jr (1991) Secretory immunity of the prostate gland. Infection Suppl 3:131–138

Fowler JE, Mariano M (1984) Longitudinal studies of prostatic fluid immunoglobulin in men with bacterial prostatitis. J Urol 131:363–369

Henocq E, Arvis G, Delsaux MC, Bizzini B (1985) Treatment of recurrent urogenital infections by immunomodulation. Ann Urol (Paris) 19:371–375

Jecht E (1978) Levamisol-Therapie bei chronischer Prostatitis und Epididymitis. Z Hautkr 54:424–425

Oates R, Stilmant MM, Freelund MC, Siroky MB (1988) Granulomatous prostatitis following bacillus Calmette-Guérin immunotherapy of bladder cancer. J Urol 140:741–744

Pinsky CM, Camacho FJ, Kerr D et al. (1985) Intravesical administration of bacillus Calmette-Guérin in patients with recurrent superficial carcinoma of the urinary bladder: report of a prospective, randomized trial. Cancer Treat Rep 69:47–53

Stilmant M, Siroky MB, Johnson KB (1985) Fine needle aspiration cytology of granulomatous prostatitis induced by BCG immunotherapy of bladder cancer. Acta Cytol 29:961–966

Torres GM, Kaude JV, Drylie D (1990) Bacille-Calmette-Guérin vaccine-induced granulomatous prostatitis: another hypoechoic nonneoplastic lesion. AJR 155:195–196

Vozianov AF, Krivoshein IS, Pasechnikov SP (1990) The effect of miramistin on the phagocytic activity of the urethral neutrophilic granulocytes in patients with chronic urethroprostatitis. Vrach Delo 210:113–115

Zhu YK (1989) Treatment of 133 cases of chronic prostatitis by seminal consolidation and turbidity excretion. J Tradit Chin Med 9:272–274

V. Nonbacterial Prostatitis

The Diagnosis, Aetiology and Pathogenesis of Chronic Abacterial Prostatitis

A. Doble and D. Taylor-Robinson

Introduction

Although John Hunter described prostatic inflammation in his treatise on venereal diseases in 1786, the first accurate description of prostatitis is attributed to Verdier in 1838 (von Lackum 1933). Later, Thompson (1861) classified the prostatitides as acute and chronic, but the inability to attribute infection and inflammation to the prostate on clinical grounds alone necessitated a further way of making a diagnosis. Several authors (von Sehlen 1893; Krotoszyner and Spencer 1894) described a three-glass test, collecting first void and mid-stream urine along with prostatic fluid, and submitting the specimens to microscopy and culture. However, the possible contamination of prostatic fluid by urethral organisms or infected urine hindered interpretation of the observations. The localisation technique was refined by Stamey et al. (1965; Fig. 1) who added a step in which a specimen of urine was collected after prostatic massage. A classification of the prostatitides was then constructed (Drach et al. 1978), allowing sub-groups of patients to be defined (Table 1). Although this localisation technique has limitations, as a dry expressate may result in the contribution from the prostate being underestimated, it does take into account the role played by urethral and bladder inflammatory cells and organisms. Thus, in any study of prostatitis, it remains a mandatory investigation, albeit time and labour intensive, as well as unpleasant for patient and clinician alike. However, more perfunctory methods of diagnosis are unacceptable and preclude comparison of data.

The incidence of prostatitis is difficult to calculate. On the basis of autopsy material (Moore 1937), 5% of men have evidence of inflammation within the prostate, and in a study of tissue obtained at prostatectomy 98% displayed inflammatory changes (Kohnen and Drach 1979). However, histological features of inflammation do not necessarily equate with clinical prostatitis. Thus, in a study of over 300 consecutive individuals presenting for the first time to an urology clinic, a 10% prevalence of prostatitis, using currently accepted criteria, was seen among normal subjects and patients with non-inflammatory urological conditions (Schaeffer et al. 1981). Among the whole cohort, a 13% prevalence of prostatitis was observed, of which 88% were categorised as having abacterial prostatitis. Although, in general terms, it is not a common condition, abacterial

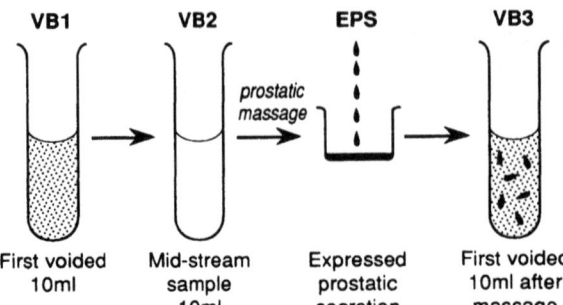

Fig. 1. The Stamey localisation technique

Table 1. Classification of prostatitis based on the Stamey localisation procedure (from Drach et al. 1978)

Category	MSU or VB2		EPS		Organisms
	WCC	Culture	WCC	Culture	
ABP	+ +	+	+ +	+	Enterobacteriaceae
CBP	+	+	+	+	Enterobacteriaceae
CABP	–	–	+	–	Nil
Pd	–	–	–	–	Nil

ABP, Acute bacterial prostatitis; CBP, chronic bacterial prostatitis; CABP, chronic abacterial prostatitis; Pd, prostatodynia; WCC, white cell count; MSU, mid-stream urine; EPS, expressed prostatic secretion

prostatitis accounts for the largest proportion of prostatitides, making its definition and understanding the more imperative.

Chronic abacterial prostatitis is a much maligned condition, due to frequent imprecision in diagnosis generating spurious and misleading data. It is exacting, therefore, from such a disadvantaged position to construct an unprejudiced view of the causative factors behind this condition. Indeed, to do so and to consider the possible mechanisms of pathogenesis logically, it is essential first to consider the way in which a correct diagnosis is achieved. Certainly, technological advances, which enable a more objective analysis of the prostate gland, together with improvements in the detection and isolation of micro-organisms, have allowed a better understanding of chronic abacterial prostatitis.

Diagnosis

The diagnosis of prostatitis rests on finding excessive numbers of leucocytes within the expressed prostatic secretion (EPS) and/or post-prostatic massage urine (VB3) over and above those found in urethral (VB1) or bladder (VB2) urine. Normal individuals undoubtedly possess leucocytes in their EPS, and the suggested upper limit of normal varies from 2 (Anderson and Weller 1979) to 20 (Drach et al. 1978) leucocytes per high-power field. Although various authors have submitted values within this range (Blacklock and Beavis 1974; Pfau et al. 1978; Stamey 1980; Schaeffer et al. 1981), a compromise has been made and a consensus reached on the number of leucocytes within the EPS that is considered the upper limit of normal; this has been set at 10 per high-power field. All too often, however, EPS cannot be obtained, and the diagnosis rests on finding excessive numbers of leucocytes in the VB3 specimen. In centrifuged urine 4 or more leucocytes per high-power field ($\times$400) over and above those found in VB1 or VB2 specimen is highly suggestive of prostatitis, whereas a figure of 10 is pathognomonic (Weidner and Ebner 1985).

Microbiology

The urethra has a rich collection of commensals which may result in misinterpretation of localisation studies. With this in mind, Meares and Stamey (1968), in studying patients with bacterial prostatitis, advised that the bacterial colony count for the VB3 sample and/or EPS should be at least ten-fold more than that for VB1 and VB2 samples. Assessment simply of numbers of organisms, as suggested by Drach (1975), is less specific and probably inaccurate. In attempting to assign an organism to the prostate, and thereby suggest an aetiological role for micro-organisms in abacterial prostatitis, it would seem appropriate to adopt the localisation criteria of Meares and Stamey (1968).

Serology

It would be perilous practice to implicate a micro-organism in prostatitis on the basis of serology alone, a reservation voiced by others (Tarizzo et al. 1968; Treharne et al. 1983). Serological data, however, may provide supportive evidence either to corroborate or refute the role of a micro-organism. This also applies to the analysis of EPS for micro-organism-specific antibodies. In chronic bacterial prostatitis, total and organism-specific immunoglobulins have been measured (Fowler et al. 1982; Fowler and Mariano 1984; Shortliffe et al. 1981; Wishnow et al. 1982; Shortliffe and Wehner 1986); IgA and IgG levels are elevated in patients with prostatitis, compared to those of controls, and the levels reflect the response to treatment. In chronic abacterial prostatitis, although both the total IgA and IgG immunoglobulins are elevated, they are not micro-organism specific (Shortliffe and Wehner 1986). An elegant technique based on an enzyme-linked immunosorbent assay has been used to measure micro-organism-specific immunoglobulins in the urine before and after prostatic massage; this has provided a simplified and valid method to support localisation of micro-organisms to the prostate in chronic bacterial prostatitis (Shortliffe et al. 1989). A similar approach in chronic abacterial prostatitis would be useful once a micro-organism of aetiological significance, if indeed one exists, has been defined.

Ultrasound

The advent of transrectal ultrasound (TRUS) saw a breakthrough in objective assessment of the prostate. The value of TRUS in prostate cancer is undisputed (Spirnak and Resnick 1984; Lee et al. 1985), yet its role in inflammatory prostatic disease is no less valuable. Since the first report of TRUS being used specifically to address the diagnostic problem presented by chronic prostatitis (Griffiths et al. 1984), several authors (Wiegand and Weidner 1986; Doble and Carter 1989; Christiansen and Purvis 1991) have found the technique valuable as an aid to diagnosis. Caution must be exercised, however, in assigning pathology to particular ultrasound features in the absence of corroborative histological data.

In a study of 200 patients who had either chronic prostatitis or prostatodynia, as well as controls, seven ultrasound features were identified as having a significant correlation with chronic prostatitis (Doble and Carter 1989). The sensitivity and specificity values of each sign were calculated, and these values correlated most acceptably with the inflammatory response within the VB3 sample when there were at least 50 leucocytes per cubic millimetre. In follow-up studies a large number of ultrasound changes were observed in patients with

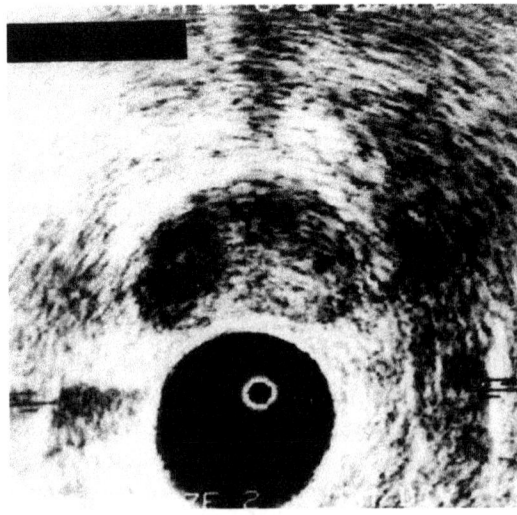

Fig. 2. An echolucent zone in a transrectal ultrasonograph of a patient with chronic abacterial prostatitis

chronic prostatitis, but there was little alteration in the prostatodynia group. Only one sign, the echolucent zone (Fig. 2), appeared to reflect the changing inflammatory status of the gland. With this possible exception, there is no single ultrasound sign which is indicative of chronic prostatitis, the diagnosis resting on a combination of ultrasound signs.

The greatest asset of TRUS is the help that it provides in the accurate placement of biopsy needle into areas of abnormality in the prostate, as seen on the scan (Harada et al. 1979; Holm and Gammelgaard 1981). The parenchymal features are amenable to biopsy in chronic prostatitis and in the above work (Doble and Carter 1989); as a result of histological examination following biopsy, they were shown to reflect inflammatory changes (in 88% of cases), fibrosis, corpora amylaceae or a combination of these pathological findings. There is no doubt, therefore, that TRUS is a valuable aid in diagnosis and enables the collection of samples directly from areas of inflammation within the prostate, without contamination by urethral cells and micro-organisms. Although ultrasound-guided prostatic biopsy is perhaps over-invasive in routine clinical practice, its niche in a research setting cannot be overstated.

Microbial Aetiology

By definition, chronic abacterial prostatitis is an inflammatory response in the absence of any detectable causative micro-organism. This classification enables the separation of those cases with infection due to the Enterobacteriaceae and *Streptococcus faecalis*, which are the main causes of chronic bacterial prostatitis, from those where these organisms cannot be isolated. Although there are a number of reports in which investigators have implicated *Chlamydia*, *Mycoplasma* and *Ureaplasma* in the aetiology of chronic abacterial prostatitis, these have been refuted by others. The situation is by no means clearly defined, and the arguments endorsing or rebutting their role are discussed below.

Chlamydia

The possibility that *Chlamydia trachomatis* may be involved in the aetiology of chronic abacterial prostatitis was first raised by Mårdh et al. (1972), who detected serum complement-fixing antibody to *C. trachomatis* at a titre of 1:5 or higher in 33% of men with chronic prostatitis, yet in only 3% of controls. However, serial estimations were not performed, nor were there any corroborative culture data. Indeed, in a later study by the same group (Mårdh et al. 1978) using a more sensitive and specific microimmunofluorescence technique, significant titres of IgG and IgM antibodies to a pooled chlamydial antigen were detected in only 14% and 8% of the patients, respectively. Furthermore, *C. trachomatis* could not be isolated from the EPS of any of the 53 patients studied.

A role for *C. trachomatis* was again favoured in one study when the organism was reported to have been cultured from 56% of cases of chronic prostatitis (Bruce et al. 1981). In a later study, *C. trachomatis* was isolated after prostatic massage from 19% of urethral swabs taken from patients, compared to 8% from controls (Weidner et al. 1983). Furthermore, 71% of the patients had serological evidence of chlamydial infection, yet only 47% of the study group had cytological evidence of prostatitis. Greater reliance can be placed on the results of chlamydial detection when they are based on the technique of direct prostatic sampling. When this biopsy procedure was undertaken in one study, albeit by blind aspiration, the *C. trachomatis* isolation rate was 33%, and rather curiously all urethral specimens were regarded as positive (Poletti et al. 1985). Further, *Chlamydia* was sought by culture and by direct immunofluorescence in urethral swabs and EPS specimens taken from six patients diagnosed by standard localisation techniques (Bruce and Reid 1989). All the urethral samples were negative, yet *Chlamydia* was reported to have been detected in the EPS; four of the group had partners who were harbouring *C. trachomatis* in the cervix.

Other investigators have also supported a chlamydial aetiology for chronic abacterial prostatitis based on the analysis of prostatic tissue. Thus, Shurbaji et al. (1988) identified chlamydial antigen, utilising a monocloncal antibody, in 31% of cases of prostatitis identified histologically. In a more recent study of patients whose prostatitis was diagnosed in a similar way, Abdelatif et al. (1991) reported that they had detected chlamydial DNA, by use of an *in situ* hybridisation technique, in 30% of specimens.

The aforementioned fragmentary but, nevertheless, cumulative support for the role of *C. trachomatis* in the aetiology of chronic abacterial prostatitis has been countered by the results of two large studies. In an extensive microbiological assessment of patients with chronic abacterial prostatitis, diagnosed in all of them by standard criteria, attempts to isolate *C. trachomatis* failed (Berger et al. 1989). In the other study (Doble et al. 1989a), direct sampling of the prostate was undertaken, with the added refinement of transrectal ultrasound guidance, in an attempt to exclude the risk of urethral contamination. Of 50 patients with chronic abacterial prostatitis, again selected using standard criteria, the demonstration of a chronic inflammatory infiltrate in 88% of the prostatic biopsies validated the sampling technique. Although *C. trachomatis* was detected by direct immunofluorescence in the urethra of one patient, the organisms could not be isolated from, nor be identified by immunofluorescence in, the prostatic tissue from any patient. These negative findings were corroborated by the detection of only low titres of anti-chlamydial IgG or IgM in the patients' sera. It was concluded that *C. trachomatis* was not implicated directly in chronic abacterial prostatitis, although the possibility could not be excluded that an original chlamydial infection, evidence for which had since disappeared, may have initiated the inflammatory process.

How is it possible to have two diametrically opposed views concerning the role of *C. trachomatis* in chronic abacterial prostatitis? The most important single factor in accounting for the discrepancy would appear to be patient selection. In four of the previously quoted studies in which there was support for a chlamydial role, there were serious deficiencies in the diagnosis of chronic abacterial prostatitis; in two the patients were selected on clinical ground alone (Bruce et al. 1981; Poletti et al. 1985), and in the two others they were selected solely on the basis of histological criteria (Shurbaji et al. 1988; Abdelatif et al. 1991). Furthermore, *C. trachomatis* was isolated from 19% of the group studied by Weidner et al. (1983), but only half of them had cytological evidence of prostatitis; as 8% of the controls apparently had *C. trachomatis* localised to their prostate, there would appear to be little difference between the two groups of subjects. Urethral contamination of specimens is a constant drawback in any study of prostatitis, and failure to take it into account will almost certainly invalidate the results. Moreover, serious doubts regarding a diagnosis of chronic abacterial prostatitis must exist when *C. trachomatis* is isolated from the urethra of many or, indeed, all of the patients (Poletti et al. 1985). It may be that the patients in the latter study had chlamydial urethritis. However, a figure of 33% for the recovery of *Chlamydia* from the prostate in chronic disease is remarkably high, comparing favourably with the isolation rate often recorded for acute urethritis (Oriel et al. 1976; Alani et al. 1977). Prostatic biopsy provides a direct route to the gland and allows sampling free from urethral contamination. Furthermore, the focal nature of chronic prostatitis (McNeal 1968) reduces the efficiency of blind sampling, a defect that is overcome by the use of an ultrasound-guided technique which allows a more precise targeting of the inflammatory lesions (Doble et al. 1989a).

In those studies in which there have been negative findings, it is important to confirm that such results are truly rather than falsely negative, having occurred possibly as a result of errors in sampling or because of poor culture or detection techniques. It is true that the sensitivity of *C. trachomatis* isolation in cell culture may be increased by blind passage (Jones et al. 1986), and that this seems not to have been done in any of the studies mentioned, whether or not *Chlamydia* was reported to have been isolated. However, those investigators who have reported negative findings (Berger et al. 1989; Doble et al. 1989a) have been well versed in the appropriate detection procedures. In one study (Doble et al. 1989a), the failure of culture to provide positive findings was supported by the negative results of testings by direct immunofluorescence, these two procedures having been shown previously (Thomas et al. 1984) to be of equal sensitivity. In addition, the inhibitory effect of prostatic tissue and secretion on the formation of chlamydial inclusions in cell cultures (Mårdh et al. 1980) was taken into account and regarded as non-contributory in producing negative data (Doble et al. 1989a).

Overall, investigators in studies (Berger et al. 1989; Doble et al. 1989a) in which the disease was diagnosed accurately by using standard methods (Meares and Stamey 1968) concur in their conclusions that *C. trachomatis* has no active role in chronic abacterial prostatitis. Those studies in which the results have prompted the investigators to hold a contrary view (Bruce et al. 1981; Weidner et al. 1983; Poletti et al. 1985; Bruce and Reid 1989), with the exception of one report (Bruce and Reid 1989), have defects in patient selection and design which may have accounted for their interpretation.

Mycoplasma and Other Micro-organisms

Other microbial agents have been cited as possible causes of chronic abacterial prostatitis, in particular *Ureaplasma urealyticum* (Weidner et al. 1980; Brunner et al. 1983) and *Mycoplasma hominis* (Brunner et al. 1983). The chief problem in assessing the relevance of these organisms is their frequent occurrence in healthy subjects (Furr and Taylor-Robinson 1987) and in those with prior sexual exposure (McCormack et al. 1973), so that quantitative studies are mandatory. The high rate of isolation from controls calls into question the view that *U. urealyticum* is causative (Weidner et al. 1980; Brunner et al. 1983) and was refuted in a large case–control study of patients and controls (Berger et al. 1989). With regard to *M. hominis*, although it was detected in 10% of patients but not in controls in one qualitative study (Mårdh and Colleen 1975), the investigators were guarded in attributing an aetiological role to it, and quantitative data seem to refute any such proposal (Brunner et al. 1983; Weidner et al. 1988; Berger et al. 1989; Doble et al. 1989b). Direct sampling of the prostate has failed to result in the isolation of either *U. urealyticum* or *M. hominis* from patients with chronic abacterial prostatitis (Doble et al. 1989b), and negative findings were also obtained in a serological study of such patients (Shortliffe et al. 1985).

The search for other agents in chronic abacterial prostatitis which might have some aetiological significance has met with conclusions of greater unanimity. No role has been found for anaerobes (Meares 1973; Nielsen and Justesen 1974; Mårdh and Colleen 1975; Doble et al. 1989b), fungi (Berger et al. 1989) or viruses (Gordon et al. 1972; Nielsen and Vestergaard 1973; Mårdh and Colleen 1975) despite repetitive examination of prostatic secretions and tissue. Thus, although the data on the aetiological significance of micro-organisms in this condition are conflicting, it seems reasonable to propose on the weight of evidence that the antigen(s) involved in maintaining the inflammatory reaction in the majority of cases is non-organismal (Doble et al. 1989b).

Pathological Features

Histology

Refined techniques of prostatic biopsy, with the aid of ultrasound guidance, have improved the accuracy of sampling the inflammatory lesions in chronic prostatitis. However, little meaningful information concerning the aetiology of chronic abacterial prostatitis has been forthcoming from routine histological analysis. It would appear that the endpoint, that is, the chronic inflammatory lesion, may be reached by a number of disparate, unconnected routes, none of which can be unravelled by a routine histological approach.

Immunopathology

In contrast to the lack of information accruing from routine histology, the study of prostatic tissue by immunological procedures has thrown some light on the inflammatory process. The use of direct immunofluorescence techniques has resulted in IgA and IgM antibodies and fibrinogen (Vinje et al. 1983; Doble et al. 1990) as well as complement C3 (Doble et al. 1990), being identified in prostatic biopsies from patients with chronic prostatitis. Furthermore, a correlation between symptoms of poor urinary flow as well as irritative voiding and immunofluorescence staining was identified, whereas none existed with histology (Doble et al. 1990). An analysis of the inflammatory cell population, using monoclonal antibodies, has also been undertaken (Doble et al. 1993). In normal prostatic tissue faint HLA-DR expression, indicative of MHC class II antigen, was observed in the basal epithelial cells, and in mononuclear, non-macrophage cells in the periglandular region and in endothelial cells. A few T-cells, comprising equal numbers of CD_4 (helper/inducer) and CD_8 (suppressor/cytotoxic) cells, were evenly distributed, but B-cells were not seen, and there were only scanty cells representative of the monocyte/macrophage series. However, within the prostatic tissue of patients with chronic abacterial prostatitis a different picture emerged. Immunoperoxidase staining showed that HLA-DR expression was most marked in the glandular structures and increased with the more severe inflammation. Quantitative estimation by the HLA-DR-glucose oxidase technique confirmed this finding. The number of T-cells also increased with the degree of inflammation, there being an increased proportion of CD_8 cells in the more severe and granulomatous forms of prostatitis. In addition, increasing numbers of antigen-presenting cells and mature tissue macrophages occurred with increasing inflammatory grade. Epithelioid cells were found only in the granulomatous form of prostatitis and monocytes in half of the more severe inflammatory lesions only. Immunofluorescence staining not only confirmed the progressive predominance of CD_8 cells with increasing inflammation but also revealed that a greater proportion of these cells expressed the CD_7 activation marker with increasing inflammatory grade. This was not the case, however, with the granulomatous reaction or with the CD_4 subset.

How may these various data be interpreted? Consistent HLA-DR expression and the presence of large numbers of T-cells and antigen-presenting cells, together with the absence of B-cells, imply that the inflammatory reaction in chronic prostatitis is cell mediated. The prominent T-cell population comprised the CD_8 subset, in contrast to rheumatoid arthritis where the CD_4 subset predominates. Also, antigen-presenting cells, although present in greater numbers with increasing inflammation, were not the predominant non-lymphoid cells, as they are in rheumatoid arthritis. The pattern in rheumatoid arthritis is consistent with immunoregulatory dysfunction, whereas that in chronic prost-atitis is compatible more with a persistent antigenic stimulus (Doble 1991). The antigen-presenting cell/mature tissue macrophage relationship in prostatitis is in keeping with a type IV hypersensitivity response. The CD_8 cell predominance might imply that the response is to a viral agent, though it is interesting to note that the immunological response in chronic abacterial prostatitis was not different from that in chronic bacterial prostatitis. We have been unable to implicate any micro-organisms in chronic abacterial prostatitis, but the intra-prostatic antibody findings described earlier raise the possibility of urine refluxing into the prostate and acting as a carrier of exogenous antigen, the nature of which is not yet known.

Conclusions and Future Considerations

To date there is no unequivocal evidence of a role for *C. trachomatis* in the aetiology of chronic abacterial prostatitis. The confusion arises from inaccurate diagnosis, the use of ill-defined groups of patients for study and the possible low specificity of detection techniques. Those investigators who have selected pa-tients using the Stamey localisation procedure, the only reputable yardstick for diagnosis, have been unable to detect *Chlamydia* in either prostatic secretions (Berger et al. 1989; Doble et al. 1989a) or prostatic tissue (Doble et al. 1989a). The same applies to *M. hominis* and *U. urealyticum* (Berger et al. 1989; Doble et al. 1989b). Investigators who perceive these micro-organisms as instrumental in causing the disease may indeed have detected their presence, yet in a hetero-genous and impure patient population, for example, in men who have an ure-thral infection as well as chronic disease of the prostate.

So far, nothing has been said about the polymerase chain reaction (PCR). This is the most sensitive way of detecting the DNA of a micro-organism. It has been developed for *C. trachomatis* (Palmer et al. 1991), has been shown to detect small numbers of chlamydial elementary bodies (Gilroy et al. 1992) and has been used to detect such bodies in the joints of patients with sexually acquired reactive arthritis (Taylor-Robinson et al. 1992). PCR must surely have a place in refuting or confirming the existence of *Chlamydia* in the prostate. The results of such an analysis in an accurately diagnosed cohort of men with chronic abacterial prostatitis are awaited. Intuitively, however, it would be surprising if more than a small proportion of cases prove to be PCR positive and unlikely, therefore, for the persistence of *C. trachomatis* to account for the maintenance of chronicity. Furthermore, by the same token, it may remain difficult to exclude fully the possibility that *C. trachomatis* initiates the chronic inflammatory response, but has long since disappeared.

In this regard, therefore, is there any further approach that would seem worthy of consideration? In view of the cell-mediated immune response in chronic abacterial prostatitis, studies to examine the role of heat-shock proteins are overdue. It is notable that a correlation between immune responsiveness to a protein of about 60 kDa and severe sequelae of chlamydial infection, such as pelvic inflammatory disease, ectopic pregnancy and tubal factor infertility, has been demonstrated (Wagar et al. 1990; Yuan et al. 1992). Although the precise involvement of the chlamydial heat-shock protein in stimulating an immuno-pathogenic response has not been determined, the development of monoclonal antibodies to the chlamydial 60-kDa protein (Yuan et al. 1992) should help not only in the identification of this antigen in tissues but also in immunoaffinity purification of the antigen for use in *in vitro* antibody and T-cell assays. Application of these techniques to the problem of chronic abacterial prostatitis would seem desirable.

Thus, although the aetiology of chronic abacterial prostatitis remains obscure, techniques are being developed which increase the likelihood of the offending antigens being identified. It is essential, however, despite the risk of labouring the point, to ensure that the search is confined to those patients for whom the diagnosis of chronic abacterial prostatitis is precise and along classical lines. Only by such means will the solution to the enigma of this disease come within reach. In the meantime, it seems clearer than ever that its treatment should be directed more towards the use of immunoregulatory agents rather than repetitive antibiotics.

References

Abdelatif OMA, Chandler FW, McGuire BS (1991) Chlamydia trachomatis in chronic abacterial prostatitis: demonstration by colorimetric in situ hybridization. Hum Pathol 22:41–44

Alani MD, Darougar S, MacD Burns DC, Thin RN, Dunn H (1977) Isolation of Chlamydia trachomatis from the male urethra. Br J Vener Dis 55:88–92

Anderson RU, Weller C (1979) Prostatic secretion leukocyte studies in non-bacterial prostatitis (prostatosis). J Urol 121:292–294

Berger RE, Krieger JN, Kessler D, Ireton RC, Close C, Holmes KK, Roberts PL (1989) Case control study of men with suspected chronic idiopathic prostatitis. J Urol 141:328–331

Blacklock NJ, Beavis JP (1974) The response of prostatic fluid pH in inflammation. Br J Urol 46:537–542

Bruce AW, Reid G (1989) Prostatitis associated with Chlamydia trachomatis in 6 patients. J Urol 142:1006–1007

Bruce AW, Chadwick P, Willett WS, O'Shaughnessy M (1981) The role of chlamydiae in genitourinary disease. J Urol 126:625–629

Brunner H, Weidner W, Schiefer H-G (1983) Studies on the role of Ureaplasma urealyticum and Mycoplasma hominis in prostatitis. J Infect Dis 147:807–813

Christiansen E, Purvis K (1991) Diagnosis of chronic abacterial prostato-vesiculitis by rectal ultrasonography in relation to symptoms and findings. Br J Urol 67:173–176

Doble A (1991) Prostatitis. In: Harris JRW, Forster SM (eds) Recent advances in sexually transmitted diseases and AIDS. Churchill Livingstone, London, pp 129–157

Doble A, Carter S StC (1989) Ultrasonographic findings in prostatitis. Urol Clin North Am 16:763–772

Doble A, Thomas BJ, Walker MM, Harris JRW, Witherow RO'N, Taylor-Robinson D (1989a) The role of Chlamydia trachomatis in chronic abacterial prostatitis: a study using ultrasound guided biopsy. J Urol 141:332–333

Doble A, Thomas BJ, Furr PM, Walker MM, Harris JRW, Witherow RO'N, Taylor-Robinson D (1989b) A search for infectious agents in chronic abacterial prostatitis using ultrasound guided biopsy. Br J Urol 64:297–301

Doble A, Walker MM, Harris JRW, Taylor-Robinson D, Witherow RO'N (1990) Intraprostatic antibody deposition in chronic abacterial prostatitis. Br J Urol 65:598–605

Doble A, Walker MM, Harris JRW, Witherow RO'N, Taylor-Robinson D, Poulter LW (1993) The immunopathology of chronic abacterial prostatitis. Clin Immun Immunopathol (in press)

Drach GW (1975) Prostatitis: man's hidden infection. Urol Clin North Am 2:499–520

Drach GW, Meares EM, Fair WR, Stamey TA (1978) Classification of benign diseases associated with prostatic pain: prostatitis or prostatodynia? J Urol 120:266

Fowler JE, Mariano M (1984) Longitudinal studies of prostatic fluid immunoglobulin in men with bacterial prostatitis. J Urol 131:363–369

Fowler JE, Kaiser DL, Mariano M (1982) Immunologic response of the prostate to bacteriuria and bacterial prostatitis. J Urol 128:158–164

Furr PM, Taylor-Robinson D (1987) Prevalence and significance of Mycoplasma hominis and Ureaplasma urealyticum in the urines of a non-venereal disease population. Epidemiol Infect 98:353–359

Gilroy CB, Thomas BJ, Taylor-Robinson D (1992) Small numbers of Chlamydia trachomatis elementary bodies on slides detected by the polymerase chain reaction. J Clin Pathol 45:531–532

Gordon HL, Miller DH, Rawls WE (1972) Viral studies in patients with non-specific prostatourethritis. J Urol 108:299–300

Griffiths GJ, Crooks AJR, Roberts EE, Evans KT, Buck AC, Thomas PJ, Peeling WB (1984) Ultrasonic appearances associated with prostatic inflammation: a preliminary study. Clin Radiol 35:343–345

Harada K, Igari D, Tanahashi Y (1979) Gray scale transrectal ultrasonography of the prostate. JC U 7:45–49

Holm HH, Gammelgaard J (1981) Ultrasonically guided precise needle placement in the prostate and the seminal vesicles. J Urol 125:385–387

Hunter J (1786) A treatise on the venereal disease, 1st edn. London

Jones RB, Katz BP, van der Pol B, Caine VA, Batteiger BE, Newhall WJ (1986) Effect of blind passage and multiple sampling on recovery of Chlamydia trachomatis from urogenital specimens. J Clin Microbiol 24:1029–1033

Kohnen PW, Drach GW (1979) Patterns of inflammation in prostatic hyperplasia: a histologic and bacteriologic study. J Urol 121:755–760

Krotoszyner M, Spencer JC (1894) Chronic prostatitis after gonorrhoea. I. Its clinical pathology. II. Its microscopic and bacteriologic aspects. JAMA 23:103–106

Lee F, Gray JM, McCleary RD, Meadows TR, Kumasaka GH, Borlaza GS, Straub WH, Lee F, Solomon MH, McHugh TA et al. (1985) Transrectal ultrasound in the diagnosis of prostate cancer: location, echogenicity, histopathology and staging. Prostate 7:117–129

Mårdh P-A, Colleen S (1975) Search for uro-genital tract infections in patients with symptoms of prostatitis. Scand J Urol Nephrol 9:8–16

Mårdh P-A, Colleen S, Holmquist B (1972) Chlamydia in chronic prostatitis. Br Med J 4:361

Mårdh P-A, Ripa KT, Colleen S, Treharne JD, Darougar S (1978) Role of Chlamydia trachomatis in non-acute prostatitis. Br J Vener Dis 54:330–334

Mårdh P-A, Colleen S, Sylwan J (1980) Inhibitory effect on the formation of chlamydial inclusions in McCoy cells by seminal fluid and some of its components. Invest Urol 17:510–513

McCormack WM, Lee Y-H, Zinner SH (1973) Sexual experience and urethral colonization with genital mycoplasmas: a study in normal men. Ann Intern Med 78:696–698

McNeal JE (1968) Regional morphology and pathology of the prostate. Am J Clin Pathol 49:347–357

Meares EM (1973) Bacterial prostatitis vs 'prostatosis'. A clinical and bacteriological study. JAMA 224:1372–1375

Meares EM, Stamey TA (1968) Bacteriologic localization patterns in bacterial prostatitis and urethritis. Invest Urol 5:492–518

Moore RA (1937) Inflammation of the prostate gland. J Urol 38:173–182

Nielsen ML, Justesen T (1974) Studies on the pathology of prostatitis. A search for prostatic infections with obligate anaerobes in patients with chronic prostatitis and chronic urethritis. Scand J Urol Nephrol 8:1–6

Nielsen ML, Vestergaard BF (1973) Virological investigations in chronic prostatitis. J Urol 109:1023–1025

Oriel JD, Reeve P, Wright JT, Owen J (1976) Chlamydial infection of the male urethra. Br J Vener Dis 52:46–51

Palmer HM, Gilroy CB, Thomas BJ, Hay PE, Gilchrist C, Taylor-Robinson D (1991) Detection of Chlamydia trachomatis by the polymerase chain reaction in swabs and urine from men with non-gonococcal urethritis. J Clin Pathol 44:321–325

Pfau A, Perlberg S, Shapira A (1978) The pH of the prostatic fluid in health and disease: implications of treatment in chronic bacterial prostatitis. J Urol 119:384–387

Poletti F, Medici MC, Alinovi A, Menozzi MG, Sacchini P, Stagni G, Toni M, Benoldi D (1985) Isolation of Chlamydia trachomatis from the prostatic cells in patients affected by nonacute abacterial prostatitis. J Urol 134:691–693

Schaeffer AJ, Wendel EF, Dunn JK, Grayhack JT (1981) Prevalence and significance of prostatic inflammation. J Urol 125:215–219

Shortliffe LMD, Wehner N (1986) The characterization of bacterial and nonbacterial prostatitis by prostatic immunoglobulins. Medicine (Baltimore) 65:399–414

Shortliffe LMD, Wehner N, Stamey TA (1981) The detection of a local prostatic immunologic response to bacterial prostatitis. J Urol 125:509–515

Shortliffe LMD, Elliott KM, Sellers RG, Stamey TA, Schachter J (1985) Measurement of chlamydial and ureaplasmal antibodies in serum and prostatic fluid of men with nonbacterial prostatitis. J Urol 133:276A

Shortliffe LMD, Elliott K, Sellers RG (1989) Measurement of urinary antibodies to crude bacterial antigen in patients with chronic bacterial prostatitis. J Urol 141:632–636

Shurbaji MS, Gupta PK, Myers J (1988) Immunohistochemical demonstration of chlamydial antigens in association with prostatitis. Mod Pathol 1:348–351

Spirnak JP, Resnick MI (1984) Transrectal ultrasonography. Urology 23:461–467

Stamey TA (1980) Urinary infections in males. In: Stamey TA (ed) Pathogenesis and treatment of urinary tract infections. Williams and Wilkins, Baltimore, pp 342–429

Stamey TA, Govan DE, Palmer JM (1965) The localization and treatment of urinary tract infections: the role of bactericidal urine levels as opposed to serum levels. Medicine (Baltimore) 44:1–36

Tarizzo ML, Nabli B, Labonn J (1968) Studies on trachoma. II. Evaluation of laboratory diagnostic methods under field conditions. Bull WHO 38:897–905

Taylor-Robinson D, Gilroy CB, Thomas BJ, Keat ACS (1992) Detection of Chlamydia trachomatis DNA in joints of reactive arthritis patients by polymerase chain reaction. Lancet 340:81–82

Thomas BJ, Evans RT, Hawkins DA, Taylor-Robinson D (1984) Sensitivity of detecting Chlamydia trachomatis elementary bodies in smears by the use of a fluorescein labelled monoclonal antibody: comparison with conventional chlamydial isolation. J Clin Pathol 37:812–816

Thompson H (1861) Inflammation of the prostate: acute and chronic. In: The diseases of the prostate and their pathology and treatment. John Churchill, London, pp 50–66

Treharne JD, Forsey T, Thomas BJ (1983) Chlamydial serology. Br Med Bull 39:194–200

Vinje O, Fryjordet A, Bruu A-L, Møller P, Mellbye OJ, Kåss E (1983) Laboratory findings in chronic prostatitis – with special reference to immunological and microbiological aspects. Scand J Urol Nephrol 17:291–297

Von Lackum WH (1933) Focal infections in urology – prostatitis. In: Ballenger EG, Frontz WA, Hamer HG, Lewis B (eds) History of urology. Williams and Wilkins, Baltimore, pp 224–235

Von Sehlen (1893) Zur Diagnostik und Therapie der Prostatitis chronica. Int Centralbl Physiol Pathol Harn Sex Org 4:117–132

Wagar EA, Schachter J, Bavoil P, Stephens RS (1990) Differential human serologic response to two 60,000 molecular weight Chlamydia trachomatis antigens. J Infect Dis 162:922–927

Weidner W, Ebner H (1985) Cytological analysis of urine after prostatic massage (VB3) – a new technique for a discriminating diagnosis of prostatitis. In: Brunner H, Krause W, Rothauge CF, Weidner W (eds) Chronic prostatitis. Schattauer, Stuttgart, pp 141–151

Weidner W, Brunner H, Krause W (1980) Quantitative culture of Ureaplasma urealyticum in patients with chronic prostatitis or prostatosis. J Urol 124:622–625

Weidner W, Arens M, Krauss H, Schiefer HG, Ebner H (1983) Chlamydia trachomatis in 'abacterial' prostatitis: microbiological, cytological and serological studies. Urol Int 38:146–149

Weidner W, Schiefer HG, Krauss H (1988) Role of Chlamydia trachomatis and mycoplasmas in chronic prostatitis. A review. Urol Int 43:167–173

Wiegand S, Weidner W (1986) Per rectal ultrasonography of the prostate in the diagnosis of chronic prostatitis and prostatodynia. In: Weidner W, Brunner H, Krause W, Rothauge CF (eds) Therapy of prostatitis. Zuckschwerdt, Munich, pp 177–180

Wishnow KI, Wehner N, Stamey TA (1982) The diagnostic value of the immunologic response in bacterial and nonbacterial prostatitis. J Urol 127:689–694

Yuan Y, Lyng K, Zhang Y-X, Rockey DD, Morrison RP (1992) Monoclonal antibodies define genus-specific, species-specific, and cross-reactive epitopes of the chlamydial 60-kilodalton heat shock protein (hsp60): specific immunodetection and purification of chlamydial hsp60. Infect Immun 60:2288–2296

Prostatic Infection by Unconventional, Fastidious Pathogens

H.G. Schiefer

Prostatitis syndrome is not a definite nosologic entity, but includes various inflammatory and noninflammatory conditions affecting the prostate.

A widely accepted clinical classification system of benign diseases associated with prostatic pain had been based on cytologic and microbiologic examinations of the expressed prostatic secretions (EPS), on medical history, and on clinical findings by rectal palpation of the prostate. Four categories have been suggested: (1) acute bacterial prostatitis, (2) chronic bacterial prostatitis, (3) nonbacterial prostatitis, and (4) prostatodynia (Drach et al. 1978; Meares 1992).

This classification system proved to be an excellent basis for correct etiologic and clinical diagnosis and adequate therapeutic approach in most cases of prostatitis syndrome. However, some critical objections should not be ignored. Drach et al. (1978) took only common uropathogens into consideration as etiologic agents for categories (1) and (2). Furthermore, although widely used, the term "nonbacterial prostatitis" must be regarded as a misnomer, since its definition, i.e., the finding of prostatic inflammation with increased leukocytes in EPS, but no evidence of the common uropathogens, excludes a priori infectious agents which are usually not covered by routine diagnostic bacteriology. Since recent evidence suggests that, beyond the uropathogens, obligately pathogenic as well as opportunistic bacteria, fungi, viruses, and parasites may occasionally infect the prostate, a more comprehensive classification system (Brunner and Weidner 1985) has been proposed to include the following:

1. Acute bacterial prostatitis
2. Chronic bacterial prostatitis due to
   a) common urinary tract pathogens
   b) *Ureaplasma urealyticum*
   c) *Mycobacterium tuberculosis*
3. Mycotic prostatitis
4. Urethroprostatitis due to *Neisseria gonorrhoeae*, *Trichomonas vaginalis*, and *Candida* spp
5. Chronic prostatitis of unknown etiology
6. Prostatodynia

We considered it appropriate to present a review of the literature on prostatic infections by unconventional, fastidious microorganisms. Their true incidence as etiologic agents in prostatitis is unknown, since routine bacteriologic studies on prostatic secretions or prostatic biopsy samples concentrate on common pathogens in bacterial prostatitis, i.e., *E. coli* and other gram-negative rods, *Enterococcus* spp, and, still not definitely proved, coagulase-negative staphylococci. However, in most studies on prostatic infections by unconventional pathogens, their true localization to the prostate and their pathogenic role are far from being settled. Most data are merely based on their isolation from secretions obtained after prostatic massage or on prostatic tissue samples which showed a more or less distinct inflammatory reaction. Thus, in most cases the stringent criteria established by Drach et al. (1978), i.e., recurrent urinary tract infection, repeated isolation of the same pathogen from EPS, evidence of increased leukocyte numbers in EPS, and specific immune response, have not been met.

Therefore, many unconventional pathogens isolated from the prostatic secretions and biopsy samples can at best be considered to be associated with prostatitis. These reservations kept in mind, the following sections review bacterial, fungal, viral, and parasitic agents presumably involved as etiologic agents in some cases of prostatitis.

Bacteria

Haemophilus Species

Haemophilus spp are usually considered to be respiratory tract pathogens. However, genital tract infections due to *Haemophilus influenzae*, were described in the early 1900s, but the number of cases remained low and has increased only recently. *Haemophilus* spp have been isolated from females suffering from genital tract infections and from perinatally infected newborns. Serologically nontypeable and biotype II *Haemophilus influenzae* were the most frequent urogenital isolates. In female pelvic inflammatory diseases and in perinatally acquired neonatal infections, biotypes I and IV prevailed. Large numbers of plasmids were found in genitourinary strains of *Haemophilus influenzae*. Colonization of the female genital tract may occur via fecal carriage. *Haemophilus* spp are assumed to be sexually transmitted and may be rare, but more important pathogens than generally thought, also in the male urogenital tract. Thus, *Haemophilus influenzae* and *Haemophilus parainfluenzae* have been isolated from ejaculates, and a single case report of prostatitis due to *Haemophilus influenzae* has been described (Goetz and Craig 1982; Quentin et al. 1989; Wallace et al. 1983).

Treponema pallidum

No tissue of the body is immune to the late manifestations of syphilis, and literally every organ of the body has been reported to be the site of either the proliferative or the gummatous lesion. The late manifestations of syphilis appear only some 8–10 years following infection. The urogenital tract may occasionally be involved, resulting in gummatous lesions of the penis, testis, and prostate. A historical review on *Syphilis of the Prostate* was published in 1920. From 24 cases purported to be syphilis of the prostate, 12 were accepted as undoubted prostatic syphilis. The most frequent symptom was pain described as "slight" to "violent," pollakisuria, urethral discharge, and cloudy urine which contained pus, mucus, and sometimes red blood cells. In all, prostatic syphilis may occur, but is an extremely rare disease manifestation (Kampmeier 1964; Thompson 1920).

Brucella Species

Worldwide, brucellosis remains one of the most widespread zoonoses, and human infections are common. Before assuming that human brucellosis is now a rare disease in industrialized countries, one must remember that the disease is vastly underdiagnosed and underreported. The clinical complaints and physical findings in human brucellosis are often nonspecific and present for prolonged periods. Urogenital involvement (epididymitis) in brucellosis is common, and, at certain stages of the disease, 20%–50% of patients may have organisms cultured from urine. Proven cases of prostatitis are rare complications and, due to the granulomatous changes, may easily be mistaken for tuberculosis or carcinoma. *Brucella abortus* and *Brucella melitensis* have been cultured from transurethrally resected prostates which showed evidence of chronic inflammation. In one further case of chronic prostatitis, *Brucella abortus* was cultured from prostatic secretions. Prostatitis due to *Brucella* spp is a rare disease. Although of infrequent occurrence, one should be aware of brucellosis and its genitourinary complications, particularly in endemic regions (Forbes et al. 1954; Kelalis et al. 1962; Young 1983).

Neisseria gonorrhoeae

In the preantibiotic era, the prostate was involved in over 90% of male gonorrheal infections causing urethroprostatitis and prostatic abscess. Antimicrobial treatment reduced the figure, and today, at least in developed countries, clinically evident prostatitis complicating gonorrheal urethritis is considered an uncommon condition. However, in a thorough search for traces of gonorrheal prostatitis, the secretions obtained after prostatic massage of 33 males adequately treated for uncomplicated gonorrheal urethritis were examined 2–3 weeks after the end of treatment: in 67% *Neisseria gonorrhoeae*-like organisms were seen by direct microscopy, and in 40% a specific identification was achieved using fluorescent antibody techniques (immunofluorescence test, IFT); bacteriologic cultures were negative; and an immune response to gonococcal antigen was positive in 78% of males with positive IFT compared with 27%

with negative IFT. The authors concluded that gonococci may invade the prostate during acute urethral infection and that conventional therapy may fail to clear *Neisseria gonorrhoeae* from male accessory glands. Thus, symptomatic prostatitis may develop despite negative cultures for *Neisseria gonorrhoeae* (Danielsson and Molin 1971).

Mycobacterium tuberculosis

Genital tuberculosis occurs most frequently in men aged 20–40 years. A large number of genitourinary cases represent instances of reactivation tuberculosis. Systemic symptoms are frequently absent. The concomitant and/or sequential involvement of more than one genital site is common. The prostate is involved in 70%–100% of cases of genital tract infection and is the sole site of genital infections in 13%–32% of urogenital tuberculosis in males (Gorse and Belshe 1985).

Tuberculous prostatitis develops as a sequela of hematogenous dissemination from pulmonary sites. Infection of the prostate may occur directly, more likely to occur in children than in adults, or via a descending route from tuberculous kidneys. In the presence of caseating or cavitating renal lesions, the likelihood of concomitant genital involvement (most commonly prostatic) is five times greater than in the presence of noncaseating miliary renal tubercles (Gorse and Belshe 1985).

Rectal digital examination fails to detect all cases of prostatitis, because prostatic disease must be extensive to allow clinical detection. When the disease is advanced, the prostate may be enlarged to two to three times its usual size and has irregular, firm, and nodular regions (granulomatous prostatitis). Caseation necrosis is detectable as softened areas.

The results of urinalysis are most likely to be abnormal in prostatic tuberculosis. "Sterile" pyuria and increased leukocyte numbers in prostatic secretions are guiding symptoms. Diagnosis is verified by tuberculin skin test reaction, radiologic and sonographic examination (calcifications in tuberculous prostates), urographic findings, and results of mycobacterial cultures from urine, prostatic secretions, and ejaculate (Gorse and Belshe 1985).

The onset of symptoms in male genital tuberculosis is usually insidious and progressive.

Nontuberculous mycobacteria occasionally cause prostatitis. Organisms isolated from involved prostates include *M. kansasii, M. avium-intracellulare* (MAC), *M. xenopi,* and *M. fortuitum.* One case of granulomatous prostatitis associated with *M. kansasii* and *M. fortuitum* infection is of considerable interest because of normal chest roentgenograms and lack of symptoms. In order to prove the etiologic significance of these "atypical" mycobacteria in urogenital infections the following criteria must be met: (a) symptoms of chronic or recurrent urinary tract infection; (b) endoscopic and/or radiologic evidence of genitourinary infection; (c) abnormal urine sediment; (d) absence of common uropathogens; (e) repeated cultural detection of identical mycobacteria; and (f) granulomatous tissue histology, ideally showing the presence of acid-fast bacteria.

Tuberculous and nontuberculous mycobacterial diseases are common manifestations of human immunodeficiency virus (HIV) infection, affecting 2%–10% (tuberculous) and 25%–50% (nontuberculous) of patients, respectively. Extrapulmonary dissemination is found in over 50% of autopsied cases (Brooker and Aufderheide 1980; Lee et al. 1977; Mikolich and Mates 1992).

Chlamydia trachomatis and Urogenital Mycoplasmas

Chlamydia trachomatis and/or *Ureaplasma urealyticum* are the main pathogens causing non- and postgonococcal urethritis (Grant et al. 1985; Hofstetter 1973; O'Leary 1990; Taylor-Robinson 1985; Taylor-Robinson and Thomas 1980). The assumption appears plausible that, by way of intracanalicular ascension, they might subsequently infect the prostate (Weidner et al. 1988). However, their etiologic role in prostatitis (Berger et al. 1989; Brunner et al. 1983; Doble et al. 1989; Grant et al. 1985; Johannisson 1981; Krieger and Egan 1991; Mårdh et al. 1978; O'Leary 1990; Peeters et al. 1985; Poletti et al. 1985; Pust et al. 1986; Taylor-Robinson 1985; Taylor-Robinson and Thomas 1980; Weidner et al. 1988; Weidner et al. 1991) is still unclear, since, in most studies, contamination of prostatic specimens by urethral microorganisms could not be excluded. At least part of the discrepant results may be due to different selection criteria of the patients included: in some studies, for example, the majority of patients examined had no cytologic signs of prostatitis.

Following an approach analogous to that previously developed for the diagnosis of chronic bacterial prostatitis, Weidner et al. (1988) applied the localization protocol of the four-specimen technique and combined quantitative determinations of microorganisms plus quantitative cytologic analysis and, in chlamydial infections, serologic investigations. In 82 out of 597 (13.7%) males with signs and symptoms of chronic prostatitis, a typical prostatitis configuration for *Ureaplasma urealyticum* was observed. A prostatitis configuration could not be assigned to *Mycoplasma hominis*. Cytologic analysis of urine voided after prostatic massage (VB3) gave further evidence for the pathogenic role of *Ureaplasma urealyticum* in prostatitis: in most cases, the leukocyte pattern was in accordance to that seen in chronic prostatitis due to conventional pathogens (Brunner et al. 1983; Weidner et al. 1991). Similarly, Hofstetter (1973) found a good correlation between excessive numbers of *Ureaplasma urealyticum* and increased numbers of leukocytes in EPS. In 15 cases, a perineal biopsy was taken from the prostate, and in 12 out of 15 cases, *Ureaplasma urealyticum* were cultured from the prostatic tissue.

After intraurethral self-inoculation of *Ureaplasma urealyticum*, prostatitis developed in one of two men; the largest portion of *Ureaplasma urealyticum* was detected in the prostatic part of the split ejaculate (Taylor-Robinson et al. 1977).

However, Shortliffe et al. (1985) found low antibody elevations against *Ureaplasma urealyticum* in their patients with nonbacterial prostatitis and, therefore, doubt the etiologic role of *U. urealyticum* in prostatitis.

The most controversial putative causative agent in prostatitis is *Chlamydia trachomatis*. Because this organism is the causative agent in about 40% of cases of male nongonococcal urethritis and in most cases of acute epididymitis in men under the age of 35 years, an etiologic role in prostatitis seems plausible. Unfortunately, reported studies still leave considerable doubt as to whether *C. trachomatis* really is an important pathogen in prostatitis (Berger et al. 1989; Doble et al. 1989; Grant et al. 1985; Johannisson 1981; Krieger and Egan 1991; Mårdh et al. 1978; Peeters et al. 1985; Poletti et al. 1985; Taylor-Robinson and Thomas 1980; Weidner et al. 1988; Weidner et al. 1991).

By critically correlating results of cultural isolation of *Chlamydia trachomatis* from EPS, cytologic studies of leukocytes in VB3, and microimmunofluorescence tests, Weidner et al. (1988, 1991) found that positive chlamydial cultures from EPS and high leukocyte counts in VB3 correlate with a specific humoral antibody response to *Chlamydia trachomatis*. When *Chlamydia trachomatis* is the only microorganism isolated from EPS of patients with high granulocyte counts in VB3, it is considered to be a possible etiologic agent.

Recently, Bruce and Reid (1989) reported on a new attempt to exclude urethral contamination. Chlamydial elementary bodies were stained by direct immunofluorescence in prostatic secretions, and chlamydial infection was diagnosed in cases of chlamydia-free urethral samples.

Some authors (Table 1) have tried to establish chlamydial infection of prostatic epithelial cells directly in prostatic tissue taken by biopsy. Cultural and immunofluorescent tests were applied. Here again, discrepant results are obvious, possibly due to the different techniques applied for gaining prostatic material: tissue taken by transrectal biopsy or transurethral resection of the prostate may contain urethral epithelial cells.

Evidence for the etiologic significance of *U. urealyticum* and *C. trachomatis* was obtained in a prospective study on patients suffering from urethritis (Schiefer et al. 1985). A total of 69 patients with nongonococcal urethritis were examined for the development of prostatitis. After initial diagnostic procedures and etiologic classification, all patients were treated with tetracycline, since a longer observation of untreated patients was considered unethical. All patients were re-examined 4 weeks after their first visit to the clinic. Prostatitis was diagnosed when more than four polymorphonuclear leukocytes (PML) were seen per microscopic field at 400-fold magnification in the sediment of 3 ml urine voided after prostatic massage (VB3). Prostatitis as sequela of nongonococcal urethritis was observed in 18 (26%) of 69 patients: in 12 of 31 patients who had *Chlamydia trachomatis*-positive urethritis, in four of 22 patients with *Ureaplasma urealyticum*-positive urethritis, in two of eight patients who had *Chlamydia trachomatis*- and *Ureaplasma urealyticum*-positive nongonococcal urethritis, and in none of the eight patients with common bacterial infection.

Table 1. Detection of *Chlamydia trachomatis* in prostatic specimens from patients with nonbacterial prostatitis

Author	Patients (*n*)	Positive chlamydial findings in		Type of operation	Method
		Prostatic urethra	Prostate		
Poletti et al. (1985)	30	not done	10	Transrectal biopsy	Culture
Pust et al. (1986)	32	6	1	Urethral and perineal biopsy	Immunofluorescence
Shurbaji et al. (1988)	16	not done	5	TURP, open operation	Immunohisto-chemistry
Doble et al. (1989)	50	not done	none	Perineal, ultrasonically guided biopsy	Culture, immunofluorescence
Abdelatif et al. (1991)	23	not done	7	TURP	In situ hybridization
Weidner et al. (1991)	22	4	none	Perineal, ultrasonically guided biopsy	Culture
Dan et al. (1991)	100	not done	3	TURP	Culture

TURP, transurethral resection of the prostate.

In a recent paper, Lomas et al. (1993) reported an observation presumably pertinent to understanding the pathogenesis of non-bacterial prostatitis. Urethral exudates obtained from patients with urethritis contained factors that induced migration of healthy neutrophils. It is appealing to hypothesize that chemotactic urethral factors might stimulate an inflammatory reaction in the prostate.

Actinomyces israelii

Urinary tract actinomycosis is rare, as is male genitourinary system infection (Ellis et al. 1979). The kidneys or bladder can be involved by direct extension from an intestinal focus, although isolated kidney, bladder, and scrotum involvement, presumably due to hematogenous dissemination from oral, pulmonary, or gastrointestinal infections, have all been reported. There is only one case report (de Souza et al. 1985) of actinomycosis of the prostate and periprostatic tissue. A 39-year-old man presented with signs and symptoms of chronic prostatitis; rectal examination revealed a large, tender prostate. An exploratory laparotomy showed a firm, whitish–tan mass that involved the prostate and adjacent tissue. Sulfur granules were noted in several abscesses extending from the prostate into the periprostatic tissue. The patient was treated with erythromycin. In this patient there was no evidence of actinomycosis outside the prostate and periprostatic tissue, indicating that the prostate was the primary site of infection. Prostatic actinomycosis is undoubtedly a rare disease. It should be considered in a patient suffering from prostatitis in whom routine cultures revealed no common pathogen, particularly when periprostatic extension of inflammation is noted.

Anaerobic Bacteria

Inspite of the fact that the resident bacterial flora of the male urethra contains a lot of microaerophilic and anaerobic bacteria, such as *Peptococci*, *Peptostreptococci*, *Bacteroides* species, and *Fusobacterium* species, thorough investigation did not provide evidence that obligately anaerobic bacteria play a major role in patients with prostatitis. It has been assumed that anaerobic bacteria might fail to adhere to uroepithelial cells and/or that prostatic secretions might destroy anaerobes (Justesen et al. 1973).

In contrast to these negative findings, high numbers of anaerobes and microaerophilic bacteria and a concomitant leukocytal reaction were detected in prostatic and vesicular secretions of some infertile men, suggesting that anaerobes might have an etiologic role in some cases of prostatitis (Colpi et al. 1985).

Mostly in combination with *Enterobacteriaceae* species, anaerobic bacteria such as *Bacteroides* spp, particularly *Bacteroides fragilis*, *Fusobacterium* spp, *Peptostreptococci*, and *Clostridium* spp were isolated from prostatic abscesses (Bartlett et al. 1978; Weinberger et al. 1988).

Emerging Pathogens

Gardnerella vaginalis was considered the etiologic agent in urinary tract infections in two thirds of male patients from whom it was isolated. It was also isolated from seminal fluid samples of four of 12 healthy volunteers (Ison and Easmon 1985; Lam et al. 1988; Smith et al. 1992) and has been incriminated as the etiologic agent in a single case of acute prostatitis (Abercrombie et al. 1978).

Mobiluncus mulieris and *Mobiluncus curtisii* have been isolated from seminal fluid samples of partners of women with bacterial vaginosis. Up to now, no signs and symptoms of male urogenital tract disease were found (Holst 1990).

Corynebacterium spp have often been found in urine, prostatic fluid samples, and ejaculates, sometimes in high numbers. They are routinely considered to be commensals. However group JK corynebacterium, group D2 corynebacterium (proposed name, *Corynebacterium urealyticum*), *Corynebacterium renale*, and *Corynebacterium genitalium* have been grown from urine samples and might be responsible for urogenital tract infections in some patients, especially when grown repeatedly as the sole bacterial species in high numbers (Lipsky et al. 1982; Riegel et al. 1992).

Viruses

Viruria is a common phenomenon in many viral diseases (Arthur et al. 1988; Tyler and Field 1990; Utz 1964), including cytomegalovirus (CMV), hepatitis A virus, hepatitis B virus, mumps virus, polyomaviruses (JC and BK virus), and human immunodeficiency virus (HIV). Viruria may be the result of viral passage through the kidney, but may also be the result of viral multiplication in the kidney or, perhaps, elsewhere in the genitourinary tract. No evidence has been provided that, by the descending route, the male adnexa might be infected during viruria. Obviously, prostatic infection occurs during systemic dissemination.

Mumps virus, herpes simplex virus type 2 (HSV II), CMV, and varizella-zoster virus (VZV) have been detected in prostatic cells and secretions. In only a few cases was virus-associated prostatitis diagnosed (Boldogh et al. 1983; Centifanto et al. 1973; Clason et al. 1982; Rapp et al. 1975; Webber and Bouldin 1977; Webber et al. 1973; Wolinski and Waxham 1990). Mumps virus infection may be accompanied by prostatitis, which is obviously not a major manifestation of the disease (Wolinsky and Waxham 1990).

HSV II genomic material has been detected in one of 13 normal prostates, in two of ten prostatic adenocarcinoma biopsies, and in none of nine benign prostate hypertrophy samples (Boldogh et al. 1983). HSV II was cultured from the EPS of a patient suffering from prostatodynia (Doble et al. 1991). Some authors have claimed to have detected HSV II in two and perhaps a further four out of 12 patients with prostatitis (Deardourff et al. 1974; Morrisseau et al. 1970). In contrast, Nielsen et al. (1973) and Mertens et al. (1985) were unable to isolate HSV II from urine or prostatic secretions.

CMV was isolated from the prostatic cells of a 3-year-old boy and has often been isolated from semen (Rapp et al. 1975). CMV DNA homologous sequences were detected in two of 13 normal prostates, two of nine benign prostate hypertrophy, and three of ten prostate adenocarcinoma biopsy specimens (Boldogh et al. 1983). Extensive CMV prostatitis has recently been described in a homosexual patient with AIDS (Benson and Smith 1992).

Granulomatous prostatitis has been observed in patients suffering from sacral herpes zoster infection (Clason et al. 1982). Histopathologically, granulomatous areas with focal necrosis, surrounding palisades of epithelioid cells, and lymphocytic infiltration were seen and diagnosed as typical of vesical herpes zoster.

Fungi

Candida Species

Candida species are opportunistic pathogens in humans. The prevalence of candiduria (> 1000 organisms/ml urine) ranges from 0.2% to 4.8%. Factors predisposing subjects to candidal infection are diabetes mellitus, extensive antibiotic and corticosteroid therapy, and disturbances of urinary flow, e.g., by obstructive uropathy, neurogenic bladder, foreign bodies, and indwelling urinary catheters. In immunocompromised patients, systemic transient or recurrent candidal fungemia, which often originates from heavily colonized intravenous catheters, induces disseminated candidiasis manifesting in liver, spleen, and kidney, whereas the prostate is seldom involved. This is presumably due to the fungistatic effect of prostatic secretions. Localized candidal infection of the prostate is often due to indwelling urinary catheters (Fisher et al. 1982; Wise 1992). Due to metabolically produced gas, candidal prostatitis may appear as prostatitis emphysematosa (Bartkowski and Lanesky 1988).

Cryptococcus neoformans

Cryptococcal infection is acquired by inhalation of fungus-contaminated dust. Pulmonary infection is often asymptomatic, but hematogenous spread may occur, mostly in patients suffering from lymphoma, sarcoidosis, or AIDS. In autopsy studies of 39 patients with disseminated cryptococcosis, 20 out of 39 patients (51%) had renal involvement and six of the 23 male patients (26%) had prostatic infection. The prostatic lesions ranged from small chronic inflammatory changes to large granulomata with caseation (Salyer and Salyer 1973; Schwarz 1982; Wise 1992).

Granulomatous prostatitis due to *Cryptococcus neoformans* has been observed in patients without evidence of systemic infection (Adams et al. 1992; Hinchey and Someren 1981; Wise 1992).

In patients with AIDS, prostatic infection is a common site of persistent cryptococcal infection after apparently effective therapy for cryptococcal meningitis. In the urine of nine out of 41 patients *C. neoformans* still grew; none had urinary symptoms. Fungi were demonstrated in EPS from four men, and the urine culture of a further four patients were positive only after prostatic massage. Two patients had positive urine cultures both before and after prostatic massage. The persistence of *C. neoformans* after adequate therapy for meningitis suggests that the prostate must be regarded as a sequestered reservoir from which systemic relapse may occur (Bailly et al. 1991; Larsen et al. 1989).

Histoplasma capsulatum

Infection with *Histoplasma capsulatum* is encountered in many areas of the world. In heavily endemic areas, virtually the entire population is infected. Pulmonary infections may be clinically asymptomatic and self-limiting. Disseminated disease occurs in immunosuppressed persons. Liver, spleen, and lymph nodes are the major sites of extrapulmonary histoplasmosis. Genitourinary sites are rarely involved (Orr et al. 1972; Schwarz 1982; Wise 1992). Thus, in an autopsy study of 17 patients with generalized histoplasmosis, the kidney was infected in three and the prostate in one patient (6%).

Blastomyces dermatitidis

Blastomyces dermatitidis is found in the midwest of the USA, in Canada, in Central/South America, and Africa. Pulmonary infection may heal spontaneously or become chronic. Progressive infection spreads hematogenously to extrapulmonary sites, e.g., skin, bones, and genitourinary system. Genitourinary involvement occurs in 15%–30% of patients with disseminated blastomycosis. Prostatic infection was found in 14 of 37 disseminated cases; other data vary from one of 36, through one of 13, four of 40, six of 31, and ten of 40, to nine of 25. Morphologically, in some prostates innumerable yeast cells are seen in the dilated ducts and glands of the prostate, with or without inflammatory reactions. Granulomatous reactions are found with or without caseation necrosis. Suppuration sometimes occurs and sexual transmission has been observed (Eickenberg et al. 1975; Inoshita et al. 1983; Orr et al. 1972; Schwarz 1982; Wise 1992).

Coccidioides immitis

Coccidioides immitis is indigenous to the semiarid regions of western USA, Mexico, and Central/South America. Following inhalation, an asymptomatic and transient pulmonary infection may develop. In some cases, pulmonary infiltration and cavitation are observed. Fewer than 1% of patients, frequently immunosuppressed, develop extrapulmonary multiorgan dissemination. However, a more virulent form of coccidioidomycosis is observed among individuals with AIDS, particularly in Arizona, USA, where one-fourth of these patients test positively for the fungus. It can give rise to a diffuse pulmonary disease combined with widespread dissemination (Anonymous 1992). In disseminated coccidioidomycosis, kidneys are involved in 35%–60%, the prostate in 6%. The patient may present with symptoms indicative of bladder outlet obstruction. Physical findings may reveal a boggy prostate or even induration suggestive of neoplasia (Kuntze et al. 1988; Price et al. 1982; Schwarz 1982; Wise 1992).

Paracoccidioides brasiliensis

Pulmonary infection produces few symptoms initially. Hematogenous spread to the mucous membranes of the mouth and nose, the lymph nodes, and various organs brings the patient to medical attention. Paracoccidioidomycotic prostatitis has been described in a few case reports from autopsy studies (Pena 1967; Schwarz 1982; Wise 1992).

Aspergillus Species

Inhalation of *Aspergillus* spores is extremely common, but disease is rare. Invasion of the lung is almost entirely confined to immunosuppressed patients. In patients debilitated by malignant tumors, diabetes mellitus, or immunosuppression, infection may progress by hematogenous dissemination afflicting the gastrointestinal tract (23% of cases), the brain (21%), the liver (13%), and the kidney (13%). Prostatic aspergillus infection has been described in a few case reports (Wise 1992).

Parasites

Trichomonas vaginalis

Trichomoniasis was diagnosed in 5%–20% of males attending sexually transmitted disease clinics or suffering from nongonococcal urethritis. The urethra is the most common site of trichomonal infection in males. Involvement of other parts of the male urogenital tract is less frequently documented. The prostate has been reported to be involved in up to 40% of infected patients. Two of five experimentally inoculated men developed clinical signs of prostatitis. Using immunoperoxidase procedures, Gardner et al. have identified *Trichomonas vaginalis* in the prostatic urethra, glandular lumina, submucosa, and stroma of the prostate. Foci of nonspecific acute and chronic inflammation and intraepithelial vacuolization were associated with prostatic infection. Most urogenital trichomonal infections in men remain clinically asymptomatic (Gardner et al. 1986; Ohkawa et al. 1992).

Schistosoma haematobium

Schistosoma haematobium occurs in Africa, Lebanon, Syria, Iran, and Arabia, where it causes urinary schistosomiasis (Cheever et al. 1977; Smith et al. 1974; Smith et al. 1992). Adult worm pairs reside in the venous plexus of the bladder; their eggs move through the wall of the bladder and pass in urine. Accumulation of eggs in the bladder wall leads to T cell-dependent granulomatous host response. Prostatic oviposition is lower than in seminal vesicles and urinary bladder. The egg burden in the prostate amounts to about 8000–10 000/g tissue, as compared to about 20 000/g tissue in seminal vesicles and about 50 000/g tissue in urinary bladder. Clinical studies consistently report cystoscopic, urodynamic, and isotope clearance abnormalities and high residual urine, indicating functional bladder outlet obstruction. Schistosomal eggs may appear in ejaculate. By radiography, calcifications are revealed within the urinary tract, including the seminal vesicles, prostate, urethra posterior, and distal ureters.

References

Abdelatif OMA, Chandler FW, McGuire BS (1991) Chlamydia trachomatis in chronic abacterial prostatitis: demonstration by colorimetric in situ hybridization. Human Pathol 22:41–44

Abercrombie GF, Allen J, Maskell R (1978) Corynebacterium vaginale urinary tract infection in a man. Lancet I:766

Adams JR, Fowler M, Mata JA, Venable DD, Culkin DJ (1992) AIDS manifesting as prostate nodule secondary to cryptococcal infection. Urology 39:289–291

Anonymous (1992) Coccidioidomycosis in AIDS patient specimen. ASM News 58:532

Arthur RR, Shah KV, Charache P, Saral R (1988) BK and JC virus infections in recipients of bone marrow transplants. J Inf Dis 158:563–569

Bailly MP, Boibieux A, Biron F, Durie I, Piens MA, Peyramond D, Bertrand JL (1991) Persistence of Cryptococcus neoformans in the prostate: failure of fluconazole despite high doses. J Inf Dis 164:435–436

Bartkowski DP, Lanesky JR (1988) Emphysematous prostatitis and cystitis secondary to Candida albicans. J Urol 139:1063–1065

Bartlett JG, Weinstein WM, Gorbach SL (1978) Prostatic abscesses involving anaerobic bacteria. Arch Int Med 138:1369–1371

Benson PJ, Smith CS (1992) Cytomegalovirus prostatitis. Urology 40:165–167

Berger RE, Krieger JN, Kessler D, Ireton RC, Close C, Holmes KK, Roberts PL (1989) Case-control study of men with suspected chronic idiopathic prostatitis. J Urol 141:328–331

Boldogh I, Baskar JF, Mar EC, Huang ES (1983) Human cytomegalovirus and Herpes simplex type 2 virus in normal and adenocarcinomatous prostate glands. J Natl Canc Inst 70:819–826

Brooker WJ, Aufderheide AC (1980) Genitourinary tract infections due to atypical mycobacteria. J Urol 124:242–244

Bruce AW, Chadwick P, Willet WS, O'Shaughnessy M (1981) The role of chlamydiae in genitourinary disease. J Urol 126:625–629

Bruce AW, Reid G (1989) Prostatitis associated with Chlamydia trachomatis in 6 patients. J Urol 142:1006–1007

Brunner H, Weidner W (1985) Acute and chronic prostatitis. In: Taylor-Robinson D (edit) Clinical problems in sexually transmitted diseases. Nijhoff, Dordrecht, pp 37–59

Brunner H, Weidner W, Schiefer HG (1983) Studies on the role of Ureaplasma urealyticum and Mycoplasma hominis in prostatitis. J Inf Dis 147:807–813

Centifanto YM, Kaufman HE, Zam ZS, Drylie DM, Deardourff SL (1973) Herpesvirus particles in prostatic carcinoma cells. J Virol 12:1608–1611

Cheever AW, Kamel IA, Elwi AM, Mosimann JE, Danner R (1977) Schistosoma mansoni and Schistosoma haematobium infection in Egypt. Quantitative parasitological findings at necropsy. Am J Trop Med Hyg 26:702–716

Clason AE, McGeorge A, Garland C, Abel BJ (1982) Urinary retention and granulomatous prostatitis following sacral herpes zoster infection. J Urol 54:166–169

Colpi GM, Zanollo A, Roveda M, Tommasini-Degna A, Beretta G (1985) Bacterial flora in expressed prostatic and vesicular secretions of infertile subjects. In: Brunner H, Krause W, Rothauge CF, Weidner W (eds) Chronic prostatitis. Schattauer, Stuttgart, pp 93–100

Dan M, Samra Z, Siegel YI, Korczak D, Lindner A (1991) Isolation of Chlamydia trachomatis from prostatic tissue of patients undergoing transurethral prostatectomy. Infection 19:162–163

Danielsson D, Molin L (1971) Demonstration of Neisseria gonorrhoeae in prostatic fluid after treatment of uncomplicated gonorrhoeal urethritis. Acta Dermatovener (Stockholm) 51:73–76

Deardourff SL, Deture FA, Drylie DM, Centifanto Y, Kaufman H (1974) Association between herpes hominis type 2 and the male genitourinary tract. J Urol 112:126–127

Doble A, Harris JRW, Taylor-Robinson D (1991) Prostatodynia and herpes simplex virus infection. Urology 38:247–248

Doble A, Thomas BJ, Walker MM, Harris JRW, Witherow RO'N, Taylor-Robinson D (1989) The role of Chlamydia trachomatis in chronic abacterial prostatitis: a study using ultrasound guided biopsy. J Urol 141:332–333

Drach GW, Fair WR, Meares EM, Stamey TA (1978) Classification of benign diseases associated with prostatic pain: prostatitis or prostatodynia? J Urol 120:266

Eickenberg HU, Amin M, Lich R (1975) Blastomycosis of the genitourinary tract. J Urol 113:650–652

Ellis LR, Kenny GM, Nellans RE (1979) Urogenital aspects of actinomycosis. J Urol 122:132–133

Fisher JF, Chew WH, Shadomy S, Duma RJ, Mayhall CG, House WC (1982) Urinary tract infections due to Candida albicans. Rev Inf Dis 4:1107–1118

Forbes KA, Lowry EC, Gibson TE, Soanes WA (1954) Brucellosis of the genito-urinary tract: review of the literature and report of a case in a child. Urol Surv 4:391–412

Gardner WA, Culberson DE, Bennett BD (1986) Trichomonas vaginalis in the prostate gland. Arch Pathol Lab Med 110:430–432

Goetz MB, Craig WA (1982) Haemophilus influenzae prostatitis. J Am Med Ass 247:3118

Gorse GJ, Belshe RB (1985) Male genital tuberculosis. Rev Inf Dis 7:511–524

Grant JBF, Brooman PJC, Chowdhury SD, Sequeira P, Blacklock NJ (1985) The clinical presentation of Chlamydia trachomatis in a urological practice. Br J Urol 57:218–221

Hinchey WW, Someren A (1981) Cryptococcal prostatitis. Am J Clin Pathol 75:257–260

Hofstetter A (1973) Mykoplasmen bei entzündlichen Erkrankungen des Urogenitaltraktes. Infection 1:247–249

Holst E (1990) Reservoir of four organisms associated with bacterial vaginosis suggests lack of sexual transmission. J Clin Microbiol 28:2035–2039

Inoshita T, Youngberg GA, Boelen LJ, Langston J (1983) Blastomycosis presenting with prostatic involvement: report of 2 cases of review of the literature. J Urol 130:160–162

Ison CA, Easmon CSF (1985) Carriage of Gardnerella vaginalis and anaerobes in semen. Genitourin Med 61:120–123

Johannisson G (1981) Studies on Chlamydia trachomatis as a cause of lower urogenital tract infection. Acta Dermato-Venereol. Suppl 93

Justesen T, Nielsen ML, Hattel T (1973) Anaerobic infections in chronic prostatitis and chronic urethritis. Med Microbiol Immunol 158:237–248

Kampmeier RH (1964) The late manifestations of syphilis: skeletal, visceral and cardiovascular. Med Clin North America 48:667–697

Kelalis PP, Greene LF, Weed LA (1962) Brucellosis of the urogenital tract: a mimic of tuberculosis. J Urol 88:347–353

Krieger JN, Egan KJ (1991) Comprehensive evaluation and treatment of 75 men referred to chronic prostatitis clinic. Urology 38:11–19

Kuntze JR, Herman MH, Evans SG (1988) Genitourinary coccidioidomycosis. J Urol 140:370–374

Lam MH, Birch DF, Fairley KF (1988) Prevalence of Gardnerella vaginalis in the urinary tract. J Clin Microbiol 26:1130–1133

Larsen RA, Bozzette S, McCutchan JA, Chiu J, Leal MA, Richman DD, Californian Collaborative

Treatment Group (1989) Persistent Cryptococcus neoformans infection of the prostate after successful treatment of meningitis. Ann Intern Med 111:125–128

Lee LW, Burgher LW, Price EB, Cassidy E (1977) Granulomatous prostatitis: association with isolation of Mycobacterium kansasii and Mycobacterium fortuitum. J Am Med Assoc 237:2408–2409

Lipsky BA, Goldberger AC, Tompkins LS, Plorde JJ (1982) Infections caused by nondiphtheria corynebacteria. Rev Inf Dis 4:1220–1235

Lomas DA, Natin D, Stockley RA, Shahmanesh M (1993) Chemotactic activity of urethral secretions in men with urethritis and the effect of treatment. J Inf Dis 167:233–236

Mårdh PA, Ripa KT, Colleen S, Treharne JD, Darougar S (1978) Role of Chlamydia trachomatis in non-acute prostatitis. Br J Ven Dis 54:330–334

Meares, EM (1992) Prostatitis and related disorders. In: Walsh PC, Retik AB, Stamey TA, Vaughan ED (eds), Campbell's urology, 6th edn, vol 1. Saunders, Philadelphia, pp 807–822

Mertens T, Lanvers A, Eggers HJ (1985) Can Herpesvirus hominis be isolated from the genitourinary tract of men having no manifest symptoms of herpesvirus infection? In: Brunner H, Krause W, Rothauge CF, Weidner W (eds) Chronic prostatitis. Schattauer, Stuttgart, pp 101–105

Mikolich DJ, Mates SM (1992) Granulomatous prostatitis due to Mycobacterium avium complex. Clin Inf Dis 14:589–591

Morrisseau PM, Phillips CA, Leadbetter GW (1970) Viral prostatitis. J Urol 103:767–769

Nielsen ML, Vestergaard BF (1973) Virological investigations in chronic prostatitis. J Urol 109:1023–1025

Ohkawa M, Yamaguchi K, Tokunaga S, Nakashima T, Fujita S (1992) The incidence of Trichomonas vaginalis in chronic prostatitis patients determined by culture using a newly modified liquid medium. J Inf Dis 166:1205–1206

O'Leary WM (1990) Ureaplasmas and human disease. Crit Rev Microbiol 17:161–168

Orr WA, Mulholland SG, Walzak MP (1972) Genitourinary tract involvement with systemic mycosis. J Urol 107:1047–1050

Peeters M, Polak-Vogelzang A, Debruyne F, van der Veen J (1985) Abacterial prostatitis: microbiological data. In: Brunner H, Krause W, Rothauge CF, Weidner W (eds) Chronic prostatitis. Schattauer, Stuttgart, pp 55–62

Pena CE (1967) Deep mycotic infections in Colombia. Am J Clin Pathol 47:505–520

Poletti F, Medici MC, Alinovi A, Menozzi MG, Sacchini P, Stagni G, Toni M, Benoldi D (1985) Isolation of Chlamydia trachomatis from the prostatic cells in patients affected by nonacute abacterial prostatitis. J Urol 134:691–692

Price MJ, Lewis EL, Carmalt JE (1982) Coccidioidomycosis of prostate gland. Urology 19:653–655

Pust R, Schäfer R, Stumpf C, Leitenberger A, Engstfeld JE, Meyer-Ewert H (1986) Urethritis posterior. In: Weidner W, Brunner H, Krause W, Rothauge CF (eds) Therapy of prostatitis. Klinische und experimentelle Urologie 11. Zuckschwerdt, Munich, pp 102–109

Quentin R, Musser JM, Mellouet M, Sizaret PY, Selander RK, Goudeau A (1989) Typing of urogenital, maternal, and neonatal isolates of Haemophilus influenzae and Haemophilus parainfluenzae in correlation with clinical source of isolation and evidence for a genital specificity of Haemophilus influenzae biotype IV. J Clin Microbiol 27:2286–2294

Rapp F, Geder L, Murasko D, Lausch R, Ladda R, Huang ES, Webber MM (1975) Long-term persistence of cytomegalovirus genome in cultured human cells of prostatic origin. J Virol 16:982–990

Riegel P, Grimont PAD, de Briel D, Ageron E, Jehl F, Pelegrin M, Monteil H, Minck R (1992) Corynebacterium group D2 ("Corynebacterium urealyticum") constitutes a new genomic species. Res Microbiol 143:307–313

Salyer WR, Salyer DC (1973) Involvement of the kidney and prostate in cryptococcosis. J Urol 109:695–698

Schiefer HG, Weidner W, Krauss H, Gerhardt U, Krause W (1985) Prostatitis as sequela of nongonococcal urethritis: a prospective study. In: Brunner H, Krause W, Rothauge CF, Weidner W (eds) Chronic prostatitis. Schattauer, Stuttgart, pp 75–83

Schwarz J (1982) Mycotic prostatitis. Urology 19:1–5

Shortliffe LMD, Elliott KM, Sellers RG, Stamey TA (1985) Measurement of chlamydial and ureaplasmal antibodies in serum and prostatic fluid of men with nonbacterial prostatitis. J Urol 133:276A

Shurbaji MS, Gupta PK, Myers J (1988) Immunohistochemical demonstration of chlamydial antigens in association with prostatitis. Modern Pathol 1:348–351

Smith JH, Kamel IA, Elwi A, von Lichtenberg F (1974) A quantitative post mortem analysis of urinary schistosomiasis in Egypt. Pathology and pathogenesis. Am J Trop Med Hyg 23:1054–1071

Smith JH, von Lichtenberg F, Lehman JS (1992) Parasitic diseases of the genitourinary system. In: Walsh PC, Retik AB, Stamey TA, Vaughan ED (eds) Campbell's urology, 6th edn, vol 1. Saunders, Philadelphia, pp 883–927

Smith SM, Ogbara T, Eng RHK (1992) Involvement of Gardnerella vaginalis in urinary tract infections in men. J Clin Microbiol 30:1575–1577

de Souza E, Katz DA, Dworzack DL, Longo G (1985) Actinomycosis of the prostate. J Urol 133:290–291

Taylor-Robinson D (1985) Mycoplasmal and mixed infections of the human male urogenital tract and their possible complications. In: Razin S, Barile MF (eds), The mycoplasmas, vol 4. Academic, Orlando, pp 27–63

Taylor-Robinson D, Csonka GW, Prentice MJ (1977) Human intraurethral inoculation of ureaplasmas. Q J Med 46:309–326

Taylor-Robinson D, Thomas BJ (1980) The rôle of Chlamydia trachomatis in genital-tract and associated diseases. J Clin Pathol 33:205–233

Thompson L (1920) Syphilis of the prostate. Am J Syph 4:323–341

Tyler KL, Field BN (1990) Pathogenesis of viral infections. In: Fields BN, Knipe DM (eds) Virology, 2nd edn. Raven, New York, pp 191–239

Utz JP (1964) Viruria in man. Progr Med Virol 6:71–81

Wallace RJ, Baker CJ, Quinones FJ, Hollis DG, Weaver RE, Wiss K (1983) Nontypable Haemophilus influenzae (biotype 4) as a neonatal, maternal, and genital pathogen. Rev Inf Dis 5:123–136

Webber MM, Bouldin TR (1977) Ultrastructure of human prostatic epithelium. Secretion granules or virus particles? Invest Urol 14:482–487

Webber MM, Stonington OG, Lehman J (1973) Virus in prostatic epithelium of man. Urology 1:561–567

Weidner W, Schiefer HG, Krauss H (1988) Role of Chlamydia trachomatis and mycoplasmas in chronic prostatitis. A review. Urol Int 43:167–173

Weidner W, Schiefer HG, Krauss H, Jantos C, Friedrich HJ, Altmannsberger M (1991) Chronic prostatitis: a thorough search for etiologically involved microorganisms in 1461 patients. Infection 19:S119–S125

Weinberger M, Cytron S, Servadio C, Block C, Rosenfeld JB, Pitlik SD (1988) Prostatic abscess in the antibiotic era. Rev Inf Dis 10:239–249

Wise GJ (1992) Fungal infections of the urinary tract. In: Walsh PC, Retik AB, Stamey TA, Vaughan ED (eds), Campbell's urology, 6th edn, vol 1. Saunders, Philadelphia, pp 928–950

Wolinski JS, Waxham MN (1990) Mumps virus. In: Fields BN, Knipe DM (eds) Virology, 2nd edn. Raven, New York, pp 989–1011

Young EJ (1983) Human brucellosis. Rev Inf Dis 5:821–842

Trichomonas vaginalis

N. Kawamura

It is often believed that "prostatitis caused by *Trichomonas vaginalis*" is a disease that has been in existence for a long time. Actually, *T. vaginalis* is sometimes detected in patients with prostatitis, and therapeutic eradication of *T. vaginalis* ameliorates prostatitis in many cases. However, the causal relationship is still uncorroborated because *T. vaginalis* has never been detected in human prostate tissue. I support the view that "prostatitis caused by *T. vaginalis*" is an actually existing condition. The evidence is described below.

Clinical Investigation

In some cases of so-called venereal prostatitis, the expressed prostatic secretion (EPS) evidently contains leukocytes, and *T. vaginalis* is actually detected in the expressed prostate secretion (EPS; Kawamura 1973; Table 1). However, the detection rate is higher in the EPS-containing urine collected following prostatic massage (VB₃) than in the EPS alone (Table 2). The possibility therefore arises that the *T. vaginalis* may originally be present in the urethra rather than the prostate. In many cases, however, *T. vaginalis* is not detected in the VB_1 from the same patient. In addition, the detection rate of *T. vaginalis* is higher in cases of prostatitis than in those of nongonococcal urethritis, providing sufficient evidence to suspect that the prostate may be infected with *T. vaginalis*. *T. vaginalis* is occasionally detected in the urine from inpatients and frequently disappears without any specific treatment during their hospitalization. In such cases *T. vaginalis* seems to be present in the urethra. In my opinion, the organisms may be present in certain nutrient-rich tissues such as the prostate and seminal vesicle in cases where the organisms are persistently detected.

Evidence from Animal Experiments

Experimental inoculation of *T. vaginalis* into the rat prostate led to the development of abscesses, as shown in Fig. 1. At this stage, fructose concentration was found to be smaller in the infected lobe of the prostate when separate

Table 1. Frequency of *T. vaginalis* detection in secretions collected by massaging the prostate and the seminal vesicles

Diagnosis	No. of cases examined	No. of culture-positive cases
Chronic prostatitis	30	10
Nongonococcal urethritis	16	4
Male sterility	5	1
Movable kidney	2	1
Acute cystitis	1	1
Prostatic hypertrophy	2	
Urethral bleeding	2	
Bladder neurosis	1	
Bilateral hydronephrosis	1	
Chronic epididymitis	1	
No abnormalities	17	1
Total	78	18

Table 2. Incidence of *T. vaginalis* from special materials

	No. of specimens	No. of culture-positive cases
Secretion obtained by massaging the seminal vesicles and prostate	109	13
Urine collected after the seminal vesicles and prostate were massaged	33	4
First urine specimen collected early in the morning	12	0
Seminal fluid	12	0
Secretion obtained by massaging the seminal vesicles	3	0
First glass of urine alone	38	4
Second glass of urine alone	2	0
First urine specimen collected early in the morning from inpatients at mental hospitals	102	0

measurements were taken in the right and left lobes (Kawamura 1979; Table 3). When *T. vaginalis* and a fructose-containing medium (Table 4) were incubated, the organisms consumed fructose, grew, and increased in number (Kawamura 1969a; Fig. 2). These findings suggest that *T. vaginalis* would be viable and able to grow in the seminal vesicle and the prostate, both of which contain a large amount of fructose. Based on these experimental findings and clinical data, I

Table 3. Amounts of fructose (μm) in the bilateral prostate lobe after inoculation of *T. vaginalis* in right lobe

Rat no.	Right	Left
T. vaginalis inoculable		
13	100	500
20	500	740
18	500	560
17	660	700
T. vaginalis noninoculable[a]		
14	600	660
16	140	220
15	480	360
22	800	760
24	600	500
21	560	400
43	500	440

[a] Not detected after inoculation.

Table 4. Composition of fructose-containing medium

Meat extract	40 mg	Agar	2 mg
Peptone	40 mg	0.1% methylene blue	0.008 ml
Cysteine-HCl	4 mg	Aq. dil. 4 ml	
Fructose	20 mg	Human serum	1 ml
Streptomycin	20 mg		
Kanamycin	20 ~ 40 mg		
Penicillin	10 000 U		

believe that the prostate and seminal vesicle may be infected with *T. vaginalis*, and that the organisms remain alive there for a long time. *T. vaginalis* inoculated in the rat urethra did not show a long-time viability (Table 5).

Nevertheless, it cannot definitely be determined whether the prostate or the seminal vesicle is actually infected. This is because: (a) the structures of the prostate and seminal vesicle vary slightly between humans and rats; (b) in humans the seminal vesicles are unavoidably massaged; (c) urethral factors can hardly be excluded; and (d) in humans the above changes in tissue fructose concentration cannot be confirmed because the prostate and seminal vesicle cannot be infected with *T. vaginalis* for ethical reasons. Furthermore, even if the prostate has actually been infected, the clinical symptoms are not always manifested. In one study we attempted to see whether *T. vaginalis* could be detected in prisoners who had had no chance to have sexual intercourse with

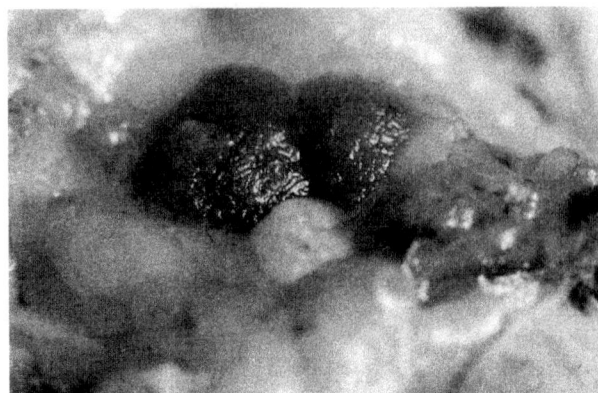

Fig. 1. Abscess developed after experimental inoculation of *T. vaginalis* into rat prostate

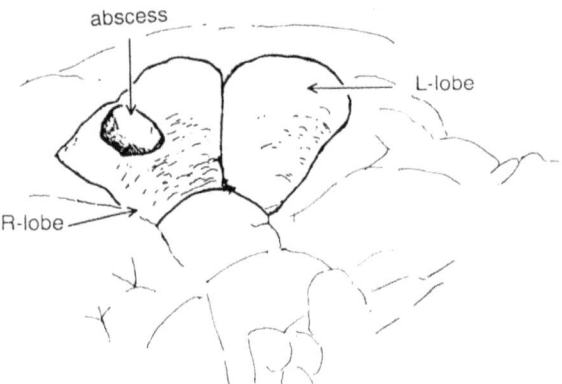

women for a prolonged period of time (Kawamura 1969b; Kawamura and Kinoshita 1979; Table 6). Prisoners whose urine specimens were *T. vaginalis* positive were free of urethritic symptoms and almost entirely asymptomatic except for a few who had indurations in the prostate. As shown in Table 6, *T. vaginalis* was detected in urine specimens from 44 prisoners. Twenty-three of them had been in prison for more than 300 days, to a maximum of 1311 days. This persistence of subclinical infections over such a long period of time suggests that the urethra, which is a rather unsuitable habitat for the causative protozoans to survive for any length of time, was not the only location of their residence, and that they were instead harbored long in the nutrient-rich prostate and/or seminal vesicles. In experimental conditions they can survive in the prostate for a considerable period of time, as shown in Table 7 (Lanceley 1953; Nakano 1957; Kimura 1965; Kawamura 1973).

From these findings, I believe that *T. vaginalis* can survive in the prostate for a long time, even causing inflammation in some cases.

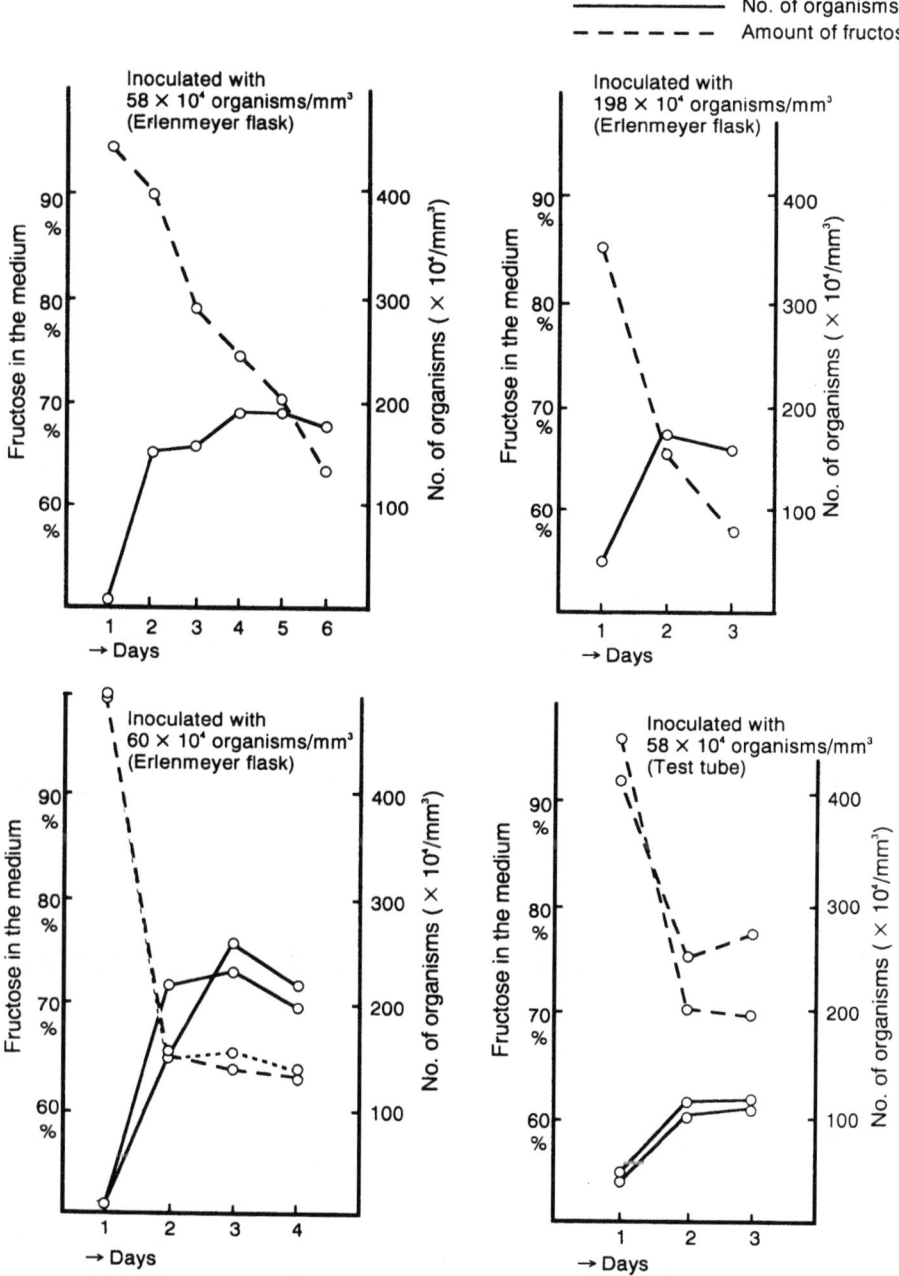

Fig. 2. Fructose consumption by *T. vaginalis*

Table 5. Experimental inoculation of *T. vaginalis* into the rat prostate

Rat no.	Time	No. of organisms (×10⁴)	Dose volume (ml)	Body weight (g)	Strain used	Culture result	Gross finding
13	5 h	20	1	230	Sakata	+	
11	24 h	?		200	c	+	Abscess (+)
4	24 h	7.1	0.1		e	−	
14	24 h	20	1		Sakata	−	
12	2 h	65	0.2		Mixed	+	
5	2 days	20	0.1		a	−	
6	2 days	20	0.1		a	−	
9	4 days	173.2	0.2		Mixed	−	
16	5 days	20	0.2	230	Sakata	−	
20	5 days	10	0.5	190	Kosai	+	
19	5 days	20	0.1	230	Kosai	+	
8	5 days	20	0.1		a	−	
27	6 days	30	0.2	180	Kosai 14	+	
28	6 days	30	0.2	200	Kosai 14	+	
3	6 days	7.1	0.1	210	e	−	
15	6 days	20	0.2		Sakata	−	
10	7 days	173.2	0.2	220	Mixed	−	
22	7 days	10	0.5	270	Kosai	−	
24	7 days	20	0.3	220	f	−	
18	7 days	65	0.2	220	Mixed	+	
23	7 days	20	0.3	180	f	−	
7	7 days	20	0.1		a	−	Adhesion to the right prostate (+)
17	10 days	20	0.1	230	Sakata	+	Induration in the right prostate
21	10 days	20	0.2	220	Kosai	−	
1	10 days	?			c	−	Abscess in the right prostate
2	10 days	?			c	−	
41	16 days	50	0.2	300	Naka	−	
42	25 days	15	0.3	250	Naka	−	Abscess in the right prostate
43	25 days	125	0.5	310	Naka	−	
39	33 days	75	0.1	350	Kosai	−	
38	2 months	75	0.1	285	Kosai	−	
26	4 months	20	0.3		Kosai	−	

Table 6. Duration of *T. vaginalis* infection

Age (years)	Duration (days)
56	1311
64	1204
35	1140
47	1094
41	889
39	803
50	793
28	772
46	755
50	714
27	700
44	617
28	605
45	407
32	400
30	381
68	358
36	351
43	346
54	333
56	333
66	329
44	325

200–300 days, 4 patients; 100–200 days, 5 patients; less than 100 days, 12 patients.

Table 7. Duration of *T. vaginalis* infection of urogenital organs in experimental animals

Reference	Organ	Duration
McGreer and McNeil (1937)	Prostate	121 h
Lanceley (1953)	Human urethra	94 days
Nakano (1957)	Prostate	6 days
	Urethra	4 days
Kimura (1965)	Bladder	8 days
	Seminal vesicles	4 days
This study	Prostate	15 days

Discussion

My detection rate of *T. vaginalis* is higher than that reported by others. This does not mean that the distribution of *T. vaginalis* is particularly wide in Japan. Indeed, since 1985 decreases in *T. vaginalis* seem to be more prominent in Japan than in other countries because wide uses of anticandidal pessaries here have led to a decreased incidence of gynecological vaginal trichomoniasis in Japan.

The high detection rate in my study is due to a high sensitivity of the medium used. I routinely use Asami's medium for the detection of *T. vaginalis* in culture. The specimen (0.2–0.5 ml) is added to this medium, incubated for 2 days, and microscopically examined. A portion of the culture is taken from the bottom of the liquid medium, aliquoted onto at least three slide glasses, mounted with cover glasses, and thoroughly examined from one end to the other. Theoretically, this procedure would allow for the detection of one organism when 40 organisms exist. Microscopic examination is usually performed by the author himself. If no organism is detected, blind subculture is performed, and the same examination is repeated 2 days later. The original culture is further incubated as well, and microscopically examined after another 2 days. Experimentally, Asami's medium allows for the detection of the organism even when only two organisms exist. When examined as described above, even a single organism can be detected if it is active. Previous experimental evidence indicates that repetitive blind subculturing through three generations or more is not meaningful for detection purposes. Instead, close attentive microscopic examination of each slide is a surer method; examining each slide for about 5 min and targeting active organisms are recommended.

It may be debatable whether the presence of only a few organisms detected by such a minutely meticulous examination is pathogenically significant or not.

I regard *T. vaginalis* as a pathogen involved in sexually transmitted diseases, the transmission of which should be blocked, and therefore consider that detection of *T. vaginalis*, even if a single organism, is important and a good reason for giving medical treatment. However, still unknown is the smallest number of *T. vaginalis* organisms that cause nongonococcal urethritis or prostatitis. *T. vaginalis* shows varied growth potentials from strain to strain, and its growth is accelerated after it acclimatizes to the culture medium. Accordingly, the doubling time is different from strain to strain, and quantitative culture methods, such as those for bacteria, have not been established yet for *T. vaginalis*. Thus, I cannot specify the smallest number of organisms which may cause prostatitis. The only evidence for pathogenic involvement of *T. vaginalis* is that its eradication results in the cure of prostatitis. I believe that *T. vaginalis*, if detected, should be eradicated because its pathogenic potential has experimentally been demonstrated, and because it is a pathogen involved in sexually transmitted diseases.

References

Kawamura N (1969a) Studies on Trichomonas vaginalis in urological field, 3rd report. Jpn J Urol 60:29–35

Kawamura N (1969b) Studies on Trichomonas vaginalis in urological field, 2nd report. Jpn J Urol 60:25–28

Kawamura N (1973) Trichomoniasis of the prostate. Jpn J Clin Urol 27:635–643

Kawamura N (1979) Parasitic infection of urogenital organs. Jpn J Urol 70:986–988

Kawamura N, Kinoshita H (1979) The incidence of Trichomonas vaginalis and the length of asymptomatic infections among male prisoners in a reformatory. Acta Urol Jpn 25:1023–1026

Kimura S (1965) Studies on Trichomoniasis vaginalis in urological patients. Jpn J Urol 56:455–475

Lanceley F (1953) Br J Vener Dis 29:213

McGreer CF, McNeil E (1937) Experimental inoculations of trichomonads from man into the prostate gland of rats. Proc Soc Exp Biol Med 36:587–589

Nakano M (1957) The experimental studies on the Trichomonas vaginalis infestation in the male genito-urinary tract. Jpn J Urol 48:16–26

Therapy of Nonbacterial Prostatitis

R.N.T. Thin

Introduction

Chronic nonbacterial prostatitis is diagnosed when there is an excess of polymorphonuclear leucocytes in the expressed prostatic secretion (EPS) and/or voided bladder urine 3 (VB3), but no urinary tract pathogenic bacterium is cultured. This contrasts with chronic bacterial prostatitis, wherein a pure growth of a urinary pathogen is cultured from the EPS and/or VB3, and prostatodynia, where there are symptoms of prostatitis, but there is no excess of polymorphonuclear leucocytes in EPS or VB3 and no pathogen is cultured (Drach et al. 1978). In the latest of a series of publications Weidner et al. (1991a) have shown a link between *Ureaplasma urealyticum* and prostatitis (*Ureaplasma*-associated prostatitis) but, as others, concluded that the role of *Chlamydia trachomatis* in prostatitis is debatable. Transrectal ultrasound scanning (TRUS) may show evidence of prostatitis; this technique also allows guided needle aspiration to obtain material for culture (Thin 1991).

One problem in the diagnosis of chronic prostatitis by culture of the EPS is that the focal inflammatory process may block the ducts, preventing drainage of organisms during prostatic massage and leading to negative culture results. This is shown diagrammatically in Fig. 1. Though the organisms may not drain, there is a surrounding inflammatory cell reaction which may drain down patent ducts. The EPS then shows excess leucocytes but no organisms, suggesting nonbacterial prostatitis when the true diagnosis is bacterial prostatitis. Despite ultrasound control needle aspiration may miss small foci of organisms. There is thus a basis for prescribing antimicrobials in the absence of positive culture results.

Though chronic nonbacterial prostatitis is common there is little information, especially recent data, on its treatment.

Treatment

General Therapeutic Measures

A wide variety of general measures have been suggested for the treatment of chronic nonbacterial prostatitis, including general health measures such as

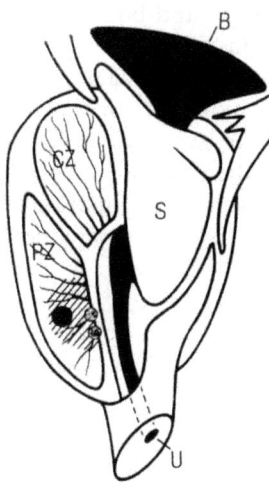

Fig. 1. Diagrammatic representation of a sagittal section of the prostate showing the drainage of the prostatic ducts into the urethra. *Black area*, a focus of inflammation which may contain bacteria; *hatched area* (around this), the zone of cellular reaction; *two stippled areas*, obstruction of the ducts as they enter the urethra. The other ducts are patent. *B*, Bladder; *CZ*, central zone; *S*, internal sphincter; *PZ*, peripheral zone; *U*, urethra. (After Blacklock 1990)

regular habits and regular bowel movements, reduction of excess weight and fresh air (Murnaghan 1980; Krieger 1984). These appear to be suggested simply as advice on healthy living as there are no data to indicate their benefit in nonbacterial prostatitis.

Measures Directed at the Prostate

More specific measures include a high fluid intake (at least 3 l daily) on the basis that inflammatory secretions draining down the prostatic ducts are less likely to irritate or inflame the urethra if they are swiftly washed away. Further, a low fluid intake leads to crystalluria which irritates the urethra predisposing to inflammation or infection of the urethra and prostatic ducts. Anecdotally many patients volunteer symptomatic benefit from a high fluid intake. In one observer-blind study 60% of 32 patients on 3 l of fluids daily for 90 days showed more symptomatic benefit and a greater reduction in their EPS polymorph count than 29 patients taking added fibre with a normal fluid intake (Thin 1986, and unpublished observations).

It appears logical to advise prostatic drainage. In the past prostatic massage has been suggested for this, including massage over a sound to dilate the prostatic ducts (Murnaghan et al. 1973), but treatment by trauma of an inflamed organ must be questioned (Colleen and Mardh 1990). Without a sound the volume of EPS obtained is small. Ejaculation produces a larger volume mixed with semen. Some clinicians have recommended frequent ejaculation while others advise abstinence (Krieger 1984), though there are no data to support either regimen. Anecdotally patients report symptomatic benefit with ejaculation once or twice weekly, rather than more or less frequently. One problem is that foci most requiring drainage may be unable to empty because of obstructed ducts. Despite this, ejaculation is preferable to complications of ill-advised

prostatic massage, which include bacteraemia, epididymitis, and bouts of syn-
ovitis, conjunctivitis and iridocyclitis (Colleen and Mardh 1990).

Counselling, support or psychotherapy are important in the management of
any chronic condition. The physician should explain the nature of nonbacterial
prostatitis, the lack of specific therapy, measures that are available and their
value, and that prostatitis is not life threatening. Many patients cope better with
their symptoms after positive reassurance, especially when it is reinforced at
intervals. Others respond less well and benefit from referral to a sympathetic
psychologist or psychiatrist.

Drug Therapy

Antimicrobials

As described above, obstructed ducts or failure to aspirate foci may lead to an
incorrect diagnosis of nonbacterial prostatitis instead of bacterial prostatitis. It
is logical to consider antimicrobials which may improve symptoms and urodynamic and secretory function (Colleen and Mardh 1990). Meares (1990) also
recommended at least one course of antimicrobial. A number of studies indicate
that some antimicrobials achieve a higher concentration in the prostate than in
the plasma; characteristics leading to this include low protein binding of the
antimicrobial, lipid solubility and a low pK_a (Stamey 1981). Drugs which fulfil
these criteria include trimethoprim, active against urinary pathogens (Meares
1973), minocycline (Hensle et al. 1977) and to a lesser degree doxycycline
(Garnes 1973), both active against Chlamydia and Ureaplasma, and the quinolone group of drugs of which ciprofloxacin appears to be the most actively
studied (Weidner et al. 1991b). Other antimicrobials reported to enter the
prostate selectively include azlocillin and mezlocillin (Smith et al. 1988), and
cefamandole (Kaisary 1988). Additional factors affecting penetration are hyper-
aemia and fibrosis, which may be present in chronic inflammation. In chronic
prostatitis 12 weeks of therapy may be more effective than 10 days (Smith et al.
1979).

There is a lack of comparative studies of antimicrobials in chronic prostatitis. In a randomised double-blind study of patients with chronic nonbacterial
prostatitis Simmons and Thin (1985) compared minocycline 100 mg twice daily
with diazepam 5 mg twice daily for 3 months. The percentage fall in the EPS cell
count was more marked in those receiving the antimicrobial than in the other
group, though symptomatic response was similar with the two regimens.

In another randomised double-blind trial comparing doxycycline 100 mg
twice daily with inert placebo, percentage reductions in the EPS cell count were
more marked after 3 months of active therapy than with placebo (Simmons and
Thin 1990), though, again, symptomatic improvement was similar in the two
groups. In a review of four regimens of treatment given for 3 months to patients
with chronic nonbacterial prostatitis, a greater percentage fall in EPS cell count

was observed with trimethoprim and minocycline than with diazepam or cotrimoxazole (Thin and Simmons 1985). Symptomatic improvement was similar with all treatments. Others have reported benefit with cotrimoxazole (Meares 1990), but it is only trimethoprim that has the characteristics associated with entry into the prostate. Trimethoprim alone in a larger dose than is present in conventional regimens of cotrimoxazole may be more effective.

Other Agents

Many accounts of treatment of nonbacterial prostatitis suggest anti-inflammatory agents may be beneficial without quoting supporting data (Krieger 1984; Meares 1990). Thin (1986) found them disappointing. Colleen and Mardh (1990) suggest they may have a role when pain is a prominent symptom.

Anticholinergic drugs have been recommended though data is lacking (Krieger 1984; Meares 1990). Colleen and Mardh (1990) suggest that they may help urinary frequency and urgency. Associated bladder outflow obstruction is present in 10% of patients with chronic nonbacterial prostatitis due to bladder neck dyssynergia (Mundy et al. 1984); this may be suspected from the history though the patient may consider his poor performance normal. It can be detected by TRUS supported by urodynamic studies. α-Adrenergic blocking agents have been suggested (Colleen and Mardh 1990), and there is a theoretical basis for their use in relaxing the internal sphincter. If there is no response, a surgical opinion should be obtained.

Tranquillisers and muscle relaxants may relax pelvic floor muscle tension, a source of pain in some patients. Tranquillisers also reduce anxiety, which may be a feature, and as indicated above they may reduce symptoms of prostatitis. They may also reduce frequency and urgency of micturition (Colleen and Mardh 1990). At present few clinicians in the United Kingdom prescribe tranquillisers long term without strong indications because of the problems of accumulation of the drug in the body and the danger of habituation. Testosterone has been suggested in the past, but there are no recent accounts recommending the hormone, which was apparently given for several months (Blandy 1976).

A recent publication from Japan suggests that Chinese herbal agents may have value in chronic nonbacterial prostatitis, more so when combined with conventional anti-inflammatory agents (Ikeuchi 1990). More data on this type of therapy are needed.

Physical Measures

Hot sitz baths have been recommended especially for relief of exacerbations of pain (Meares 1990; Colleen and Mardh 1990). Heat has also been suggested in the form of externally applied short-wave diathermy (Krieger 1984) though it is unlikely to produce anything more than transient relief of pain or discomfort.

Recently there have been a number of publications describing local endo-urethral microwave hyperthermia as an alternative treatment for benign prosta-tic hypertrophy (Blute et al. 1991). This has been used in patients who have had an indwelling catheter, and who probably had some prostatitis. There are also anecdotal reports of its use with less success in chronic prostatitis unrelated to benign prostatic hypertrophy.

Surgery has been suggested as a final form of treatment in patients with severe symptoms. It must be remembered that the focal pathological process is peripheral within the prostate. Both transurethral resection and radical prost-atectomy have been suggested; though initial results may be encouraging, benefit is frequently short (Blandy 1976).

Special Forms of Prostatitis

Mycotic prostatitis has been described and appears to respond to oral antifun-gal treatment such as fluconazole (Bozette et al. 1991). Granulomatous prost-atitis is uncommon, presents in patients over the age of 50 years usually with evidence of obstruction, and treatment is surgical. Allergic or eosinophilic prostatitis is another rare form seen in patients with other hypersensitivity states which usually overshadow the symptoms of bladder neck obstruction; treatment is, again, surgical (Blandy 1976).

Conclusion

In the practical management of chronic nonbacterial prostatitis a simple regimen which encourages compliance should be advised. This should include a high fluid intake, such as 3 l daily, regular drainage of the prostatic secretion by ejaculation once or twice weekly, support by psychotherapy, and a prostate-penetrating antimicrobial. If the history suggests recurrent urethritis in the past, give minocycline or doxycycline 100 mg twice daily by mouth. If previously there has been bacteriuria, prescribe trimethoprim 200 mg twice daily by mouth. The first course should continue for 3 months in chronic prostatitis. Ciprofloxa-cin 250 mg twice daily may be used as a second-line antimicrobial. In cases resistant to these regimens other measures outlined may be considered. The problem of possible bladder neck dyssynergia must be remembered and, when suspected, TRUS and urodynamics considered.

References

Blacklock NJ (1990) The prostate; surgical anatomy. In: Chisholm GD, Fair WR (eds) Scientific foundations of urology, 3rd edn. Heinemann, London, pp 340–350
Blandy J (1976) Urology. Blackwell, Oxford, pp 923–925

Blute ML, Lewis RL (1991) Local microwave hyperthermia as a treatment alternative for benign prostatic hypertrophy. J Androl 12:429–434

Bozette SA, Larsen RA, Chiu J, Leal MAE, Tilles JG, Richman DD, Leedom JM, McCutchan JA (1991) Fluconazole treatment of persistent Cryptococcus neoformans prostatic infection in AIDS. Ann Intern Med 115:285–286

Colleen S, Mardh P-A (1990) Prostatitis. In: Holmes KK, Mardh P-A, Sparling PF, Wiesner PJ (eds) Sexually transmitted diseases, 2nd edn. McGraw-Hill, New York, pp 653–661

Drach GW, Meares EM Jr, Fair WR, Stamey TA (1978) Classification of benign diseases associated with prostatic pain; prostatitis or prostatodynia? (Letter). J Urol 120:266

Garnes HA (1973) Doxycycline levels in serum and prostatic tissue in man. Urology 1:205–207

Hensle T, Prout G, Griffin P (1977) Minocycline diffusion into benign prostatic hyperplasia. J Urol 118:609–611

Ikeuchi T (1990) Clinical studies on chronic prostatitis and prostatitis-like syndrome. IV. The Kampo treatment for intractable prostatitis. Hinyokika Kyo 36:801–806

Kaisary AV (1981) A study of cefamandole prostatic tissue levels. Br J Urol 53:336–338

Krieger JN (1984) Prostatitis syndromes: pathophysiology, differential diagnosis, and treatment. Sex Transm Dis 11:100–112

Meares EM Jr (1973) Observations on activity of trimethoprim-sulfamethoxazole in the prostate. J Infect Dis 128 Suppl: S679–S685

Meares EM Jr (1990) Prostatitis. In: Chisholm GD, Fair WR (eds) Scientific foundations of urology, 3rd edn. Heinemann, London, pp 373–378

Mundy AR, Stephenson TB, Wein AJ (1984) Urodynamics – Principles, practice and application. Churchill Livingstone, Edinburgh, p 194

Murnaghan GF (1980) Prostatitis. In: Kaufman G (ed) Current urological therapy. Saunders, Philadelphia, p 287

Murnaghan GF, Tynan AP, Farnsworth RH, Harvery K (1973) Chronic prostatitis – an Australian view. Br J Urol 45:55–59

Simmons PD, Thin RN (1985) Minocycline in chronic abacterial prostatitis: a double blind prospective trial. Br J Urol 57:43–45

Simmons PD, Thin RN (1990) Abstract book. Spring Meeting of Medical Society for the Study of Venereal Diseases, Bordeaux

Smith JW, Jones SR, Reed WP, Till AD, Deupree RH, Kaijser B (1979) Recurrent urinary tract infection in men. Ann Intern Med 91:544–548

Smith RP, Wilbur HJ, Bassey C, Baltch AL (1988) Azlocillin and mezlocillin concentration in human prostatic tissue. Chemotherapy 34:267–271

Stamey TA (1981) Prostatitis. J R Soc Med 74:22–40

Thin RN (1986) Treatment of non-bacterial prostatitis. In: Weidner W, Brunner H, Krause W, Rothauge CF (eds) Therapy of prostatitis. Zuckschwerdt, Munich, pp 145–149

Thin RN (1991) The diagnosis of prostatitis: a review. Genitourin Med 67:279–283

Thin RN, Simmons PD (1985) Review of results of four regimens for treatment of chronic non-bacterial prostatitis. Br J Urol 55:519–521

Weidner W, Schiefer HG, Krauss H, Jantos C, Friedrich HJ, Altmannsberger M (1991a) Chronic prostatitis: a thorough search for etiologically involved microrganisms in 1,461 patients. Infection 19:S119–S125

Weidner W, Schiefer HG, Brähler E (1991b) Refractory chronic bacterial prostatitis: a re-evaluation of ciprofloxacin treatment after a median followup of 30 months. J Urol 146:350–352

Microwave Hyperthermia for Chronic Prostatitis and Prostatodynia

L. Baert, F. Ameye, and Z. Petrovich

Introduction

Prostatitis syndromes are relatively frequent problems seen by practising urologists. Acute and chronic bacterial prostatitis are caused mainly by gramnegative bacteria and require an appropriate, extended antimicrobial therapy. About 90% of men with prostatitis have nonbacterial prostatitis (NBP) or prostatodynia (PD), clinically characterized by a syndrome of chronic pelvic, perineal, ejaculatory pain associated with irritating or obstructive symptoms and psychological disturbances. In contrast to men with NBP, patients with PD have normally appearing expressed prostatic secretions (EPS) with no sign of an inflammatory process (Drach et al. 1978). As many as 25% of patients with PD, however, occasionally show excessive leukocytes in their EPS (Meares 1986). This suggests that NBP and PD are syndromes with numerous similarities, as demonstrated in common unclear etiologies and therapy resistance of both conditions. There are multiple hypotheses to explain their etiology, varying from infectious or inflammatory processes to neuromuscular and psychological dysfunctions; however, none of these is generally accepted (Orland et al. 1985). Numerous therapeutic approaches have been utilized, such as antibiotics, antiinflammatory agents and α-blockers. Treatment results, however, have frequently been disappointing.

Microwave hyperthermia (HT) has recently been used for the treatment of prostatic diseases, using a transrectal (TRHT) or transurethral (TUHT) approach. The use of HT in the treatment of carcinoma of the prostate was first reported by Mendecki et al. in 1980. Yerushalmi et al. (1982, 1985) reported good treatment results with TRHT in benign prostatic hyperplasia (BPH) and carcinoma patients. Sapozink et al. (1990) and Baert et al. (1990) reported significant subjective and objective improvement in BPH patients, using TUHT. These good results obtained in BPH patients encouraged the use of TRHT and TUHT in patients with nonbacterial prostatitis and prostatodynia (Servadio et al. 1987; Baert et al. 1991).

This report presents the results of a comparison between TUHT and TRHT for NBP and PD patients and reviews the literature.

Material and Methods

Forty patients with PD or prostatitis-like symptoms were treated with HT. Of these, 15 received TUHT using a helical coil microwave applicator, and the other 25 were treated with TRHT using a water-cooled rectal probe. Treatment characteristics are listed in Table 1. All were investigated according to a standardized procedure as proposed by Wedren (1987). Subjective symptoms were evaluated by qualification of standardized questions concerning previous history and symptoms during the preceding month, with special attention to pain and prostatitis-related symptoms. Detailed analysis of previous periods of prostatitis and prior treatments was performed.

Objective evaluation consisted of careful general and urological clinical examination, urine analysis with microscopic examination and culture of

Table 1. Treatment characteristics

	TUHT	TRHT
Applicator	Transurethral helical coil	Transrectal water-cooled
Frequency	915 MHz	915 MHz
Number of sessions	5	5
Duration	60 min	60 min
Temperature		
Desired	44°–46°C	42°–43°C
Mean	45.5°C	42.3°C

Table 2. Results in patients receiving TUHT and TRHT

	TUHT (n = 15)	TRHT (n = 25)
Age (years)	55 years (27–68)	53 years (23–65)
History prostatitis	7	14
Prior treatments	15	21
Duration of symptoms (months)	33 (9–60)	18 (1–24)
Subjective symptom score (points)	16 (10–20)	15 (11–19)
Uroflowmetry (cm³/s)		
Mean peak flow	11.2	12.3
Mean average flow	6.3	7.6
Residual urine (cm³)	40	30
Prostatic volume (cm³)	26 (15–37)	30 (15–43)
Follow-up (months)	6.5	6

Table 3. Symptoms in patients receiving TUHT and TRHT

	TUHT (n = 15)		TRHT (n = 25)	
	n	%	n	%
Pain	15	100	23	92
Obstruction	7	47	10	40
Urgency	6	40	13	52
Frequency	6	40	13	52
Nocturia	5	33	7	28
Impotence	4	27	3	12

fractionated urine portions and EPS, and urine cytology. Uroflowmetry, post-voiding residual urine, transrectal prostate sonography and prostate-specific antigen (PSA) determination completed this work-up. Special attention was directed to quantification of the leukocytes in EPS. This work-up classified all patients as PD patients, according to Drach et al. (1978). Once every 3 months, a follow-up was carried out according to this standardized formula, except for urine and EPS examination, which were performed just before and at the end of the treatment. Data on patient characteristic and pretreatment variables are listed in Tables 2 and 3.

Results

In the TUHT group, the symptom score decreased from 14 to 9 points (36% Fig. 1). Seven patients (47%) showed complete pain relief and decrease of dysuria. In the seven patients who presented with obstructive micturition symptoms, five (71%) had substantial improvement as confirmed objectively in improvement of mean peak flow rate from 7.2 to 14.9 cm^3/s following TUHT. Other objective parameters such as residual volume, prostatic volume, PSA, and overall flow rate for the whole group did not change significantly.

In the TRHT group, 14 of the 23 patients showed complete pain relief (61%), and the symptom score decreased from 15 to 6 (60%: Fig. 1). Especially patients with irritating symptoms showed substantial relief; 9 of the 13 patients had less frequency and urgency after TRHT. Importantly, five patients with normal pretreatment EPS (white blood cell count of less than 10/field) showed an excessive increase in white blood cells (more than 20/field) in posttreatment prostate secretions. Results of repeated cultures and transrectal sonographies, however, remained negative. Other objective parameters showed no substantial changes.

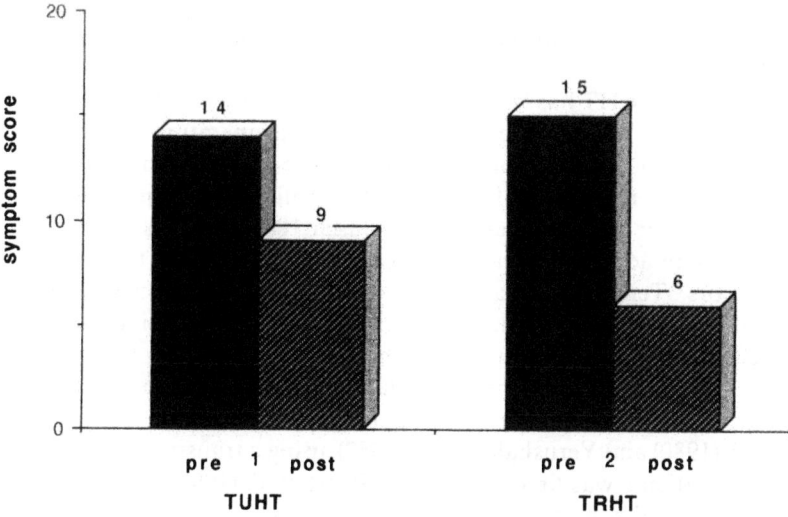

Fig. 1. Symptom scores in patients receiving TUHT and TRHT

Discussion

The etiology of NBP and PD remains unclear. It appears that NBP either is an infectious disease caused by some questionable pathogens such as *Chlamydia trachomatis*, *Mycoplasma*, or *Ureaplasma* or is a noninfectious inflammation of the prostate caused by intraprostatic reflux and secondary chemical prostatitis. Even if one accepts the putative causal role of *Chlamydia*, treatment results with tetracyclines are frequently disappointing, warranting additional treatments such as anti-inflammatory agents, anticholinergics, or other conservative means (Meares 1991). The etiology of PD is even more obscure, as demonstrated in the various terms used to describe this entity, such as tension myalgia of the pelvic floor (Segura et al. 1979), functional voiding disorders (Siroky et al. 1981), bladder neck/urethral spasm syndrome (Barbalias et al. 1983), and pelvic pain (Schmidt 1989). Psychiatric disorders, primary emotional disturbances, and stress have frequently been implicated in men with this condition. Some authors have suggested urodynamically confirmed conditions such as primary over-activity of the pelvic sympathetic nervous system at the level of the external urethral sphincter (Barbalias et al. 1983) or primary functional voiding disorders with bladder areflexia and striated sphincter spasm or bladder hyperreflexia with appropriate striated sphincter relaxation (Siroky et al. 1981). In this way previous empiric use of α-blockers, anticholinergics, muscle relaxants, and anxiolytic agents may be scientifically justified but has shown insufficient therapeutic efficacy. Other conservative physical methods such as hot sitz-bath, diathermy, pelvic musculature-relaxing biofeedback, acupuncture, neural stimulation, and sacral root stimulation have all been tested with variable success (Schmidt 1989).

Recently, microwave HT has been introduced for therapy-resistant NBP and PD. HT, or the artificial increase in human body temperature to promote healing, has been recognized and practiced since ancient times (Singh 1991). In 1866 Busch reported a regression of histologically confirmed sarcoma following an attack of high fever caused by erysipelas (Busch 1866). HT has been under intensive study as an adjuvant to radio- and chemotherapy in the treatment of malignant tumors. Temperature above 42°C is cytotoxic and neoadjuvant potentiator of radiation and chemotherapy effects. HT in combination with radio- and chemotherapy was found in numerous clinical trials to be more effective than either modality alone for advanced recurrent tumors. The first clinical applications of HT in BPH and carcinoma patients were reported by Mendecki et al. (1980) and Yerushalmi et al. (1982), using a transrectal approach. TUHT in BPH patients was first reported by Baert et al. (1990) and Sapozink et al. (1990), with good subjective and objective results.

The goal of TUHT and TRHT is to deliver electromagnetic energy at prostatic tissues, using microwaves at a frequency varying from 2450 to 915 MHz. Microwave penetration and absorption cause tissue temperature elevation to the hyperthermic range of 41°–45°C by tissue-energy interaction at molecular, cellular, and tissue levels. TRHT is delivered by a water-cooled transrectal probe with a radial penetration depth of 2 cm and temperature elevation to 42°–43°C in peripheral perirectal prostatic tissues. Periurethral prostatic tissues are concentrically heated by TUHT to 44°–45°C at a radial depth of 0.5–1 cm around a transurethral microwave applicator. Details on method and applicator characteristics and clinical treatment results in BPH and carcinoma patients are reported elsewhere (Sapozink et al. 1990; Baert et al. 1991; Astrahan et al. 1991). This clinical work was further expanded to fundamental research on pathological (Lauweryns et al. 1991), thermophysical (Astrahan et al. 1991a,b), and immunological (Szmigielski et al. 1991) mechanisms to elucidate the mechanism of action of TRHT and TUHT; these, however, remain unknown. Baert et al. (1990) hypothesize that the effect of TUHT on the BPH-obstructed urethra is probably expressed through selective shrinking and retraction of the periurethral prostatic parenchyma due to organizing localized tissue necrosis and cicatrization. The good clinical results in BPH patients as well as applicability of these experimental data in other prostatic diseases have stimulated the application of HT in patients with NBP and PD.

The first preliminary clinical results were reported by Servadio et al. (1987) in 21 patients, indicating improvement in subjective results using TRHT. This series was expanded to 45 patients, with a mean follow-up of 38.5 months. Of these patients 25% showed a sustained and complete loss of symptoms, and 50% had a partial response, especially in irritating symptoms. The remaining 25% reported no improvement (Servadio and Leib 1991). These results were confirmed in the present study group of 25 patients, in whom a major improvement was seen in 60%, with a mean follow-up of 6 months.

Preliminary results on TUHT were first reported by our group (Baert et al. 1991). Good treatment response, manifested by complete pain relief and a decrease in dysuria, was noted in 47%, with a mean follow-up of 6.5 months. A decrease in obstructive micturition problems was noted in 71% of the patients who had this symptom upon presentation. Higher treatment temperatures correlated well with good response ($p < 0.01$), which suggests a temperature-related response.

Comparing the two treatment modalities, TRHT seems to be more effective than TUHT in NBP and PD patients, with success in 60% and 47% of the patients, respectively. The evaluation of treatment response in patients with PD, however, presents a complex problem. Any assessment of such a response should consider the possibility of a strong placebo effect. The placebo factor is certainly influenced by characteristics of the selected patient group and toxicity of the applied modality. Insertion of a transurethral catheter in a selected group of anxious, hyperesthetic PD patients can influence treatment results in favor of those treated by the transrectal approach. A prospective, comparative phase III trial comparing TUHT, TRHT, and sham procedures is needed in the future to solve these questions.

On the other hand, it is difficult to claim that all good treatment results are due merely to placebo effects. All patients had a long-standing history of NBP or PD symptoms, had been treated by several urologists in various ways, but definitely showed subjective improvement lasting for many months. Actually, however, there is no evidence of a proven mechanism of action. Suggestions for possible mechanisms are derived mainly from experience in BPH and carcinoma patients. Heat-induced HT of the prostate and secondary revulsive or anti-inflammatory effects are probably the most important mechanisms. Secondly, immunological effects due to reaction of the host immune system to local HT must be considered. Most observations on immune-modulating effects were made on laboratory animals or patients treated with whole-body HT. Recently a transient, significant stimulation of the cell-mediated immune system and increase in natural killer cytotoxic activity was noted following TRHT for prostate carcinoma and BPH patients (Szmigielski et al. 1991). It is well known that local humoral and cell-mediated immunological reactions determine pathogenesis and therapy response in NBP patients.

The above mechanisms may explain response to HT in NBP patients. The exact mechanism leading to stimulation with HT of cell-mediated immunity, however, remains unclear. The presence of extensive granulocytic and lymphocytic infiltrates adjacent to zones of periurethral necrosis after TUHT indicates the existence of inflammatory reactions that might be responsible for triggering the stimulation of the host's cell-mediated immunity. The excessive amount of leukocytes in sterile posttherapy EPS compared with negative pretreatment EPS in some of our patients may substantiate this hypothesis. However, Rigatt et al. (1990) noted no differences in seminal fluid after TRHT. Finally, interactions of microwaves or heat with alpha or other neuroendocrine receptors are possible yet hypothetical mechanisms to explain the decrease in obstructive or irritating symptoms in these patients.

Conclusion

Local microwave HT is a palliative treatment modality for NBP and PD. Preliminary results of phase I clinical trials with TUHT and TRHT are promising. Phase II trials are needed to optimize treatment modalities. Prospective randomized phase III studies with long-term follow-up are needed to compare TUHT, TRHT, and placebo effects. Finally, further research should be directed to study the adjuvant effect of HT on drug therapies due to changes of pharmacokinetics of antibiotic or anti-inflammatory drugs.

References

Astrahan M, Ameye F, Oyen R et al. (1991a) Interstitial temperature measurements during transurethral microwave hyperthermia. J Urol 145:304–308

Astrahan M, Imanaka K, Jozsef G, Ameye F et al. (1991b) Heating characteristics of a helical microwave applicator for transurethral hyperthermia of benign prostatic hyperplasia. Int J Hyperthermia 71:141–155

Baert L. Ameye F, Willemen P et al. (1990) Transurethral hyperthermia for benign prostatic hyperplasia: preliminary clinical and pathological results. J Urol 144:1383–1387

Baert L, Willemen P, Ameye F et al. (1991) Transurethral microhyperthermia: an alternative treatment for prostatodynia? Prostate 19:113–119

Baert L, Willemen P, Ameye F, Petrovich Z (1991) Treatment response with transurethral hyperthermia in different forms of benign prostatic hyperplasia: a preliminary report. Prostate 18:315–320

Barbalias GA, Meares EM, Sant GR (1983) Prostatodynia: clinical and urodynamic characteristics. J Urol 130:514–517

Busch W (1866) Über den Einfluß welchen heftigere Erysipeln zuweilen auf organisierte Neubildungen ausüben. Verh Naturh Preuss Rhein Westphal 23:28

Drach GW, Fair WR, Meares EM, Stamey TA (1978) Classification of benign diseases associated with prostatic pain: prostatitis or prostatodynia? J Urol 120:266

Lauweryns J, Baert L, Vandenhove J, Petrovich Z (1991) Histopathology of prostatic tissue after transurethral hyperthermia. Int J Hyperthermia 7:221–224

Meares EM Jr (1986) Prostatodynia: clinical findings and rationale for treatment. In: Weidner W, Brunner H, Krause et al. (eds) Therapy of prostatitis. Zuckschwerdt, Munich, pp 207–212

Meares EM Jr (1991) Prostatitis. Med Clin North Am 75(2):405–424

Mendecki J, Friendenthal E, Botstein C et al. (1980) Microwave applicators for localized hyperthermia treatment of cancer of the prostate. Int J Radiat Oncol Biol Phys 6:1583

Orland SM, Hanno PM, Wein AJ (1985) Prostatitis, prostatosis and prostatodynia. Urology 25:439–459

Rigatti P, Buonaguidi A, Grasso M et al. (1990) Morphodynamic and biochemical assessment of seminal plasma in patients who underwent local prostatic hyperthermia. Prostate 16(4): 325–330

Sapozink MD, Boyd SD, Astrahan MA et al. (1990) Transurethral hyperthermia for benign prostatic hyperplasia: preliminary clinical results. J Urol 143:944

Schmidt RA (1989) Pelvic pain. In: Paulson DF (ed) Prostatic disorders. Lea and Fibiger, London, pp 139–154

Segura JW, Optiz JL, Greene LF (1979) Prostatosis, prostatitis or pelvic floor tension myalgia? J Urol 122:168–169

Servadio C, Leib Z (1991) Chronic abacterial prostatitis and hyperthermia. A possible new treatment. Br J Urol 67:308–311

Servadio C, Leib Z, Lev A (1987) Diseases of the prostate treated by local microwave hyperthermia. Urology 30:97–99

Singh BB (1991) Hyperthermia: an ancient science in India. Int J Hyperthermia 7(1):1–6

Siroky MB, Goldstein I, Krane RJ (1981) Functional voiding disorders in men. J Urol 126:200–204

Szmigielski S, Sobczynski, Sokolska et al. (1991) Effects of local prostatic hyperthermia on human NK and T cell function. Int J Hyperthermia 7(6):869–880

Wedren H (1987) Effects of sodium pentosanpolysulphate on symptoms related to chronic non-bacterial prostatitis. Sc and J Urol Nephrol 21:81–88

Yerushalmi A Servadio C, Leib Z et al. (1982) Local hyperthermia for treatment of carcinoma of the prostate: a preliminary report. Prostate 6:602

Yerushalmi A, Fishelovitz, Singer D et al. (1985) Localized deep microwave hyperthermia in the treatment of poor operative risk patients with benign prostatic hyperplasia. J Urol 133:873–876

Subject Index

Springer-Verlag
and the Environment

We at Springer-Verlag firmly believe that an international science publisher has a special obligation to the environment, and our corporate policies consistently reflect this conviction.

We also expect our business partners – paper mills, printers, packaging manufacturers, etc. – to commit themselves to using environmentally friendly materials and production processes.

The paper in this book is made from low- or no-chlorine pulp and is acid free, in conformance with international standards for paper permanency.

Lightning Source UK Ltd.
Milton Keynes UK
UKHW01f1424191018

330837UK00003B/90/P